*SURVIVING MODERN MEDICINE*

# Surviving Modern Medicine

## HOW TO GET THE BEST
## FROM DOCTORS, FAMILY, AND FRIENDS

*PETER CLARKE and SUSAN H. EVANS*

RUTGERS UNIVERSITY PRESS
*New Brunswick, New Jersey, and London*

Library of Congress Cataloging-in-Publication Data
Clarke, Peter.
    Surviving modern medicine : how to get the best from doctors,
family, and friends / Peter Clarke and Susan H. Evans.
        p.      cm.
    Includes bibliographical references and index.
    ISBN 0-8135-2555-1 (cloth: alk. paper). — ISBN 0-8135-2556-X (pbk. :
alk. paper)
    1. Medical care.   2. Consumer education.   I. Evans, Susan H.
II. Title.
RA776.5.C54    1998
362.1—dc21                                                    98-6812
                                                                CIP

British Cataloging-in-Publication data for this book is available from the
British Library

Portions of Chapter 5 also appear in "The Critical Care Choices Guide," developed
jointly by Susan H. Evans and Peter Clarke with the American Association of
Critical-Care Nurses (AACN) under a grant from the U.S. Agency for Health Care
Policy and Research. The AACN has given permission to reproduce this material.

Permission to reproduce the California Natural Death Act Declaration copyright
© 1991 document is granted by the Pacific Center for Health Policy and Ethics.

CMA's Durable Power of Attorney for Health Care Decisions copyright © 1995 by
the California Medical Association. Published with permission of and by arrangement with the California Medical Association. Copies of this form, as well as an
accompanying brochure and wallet card, may be obtained from CMA Publications
by calling 1-800-882-1-CMA.

Manufactured in the United States of America

*To Madie, Jack, and Chris*

# CONTENTS

# LIST OF TABLES

# ACKNOWLEDGMENTS

MANY INDIVIDUALS contributed to this book, sometimes without realizing it. Physicians and other health professionals, including close friends, helped test our ideas and gain access to patients whose own experiences with illness enrich these pages. We are grateful to Paul Barkopoulos, Harold Benjamin, Avrum Bluming, Larry Cone, Ed Gilbert, Ronnie Kaye, Gerald Rosen, Selma Schimmel, Mel Silverstein, Michael Van Scoy-Mosher, and David Wellisch.

Throughout our research, other people contributed their talents in such varied specialties as behavioral theory, graphics, legal review, software design, data analysis, and much more. We thank Joanna Bull, Harold Burch, Alex Capron, Bob Cialdini, Geoff Cowan, Louis Cutrona, Delores Esparza, Fawzy Fawzy, Nancy Fawzy, Sandra Holden, Mitzi Inman, Wanda Johanson, Andy Johnson, Bob Letters, Robyn Letters, Sydney Levy-Jensen, Terry Lierman, Jon Linden, Wendy Linden, Jo-Ann Luongo, Bob Pearlman, Flo Porter, Ev Rogers, Joan Salat, Renee Salick, Sarah Sanford, Doug Shook, Joel Swerdlow, James Waisman, Ellen Waisman-Smith, and Nivia Young.

Students helped us create materials to improve patient education and to evaluate their effectiveness. We want to recognize the contributions of Wei-Tsen Chen, Kevin Hoyes, Meryl Klein, Hollie Muir, Patrick O'Sullivan, Raj Patel, Mary Ann Serrano, Debbie Tan, and Joan Van Tassel.

For reading and commenting on sections of our manuscript, we owe a great debt to Jean Campbell, Cherilyn Parsons, and Carol Tavris. Gareth Esersky never flagged in her support for this project. Doreen Valentine gave us insightful editing. Teresa Carson, Marilyn Campbell, and Tricia Politi ushered the book through the production process with meticulous care.

People at many of our research sites supervised the collection of data and brought a commitment to project goals that far exceeded the norm. We are grateful to Maria Carmen Aguirre, Mary Ellen Stone Amodeo, Susan Blatt, Jeanette Kraemer, Kathy Lane, Sharon Mayell, Charlotte Newsome, Katherine Paul, Allison Porter, Anne Riley, Kathryn Stivers, and Elnora Von Verdo.

Organizations that have supported our research with grants include the U.S. Agency for Health Care Policy and Research (RO1 HS09232-02), where we thank Linda Siegenthaler and Carolyn Clancy; the IBM Corporation, thanks to Dennis Palmiero; the Ralph M. Parsons Foundation, thanks to Christine Sisley; the Xerox Corporation; and the Annenberg Foundation.

Across five years of work on a project to fight hunger and malnutrition, we came to depend on weekly meetings with Mickey Weiss to raise provocative questions about facets of this book. We thank him for his wisdom and sense of wonder.

Finally, thousands of patients, their family members, and friends talked with us about their own medical crisis or efforts to avert one. Without their candor and generosity, our studies would have ground to a halt.

*SURVIVING MODERN MEDICINE*

## INTRODUCTION

WHEN AN ISSUE makes it into the comics, everyone understands that the problem is truly widespread. Recently, we found this out firsthand when we gave a talk about how people can take better control of their own health care. We opened the discussion with a cartoon that showed a hapless patient sitting upright in his hospital bed. His doctor clutches a chart; by his side is a woman in a miniskirt holding a large, gift-wrapped package. The physician announces: "In your case, Dave, there's a choice—elective surgery, outpatient medical therapy, or whatever's in the box that our lovely Carol is holding." Our audience's burst of laughter melted into nods of recognition as we talked about common pitfalls that lie along the road to making important medical decisions. Listeners began jotting down our tips about wrestling the health-care system into submission, mobilizing family and friends during an illness or accident, relating to caregivers, and much more.

This book brings the same good news that we brought to our audience that day. Fortunately, no matter what health problems you may be fighting now or will fight in the future—minor aches or infections, an accident, a chronic condition, or a terminal illness—you can use the medical system even more intelligently than you may imagine.

The experience of Sally and Bob (all patients' names have been changed to protect their privacy), a couple we interviewed during our research with cancer patients, illustrates the difficulties that many face as they scramble to get top care. Sally, a forty-three-year-old mother of two children, was undergoing chemotherapy to fight breast cancer. Her husband, Bob, managed to get away from work to drive Sally to that day's appointment. When we talked with Sally, we learned that she was most concerned with her hair loss, even though she understood that this would be a temporary condition. Her changed appearance frightened her children and made her feel ugly and rejected. She had tried to voice these anxieties to her physician, but he dismissed them by saying that "everything will return to normal once the treatments are over."

Bob didn't have it much easier. He was sinking under an avalanche of fatigue as he put in triple time as wage earner, parent, and caregiver. He felt that no one acknowledged his situation and that family and friends focused all their attention on Sally. Bob wanted to help Sally but didn't know how. He had been demoralized when, during the initial meeting with Sally's physician, he was handed a booklet on chemotherapy that failed to answer the many pressing questions he had on *his* mind. Both partners felt that they needed more information to work their way through the labyrinth of treatments, tests, appointments, and emotional ups and downs. Doctors seemed too rushed to sit down and visit. Neither Sally nor Bob knew where to turn.

Listening to Sally and Bob, as well as to thousands of other people we have interviewed in our research, has helped us see how a lack of communication with family and friends and with the medical system can drain people of the vital edge they need to maintain or regain health, and get the quality of medical treatment that they deserve. Sally didn't know how to open up lines of communication with her physician or with her family; Bob didn't know how to mobilize empathic and effective social support to help him through his wife's illness. Neither knew how to weigh choices among treatment options.

Sally and Bob are like many consumers who have not had a chance to discover basic principles that could help them manage the medical system with greater ease and better results. Anxiety, timidity, and resignation have replaced the confidence that people used to have when dealing with their own health care. These days patients, perhaps you among them, need tools for coping with doctors, who themselves are squeezed by a cost-conscious health-care system. Managed care is cutting costs by crowding physicians' schedules, curtailing tests, and discouraging referrals and expensive procedures.

Helping health consumers unravel their confusions has driven us to write this book. Our research into new strategies for patient education at the University of Southern California's School of Medicine (in the Institute for Health Promotion and Disease Prevention) and the Annenberg School for Communication has shed light on dozens of lessons about people's experiences. We provide a detailed road map for readers determined to do everything within their power to fashion more effective and more rewarding encounters with the medical system. This book translates hundreds of sound medical and psychological research studies and personal accounts into well-grounded and practical tips.

The chapters cover five essential areas that are important whether you are healthy or ill, and whatever insurance plan or type of provider you may have. "Getting Your Doctor to Pay Attention" reviews the health hazards of the traditional, passive role that is so familiar to many patients. It introduces four different types of relationships with physicians and offers practical means for managing nonverbal and verbal communication in order to set a more constructive agenda during consultations. Simple exercises help you prepare for your office visits and get your doctors to pay attention to what's really on your mind. We also offer ways to get your insurer to pay attention to your needs.

"Making the Best Medical Decisions" helps you deal with all phases of medical choice—the initial diagnosis, second opinions, weighing alternative treatment programs, and coping with medical disappointments. We explain faulty habits of thinking that often jeopardize sound decisions, the harmful effects of rushed deadlines, and the ways emotions can limit creative problem-solving.

"Seeking the Right Kind of Social Support" documents how essential it is to enlist empathic family and friends to help during illness or accident. The prevention of illness in the first place, as well as a swift recovery from accident or disease, depend vitally on the right kind of social relationships. You can determine whether you have too little support, too much support, or support from the wrong people. We offer a plan for asking for help and for supplying quality support to others.

"Appreciating Your Caregiver" conveys the dynamics that bind patient and long-term caregiver, highlighting the stresses and strains each partner must master. We explain why family caregivers are in short supply these days, and why some caregivers become just as ill as their patients.

We offer tips to restore the caregiver's spirits and motivation to deal with another person's accident, or acute or chronic illness, whether the patient is an adult or child.

"Protecting Your Choices in Critical Care" recognizes that advanced medical technology can often sustain life even when the quality of life becomes unbearable. We show you how difficult it is to predict what life support your doctor will provide if you become too ill to make and to communicate your own medical decisions. We provide a step-by-step guide for defining your values about critical care, discussing these with family, and completing an advance directive so that your wishes will be known.

■ ■ ■

Many of us were raised to picture doctors in the Norman Rockwell model—a kindly, twinkling physician who knows all about our family, work, and hobbies. Appointments are leisurely. In this nostalgic world, decisions are clear-cut, and when they're not, we can consult with an extended family who will also be able to provide ongoing care if we need it.

If you're scoffing at this mythic picture, you're right. The medical establishment has changed, and many of our traditional assumptions are now badly out of step with today's realities.

Over the past hundred years, the general public's experience with medicine has undergone a revolution (and it hasn't stopped yet). Until the mid-nineteenth century, medicine was largely the province of country doctors, folk practitioners, and quacks. Only major cities, like New York and Boston, boasted hospitals and medical schools. Even doctors trained in such schools were not required to have state licenses to practice. Health care, for those who could afford it, depended heavily on the personal element of the doctor-patient relationship, symbolized in home visits. However, with the advent of the stethoscope, aseptic procedures, physical probing, and microscopic examination of blood, urine, and tissues, the average doctor began to label conditions with increasing precision. The twentieth century brought powerful diagnostic tools like X-ray machines and electrocardiography. The capacity to cure gained additional power from new drugs, especially with the arrival of antibiotics in the 1940s.

The curriculum of medical training marched ahead lockstep with such advances. Microbiology, immunology, and genetics gained ground, while the arts of listening closely to patients' own words and taking a physical exam fell to a lesser rank. Increasingly, technology insisted that the body speak with physicians through electrical or biochemical readings, often printed starkly on computer printouts. In competition with feedback from electrodes and scans, the human voice has lost much of its credibility. Patients' sighs grew irrelevant.

As the medical system ratcheted upward in complexity, an army of body-part and disease-specific specialists grew, while the number of generalist-physicians and family doctors shrank. These days, the cadre of specialists expands at three times the rate of primary-care doctors. Patients must now cycle through a tangle of different providers, each of whom knows little about them personally. Each specialist speaks in an elegant vocabulary but focuses on one facet of disease alone. In addition, most specialists consider themselves "fixers" with little time or interest in preventive measures. They tend to overdiagnose, charge higher fees, and order more tests than generalists, even when the patient presents an ordinary complaint. Such a piecemeal approach to health frightens many people even more than the spiraling costs of care and inadequate insurance coverage.

The new marketplace of medicine, which includes HMOs (Health Maintenance Organizations) and other forms of managed care, has further separated patients from their providers. Corporate conglomerates and professional corporations now vend medical care, replacing that Norman Rockwell figure. Uninterrupted contact with the same doctor is no longer assured. In a distressing number of cases, patients with catastrophic diagnoses learn the bad news over the phone instead of in person. Procedural guidelines to "standardize care," which large organized groups of physicians follow in an attempt to control costs, often ignore individuals' widely varying needs and personal histories.

On top of this, the way doctors and hospitals get paid for their services in the United States fails to reimburse for patient education and psychological support. Insurance companies and the government issue checks when invoiced for medical procedures, not for explaining the risks of a procedure or treatment program *one more time* or for gently helping someone cope. Decisions about what is reimbursable are rendered by health-plan managers who haggle with networks of providers and insurance companies. It goes without saying that the isolated patient does not know the names or phone numbers of any of these crucial gatekeepers who shape options for care.

It should come as no surprise, then, that relationships between many doctors and their patients have grown edgy and detached. The boun-ties of technology have come at a cost—many doctors no longer lis-ten, counsel patients about their own role in managing disease, or offer emotional support. Many patients today feel overwhelmed.

Yet, consumers have become increasingly dependent on the health-care system. In the United States, the incidence of reported conditions, acute and otherwise, has shot upward in the past fifty years by nearly 200 percent on a per-capita basis. People turn in ever-growing num-bers to the medical establishment, not only when suffering severe pain but also when experiencing minor bodily twinges. Run-of-the-mill ill-nesses now require more bedridden days away from work than a half-century ago. An avalanche of symptoms threatens to bury the medical system, even though the number of doctors per person has doubled since 1950.

Nowadays, it would seem that the state of our health seldom strays far from our minds. The mass media do their part to remind people about their physical condition. Television's most watched prime-time dramas exploit the suspense of medical crises; talk shows routinely cover dis-eases and the risks of weight gain. Large-circulation magazines stir the public's consciousness about personal health. Between one-quarter and one-third of advertising in the most popular magazines features a health-related message, usually involving a patient using an over-the-counter medication or a diet-related product.

Much of the public's preoccupation with health has solid ground-ing. Chronic conditions afflict more than half of Americans over the age of sixty-five. Even though people live longer, they spend a greater proportion of their time coping with illness. And the United States does not do well in comparison with many other developed countries, even though we spend 14 percent of our Gross Domestic Product (GDP) on health care. For example, this country fares much worse than other nations in fighting infant mortality, suicide, and obesity.

Widespread insecurity over health may have even deeper, psycho-logical roots. Some observers lay the blame on lifestyle. The breakup of traditional family structures has led to increasing levels of stress; divorce and tensions from failed personal relationships (including out-of-wed-lock pregnancies) abound. Along with this, many communities have dis-integrated in the wake of urban sprawl, with jobs scattered to new locales, including overseas. Physical decay in major cities and unplanned growth in newer places have created ugly vistas. The country's failure to rebuild its infrastructure allows grime and tumult to assault the eye and uproar to jar the ear. Relief from such conditions lies beyond the reach of many people. Anthropologists have noted the disappearance of places where people can retreat: Public parks are unkempt or unsafe, and a comforting social buffer of small-group life has also waned. Many of the cafes, beauty shops, and other neighborhood hangouts where people used to pass time between the hubbub of work and sanctity of home have given way to sterile, numbing malls.

Thus, overloaded sensory stimulation, losses in loving support, and a shriveled basis for community life afflict many people. Add to this the stagnation that the majority of families have experienced in real income since 1980, coupled with the turmoil of corporate downsizing and other job-related uncertainties. Two-income households now labor hero-ically to pay the bills and see children through school. Parents know that previous generations usually met these obligations with one paycheck. It's little wonder that these harrying conditions leave many people ill, or at least feeling that way.

The chapters that follow throw out a lifeline. In these pages you'll gain a fresh perspective to bring worry and confusion under control. Health care is something you can learn to manage, just like managing household finances, the development of children, or any other sector of life. There are practical, successful steps you can take to reduce frus-trations, pain, and disorientation.

Read chapters in any order you wish, depending on which need stands uppermost in your life right now. Each chapter offers a self-con-tained unit of ideas that can be most potent in helping you manage your care. Each chapter shares lessons from our own work in patient edu-cation and medical communication. Each also distills the best ideas for taking personal action that we have discovered from others' clinical prac-tice and research.

Wise patients are learning that they need to stand tall in order to receive the greatest quality of care possible from a range of options. As you'll see, research shows that gaining a sense of control over your life has therapeutic rewards itself. Whether you're healthy now or facing med-ical challenges, you can benefit by learning techniques to manage your medical encounters. That step alone will bring a greater sense of well-being and peace to your life.

## CHAPTER 1

# Getting Your Doctor to Pay Attention

SOMETIMES IT TAKES a novelist's insight to expose hidden or unspoken truths. Witness Pat Barker's apprehensive patient who seeks assurance from a "Dr. Yelland" before therapy begins:

> "Will it hurt?" the patient asked.
>
> Yelland said: "I realize that you did not intend to ask that question and so I will overlook it. I am sure you understand the principles of treatment, which are . . ." He paused, as if expecting the patient to supply them. "Attention, first and foremost; tongue, last and least; questions, never. I shall see you this afternoon."          (Barker 1993, 226)

This grotesque exchange may contain familiar echoes from your own office or hospital visits. Do you ever feel more estranged after a consultation than when you began? Do you wonder if your doctor's brusque or distracted manner weakens the quality of care that is provided? Does your physician's style of care leave you feeling more ill, even as he or she strives to correct some physical malady?

If so, you are not alone. The good news is that you can improve your encounters with doctors, along with your well-being. You can recognize the most damaging features of today's medical examinations. You can secure the type of relationships you want with your doctors by seeing clearly what is happening and discovering the corrective actions that build self-confidence and bolster health.

## THE CHILL BETWEEN DOCTORS AND THEIR PATIENTS

The plaque on the door of many doctors' offices nowadays includes this impersonal line: A Professional Corporation. Unintended, the announcement puts patients on notice that medical decision making has entered an era of conflict between the values of patients and the professional desires of physicians, between autonomy and health.

Consider, for example, Sandra's experience. She had been troubled by a persistent cough and was referred to a respiratory clinic for testing for asthma. As is common on a first visit, she completed a Patient Information Sheet with the requisite phone numbers, insurance information, and medical history. Then she found this brusque message in bold type: "In the interest of a good patient-doctor relationship, it is desirable to establish a good credit policy. An effective policy enables the doctor and patient to avoid misunderstandings." No doubt about this clinic's priorities, in its *first words* to new clients!

The wall of impersonality separating Sandra from her medical team didn't end with the paperwork. The arrangement of space and activities in the offices played a part as well. The staff kept a frosted pane of glass firmly shut, separating them from waiting patients, except for brief openings in order to summon people or issue instructions. As Sandra's treatment progressed, props and side dramas weakened her connection with medical authority even more. Many patients crowded the waiting area. Examining rooms lined a narrow corridor, and medical staff ducked back and forth among them, juggling several patients at a time. Phones rang constantly and were heard nearly everywhere. Appointment times always seemed scarce, with the receptionist only too willing to emphasize Sandra's good fortune in getting one, as she riffled through the calendar searching for moments when "Doctor can fit you in."

This frantic atmosphere erases a patient's individuality. The rush to process a large caseload undermines the quality of consultations. Evidence for this comes from more than just anecdotal reports. For example, experts reviewed audio recordings of patients' visits to internists (Beckman and Frankel 1984). In three-quarters of the encounters, physicians began probing for details without encouraging the patient to supply a complete account of reasons for seeking help or concerns since the last visit. Doctors commonly jumped in with yes–no questions or restated the patient's complaint in ways that narrowed the focus rather than using nonspecific conversational tools (aptly called "continuers") like "Mmm hmm," "Go on," or "I see." On average, doctors interrupted their patients eighteen seconds after patients began to speak. In the exceptional cases in which physicians kept quiet or used continuers, patients responded by talking up to sixty seconds, often supplying clinically important details. In fact, patients never rambled on longer than 150 seconds.

Haste, cutting off the patient's opening statement, shifts the focus of information gathering to a physician-centered format and away from a patient-centered one. This style also treats the earliest pieces of clinical information as the patient's most relevant complaint.

Such an early conversational interruption diminished Lydia's point of view about her condition. She was an athletic and energetic thirty-eight-year-old who had suffered from foot pain for four months, when her orthopedist recommended a foot and ankle specialist. At her first meeting, the physician entered the examination room and asked, "What's the problem?" "Well," Lydia began, "I'm frustrated and discouraged because . . ." "No," he said, "I mean, what's the problem with your foot?"

His abrupt intervention succeeded in wrenching the consultation onto his favored terrain, physical pain, and away from emotional or lifestyle consequences. That he smiled, on occasion, only softened his seizure of control. Throughout a year of treatment, the doctor never did ask how the foot condition affected Lydia's sports activities, work, or other pursuits.

Many patients respond to indifference or callousness with silent rebellion. They resist medical opinion that they or their insurers have spent good money to secure. Public alienation from medical care can surface in unsuspected ways. For example, people may put on a show of following their doctor's advice. They acknowledge symptoms and agree to curtail activities and enact other rituals of the "sick role." Then, they turn right around and neglect the treatments that have been prescribed. Two of ten people routinely fail to follow short-term and simple therapies such as taking antibiotics for bronchitis. Among cancer patients, as many as half may not stick religiously to their treatment program. For long-term and chronic conditions (such as juvenile asthma), as many as nine of ten neglect essential parts of their regimens. Across the wide range of human ailments, a shocking number of patients miss crucial appointments, ignore vital medications, evade corrective procedures, or disappear off the medical rolls entirely.

Other patients indicate their skepticism about mainstream medical providers more overtly. For a wide variety of chronic conditions, many supplement their use of traditional medicine by pursuing alternative therapies—techniques such as relaxation, chiropractic and massage, acupuncture, megavitamins, and more (Eisenberg et al. 1993). In a typical year, one of three adults relies on these means for disabilities like back problems, allergies, arthritis, headaches, other chronic pain, and depression. Clients of unconventional medicine are clustered in the upper levels of education and income. Visits to such providers actually outnumber the visits made to all the mainstream primary care physicians in the United States. Importantly, people seeking this care pay out of their own pockets because insurance plans rarely reimburse such services, and they usually keep their alternative treatments a secret from the traditional doctors they see. We will have more to say about why people use unconventional therapies in chapter 2.

## WHEN DOCTORS RETREAT

An instinctive, emotional retreat from many doctors stems from even more fundamental causes. At many medical practices, the quality of clinical services suffers from a separation between body and spirit in the actual treatment of disease. Here is Arthur Frank, an expert on two counts. He holds a Ph.D. in medical sociology from Yale and has endured two serious illnesses, a heart attack at age thirty-nine and cancer a year later:

> When the body breaks down, so does the life. Even when medicine can fix the body, that doesn't always put the life back together again. Medicine can diagnose and treat the breakdown, but sometimes so much fear and frustration have been aroused in the ill person that fixing the breakdown does not quiet them. At those times the experience of illness goes beyond the limits of medicine.
> (Frank 1991, 8)

In vivid detail, Frank reports how his medical team assumed that only his illnesses, "what is measurable and mechanical," could be discussed in office visits, in the hospital, or on the phone. His physicians, in a self-imposed exile from the emotions triggered by his failing health, placed off-limits any talk of fears and momentary victories. They pronounced their medical diagnoses and prognoses with abrupt candor, usually in cold, monotonic voices. Frank's physical conditions became the subjects and objects of dialogue, replacing the colloquial "we" and "you" of friendly conversation.

> The physician was speaking as if to himself, allowing me, the patient, to overhear. It is dangerous to avoid doctors, but it is equally dangerous to allow them to hog center stage in the drama of illness. . . . If we allow them to dominate the drama, they will script it to include only disease. By saying "This will have to be investigated," my physician claimed center stage and scripted the drama to follow; the person within my body was sent out into the audience to watch passively.                    (Frank 1991, 51, 53)

Frank interpreted the physician's cool professionalism as implicitly offering him a deal: "If my response was equally cool and professional, I would have at least a junior place on the management team" (Frank 1991, 10). But this "partnership" would be gained at the expense of any emotional recognition of what was happening to his life. Frank's wife was shunted aside even more decisively. Doctors and nurses rarely acknowledged her presence. When she was addressed, it was often with over-the-shoulder remarks deprived of the sincerity of eye contact.

The pain of this depersonalization is often inflamed by the way that acquaintances treat patients. When your body goes out of control, people tend to recoil as if *you* have lost control, with an implication of moral failure. You get the feeling that you are vaguely responsible for the condition. In order to compensate, to regain moral ground, you struggle to keep up appearances, to demonstrate courage, optimism, and cheer whenever possible. This can be hard work. Frank describes the pressures he felt to laugh and make others feel good, rather than grieving or sharing the profound sadness that he was actually feeling. Medical staffs often encourage such dissembling, knowing that it molds patients into more easily managed subjects.

Anatole Broyard, former editor of *The New York Times Book Review,* wrote feelingly about the same forces of emotional disconnection. Before succumbing to cancer, he longed for understanding from his physician:

> I wouldn't demand a lot of my doctor's time; I just wish he would *brood* on my situation for perhaps five minutes, that he would give me his whole mind just once. I would like to think of him as going through my character, as he goes through my flesh, to get at my illness, for each man is ill in his own way. . . . Just as he orders blood

tests and bone scans of my body, I'd like my doctor to scan *me*, to grope for my spirit as well as my prostate.

His insights continue: "Whether he wants to be or not, the doctor is a storyteller, and he can turn our lives into good or bad stories, regardless of the diagnosis. . . . Astute as he is, he doesn't yet understand that all cures are partly 'talking cures.' Every patient needs mouth-to-mouth resuscitation, for talk is the kiss of life" (Broyard 1990, 33, 36).

Only exceptional doctors, Broyard noted, perceive a fundamental incongruity: To physicians, each serious illness is a routine incident in their rounds, whereas, to the patient, it is the crisis of his or her life. Martha Weinman Lear echoes this concern from her husband's ordeal with heart disease. They were both perplexed and confused by the distant and impersonal manner their doctor adopted: "Roberts (the doctor) never looked at him or talked to him directly. Roberts never called him by any name—not Hal, not Harold, not Dr. Lear, nothing. Simply 'you.' He would come by twice a day, bury his head in the chart and say, 'Well, you seem to be okay.' As in the relationship between a building and a janitor" (Lear 1980, 46).

Even physicians who suffer acute illnesses slump into the deferential patient role, as we learn from Dr. Edward Rosenbaum's account of his diagnosis and treatment for cancer of the larynx. Being a physician himself provided no insulation from curt handling by the medical system. Once he took on the patient role, he was subjected to the same perfunctory consultations and the same hasty exchanges of yes–no questions that anyone else endures. On his tenth day of radiation treatment, the patient and physician met for the first time since the initial diagnosis. Rosenbaum recounts their encounter:

> "How do you feel?" he asks.
> "Okay."
> "No sore throat?"
> "No."
> "No cough?"
> "No."
> "No trouble swallowing?"
> "No."
> "Skin sore?"
> "No." I'm afraid to say yes to anything for fear that he might stop therapy.

"What's going to happen?" I ask.

And he says shortly, "You're going to feel worse."

(Rosenbaum 1988, 95)

Rosenbaum was as mystified as the rest of us often are about the course of disease and therapy, and he was just as reluctant to raise questions, to tug at the doctor's sleeve for a bit more time and emotional exposure. He recollects his understanding of the delicate balance of power between doctor and patient this way: "Don't upset the doctor or he or she won't like you and won't take good care of you" (Rosenbaum 1988, 28).

These denials of patients' human individuality strike heavy blows against the courage to defeat illness. And doctors' refusal to see connections between bodily tissues and emotional tone actually prolongs sickness.

## HEALTH HAZARDS OF THE TRADITIONAL PATIENT ROLE

The traditional patient role often works against getting well. Seeing oneself as a patient can unleash morbid thoughts of decline, weakness, and embarrassment over being dependent on others. Patients who succumb without protest to unfeeling treatment pay dearly for their submission. In an ironic twist, a health-care system that abuses people's independence manufactures unnecessary work for itself. People who feel a lack of control under adverse conditions complain of extra physical ailments. They report more headaches, upset stomach, dizziness, itchiness, and shortness of breath than people who feel more in control. People with such symptoms naturally label them as a physical malady, mixed in with the condition that brought them to seek help in the first place.

Alas, health professionals often fail to realize that their insensitive ways defeat the purposes of medical care. They focus on achieving efficiencies. By treating patients coolly, medical personnel discourage them from demanding unacceptable amounts of time, disturbing the patterned flow of treatment, disagreeing about procedures, or complaining too much about pain. Staff wield control by withholding information, so that patients cannot argue from adequate knowledge; staff explain that routines or procedures cannot be varied, thus underscoring their own professional authority (Taylor 1979).

The "good" patient cooperates, follows instructions, is passive, and seeks little information. Doctors and nurses appreciate these cheerful stoics. But this state can confound good care. The "good" patient often slumps into feelings of helplessness and refrains from disclosing emotions and sensations that would help the staff manage a condition more successfully.

"Problem" patients, on the other hand, play a consumer role in terms of right-to-know. They complain, demand attention, and can grow defiant. These patients are seen as grouchy, argumentative, over-emotional, and as requiring pampering. In fact, the more that patients preserve their autonomy and assert their individual differences, the more likely they will be labeled as "problems" by the staff. Studies in a hospital setting show that sedatives are often used to quiet problem patients, and that staff seldom resort to talking (reassuring, encouraging, explaining, ordering, chastising) with them. In fact, patients with whom staff remember taking time to talk are likely to be recalled as "problems" rather than "good patients" (Lorber 1975).

Neither helplessness nor anger is an ideal posture for any patient all the time. Furthermore, patients' style of behavior can ebb and flow: The "whiner" may suddenly withdraw; the pleasant patient may begin to terrorize the staff. In order to discriminate between life-sustaining and life-denying acts, patients need to adopt a variety of roles throughout their illness. Recognizing the range of possibilities can bring a deeper understanding of how to enact a particular patient script and what the advantages and disadvantages of different scenarios might be.

## GETTING ON THE RIGHT WAVELENGTH WITH DOCTORS

Communication between doctor and patient takes many forms. Each person "reads" the other's voice intonations, and hears sounds of confidence, despair, respect, indifference, or other emotions and judgments. Patients can be quite accurate when interpreting others' voices, and often the actual words being spoken matter very little. Many people, including physicians, fail to disguise their inner feelings, even when speaking to clients in a professional setting.

Communication also rests on facial cues, posture, gestures, and other nonverbal behavior. But right now, consider the verbal exchanges in medical consultations. What do patients and doctors talk about with one another? And can insights into these exchanges launch medical encounters along more productive and satisfying lines?

There's little question that patient and doctor coordinate their actions. At the outset, each has an idea of how matters ought to be handled between them. Each party believes that mutual accommodation is taking place, and each understands that the other is aware of it. Of course, a patient gives up more ground during this "dance" than does the physician, considering the chasm in power and status that separates them.

The words that contribute to a patient-physician relationship fall into two categories. The most obvious has to do with *medical issues*: the physical exam, complaints, and diagnostic tests. This represents the hard, scientific stuff of consultations. The second use of language concerns the patient's *personal life*: details about family, curiosity about career, sports or hobbies, vacation plans, and much more.

Four kinds of relationships between patients and doctors might evolve:

1. A *distant* relationship, in which little conversation of any type takes place
2. A *technical* relationship, in which medical questions occupy center stage and shoulder aside attention to the patient's life outside of biological events
3. A *personal* relationship, involving scant amounts of medical talk but full discussion about the patient's life
4. A *complete* relationship, where talking covers both fronts

In some consultation rooms, the two voices—one concentrating on medicine, the other on personal issues—seesaw for importance. Regardless, physicians are always at the helm of the meeting's turn-taking system, always the dominant figure. When a patient interrupts to comment about the meaning of illness or to insert an anecdote from personal experience, the doctor may rush to regain control of the interview. Doctors often use euphemisms and even concealment in order to maintain an antiseptic detachment between the illness and both parties. Sometimes, of course, both participants seek this stylized communication, or at least tacitly agree to it.

Which kind of relationship do you have with your physicians? More importantly, which relationship do you want to have? A deeper look at the dynamics of each helps show the way toward your personal answer to these questions.

The *distant relationship* is fueled by a physician's brisk greeting and bland inquiry about how "we've" felt in the past week, followed by a perfunctory "Keep on the medication" and "See the receptionist about scheduling your next appointment."

The case of Leon, a patient in a busy oncology practice, typifies the many distant relationships witnessed in our fieldwork studying doctor-patient communication. He was in his early sixties, and was being treated for liver cancer; he had received an experimental implant, about the size and shape of a hockey puck, that dripped chemotherapy directly into his diseased organ. This was one of Leon's regular, weekly visits. The consultation began with under one minute of talk, opening with pleasantries between him and the physician but moving speedily into symptoms.

"No," Leon reported, "nothing unusual this past week," whereupon the doctor wheeled out of the room to get the current X ray. He promised to be right back. After half a minute of awkward silence, Leon turned to our observer and shyly confessed that he was urinating more often than usual and was troubled by headaches that wouldn't go away.

"You should tell that to the doctor," our observer advised.

"Naw," Leon replied, "it's not important or he would have asked about it. Besides, you can see how busy he is; I don't want to bother him with little things." And he didn't. Minutes later, the consultation ended without these symptoms reaching the oncologist's ears or the patient's chart.

Subsequent questioning revealed that Leon had grown accustomed to his distant relationship with his doctor. Its superficiality comforted him, blanking out symptoms and troubles he would just as soon ignore. He was grateful for a slice of the doctor's lofty attention during visits to the clinic, and he reassured family and friends about the high quality of medical care he was receiving. He felt fortunate to be in the hands of an oncologist who was obviously distracted by other patients with more serious conditions.

In the *technical relationship*, communication covers the physical problem—perhaps about symptoms, diagnosis, treatment options, issues of compliance, and side effects. The doctor allows enough time for talk and covert observation to spot inconsistencies or omissions that might spark consideration of a different course of treatment. But a concern for the patient-as-person is superficial, at best. It might be enough to ask: "How's the wife and kids?" or "Things okay at work?"

Gerda Lerner, a professor at the University of Wisconsin, describes a classic technical performance from experiences while her husband

was being treated for a brain tumor. She summoned the doctor because
Mr. Lerner was having trouble keeping his balance:

> It was typical of Dr. Goldman that he would make a house call in
> Queens, which involved for him perhaps an hour's loss of his pre-
> cious time, charge what for a specialist was a moderate fee for such a
> service, prescribe a new course of treatment and yet would evoke in
> us not only gratitude and confidence in his ability, but outrage and
> anger. He did this by spending no more than five minutes in the
> apartment, refusing to sit down while he was there and pronouncing
> his diagnosis—which turned out to be absolutely correct—a minute
> after he entered the room and without having spoken a personal
> word to a patient who was in mental agony, thinking he had finally
> lost his ability to walk. "It's nothing but Dilantin toxicity," Dr. Gold-
> man declared, ordered Carl to bed for a week, left changed drug or-
> ders with the nurse and departed.                 (Lerner 1985, 97)

When a technical relationship is achieved instead of a merely distant one, credit is often due to the patient's own doggedness. It is legendary by now that physicians give out less medical information than
patients and their family and friends crave.

Just one study involving epilepsy illustrates the point (Faden et al.
1981). Two groups were studied: adults with epilepsy and parents of
children with epilepsy. Most of the doctors preferred to confine discussions to the benefits and risks of the dominant therapy, but the
patients and parents wanted to hear much more about alternative treatments and why they should be rejected in their case. Doctors tended
to shield the adult patients and parents from information about drugs,
believing it would "make the patient very upset and anxious." But
patients and parents consistently felt that detailed information, even
about adverse outcomes, would be a comfort, promote adherence,
strengthen trust in their doctor, and bolster confidence in the therapy
finally chosen. Furthermore, patients wanted to decide on final drug
choice, knowing the pros and cons, whereas the neurologists wished to
reserve that authority for themselves.

Gulfs like these between doctor and patient remain unbridged
unless patients read consumer guidebooks about their condition and start
asking questions. Bookstores and libraries contain many such guides,
which can be found in the Health Section or by looking in the electronic catalogue under specific conditions, such as arthritis or heart
disease. We give you help in using Internet sources below, in a section
about coping with managed care; the sources provide a wealth of infor-

mation about diseases and treatments, as well. Later in this chapter, we'll offer ideas for getting more information from doctors than they spontaneously provide.

Studies have found that doctors tend to give more information to women patients than men, in part because women are more active verbally, whether they have studied their condition or not. Patients of lower education and social class receive less information than those who are comparatively well off (Waitzkin 1984, 1985).

Patient and physician fashion a *personal relationship* out of different material. In this scenario, the physician remembers family members' names and occupations. Conversation may dwell on the patient's hobbies, a recent trip, or other personal accomplishments; the physician extends sympathy over disappointments. Time is set aside to uncover important events in the patient's life: death of a friend, trouble at work, a disorienting experience. Tests, medications, and symptoms take a back seat.

The case of June, a sixty-two-year-old, is illustrative. Three years after completing treatments following a lumpectomy, her cancer had recurred. This time around with malignancy, June had decided to refuse chemotherapy. She was determined to live a vigorous and cheerful life, without prolonging it with distressing treatments. Nevertheless, she continued to visit her oncologist weekly. They discussed recent events in the community and her interests and feelings; her doctor refrained from bullying her into treatment. June wanted a personal relationship with her physician, and he gave it to her.

Some months later, we ran into June at the airport, where she was catching a vacation flight to Hawaii. She felt fine, she said, and she had tapered off her oncological visits to once a month or so. Her physician confirmed that they still met for office consultations—no drugs, no exams, just talk. June maintained the pretense of a socially accepted role as patient for the sake of friends and for the support and attention she received from her physician, but she had narrowed the treatments she accepted to the personal side of her life.

The *complete relationship* combines elements from both the personal and medical side. Jean Craig reports such an experience in her husband's fight against cancer. After his initial diagnosis, they did considerable research on various treatment protocols and sought second and third opinions. She recounts her experience in meeting yet another physician: "He began with a question no other doctor had ever asked.

'What do you do for a living?' Ed told him about advertising, marketing automobiles, and that he was currently looking for a car-related business to buy. He continued to chat with Ed, asking about me, the children, where we lived" (Craig 1991, 32). Only after this warm and inquisitive line of questions did the physician turn to the serious medical decisions that needed to be resolved.

These four relationships may perplex some patients. When, they wonder, should I seek one of these over the others? What's gained or lost in each? The distant relationship, for example, borders on callousness. But this may be acceptable to both doctor and patient where they have already forged a therapeutic plan and there's little risk that fresh or subtle symptoms might emerge.

The priestly, technical relationship keeps in step with traditions of medical practice: a doctor doing what he or she considers best for patients, even though patients might not necessarily agree at the time. Patients may wish to settle for this instrumentalism when they are confident that their own emotions and life experience have nothing to do with the course of disease, or they just don't want to share that part of their life.

A personal relationship resembles the placebo effect in pharmaceutical experiments. The patient receives no "active ingredients" but may improve anyway. Choosing just regular consultations can encourage good health practices in general and boost morale. Mysteriously, the disease resolves itself. Or, at the least, the patient stays in good spirits during a period of decline.

Complete relationships offer a lofty standard, though constraints on a doctor's time prevent embracing both medical and social issues in every office visit. A full spectrum of talk, however, allows both parties to weigh personal values, question treatment goals, and judge the effectiveness of different plans for care every step along the way. The doctor can emerge as friend and teacher, as well as adviser.

Each patient deserves a preference among these options, and each merits the chance to switch gears during the course of care. To have a say in framing relationships, though, you need to understand the shaping forces of verbal and nonverbal communication.

Many doctors will instinctively steer the consultation toward the distant or the technical variety, unless patients take a measure of control. Seizing the conversational baton is never easy, but, simple verbal interjections can halt a preoccupation with medical talk. For example,

"Doctor ——, I need to talk about my feelings about my condition (or the test you've just advised). Can we take a few minutes for this?" "Doctor ——, I'd like you to know me better, because it will help in your treatment. My (family, work, favorite activities) are important."

Timidity in the consultation room serves both patient and physician poorly. This was clear in the case of Ethel, a woman in her sixties. She presented herself one day, a tanned and athletic figure dressed in a kelly green jump suit and striking silver brooch. We would not have guessed that her cancer had spread to a variety of organs and her bones. The most urgent topic on her mind, however, was the Jazzercise classes she was taking, and how she might tailor music and movements to her diminishing mobility.

Immediately, her oncologist began scolding her for indulging in a dangerous pastime, in light of her serious condition. In an exasperated voice, he firmly directed the conversation back to the medical side of treatment and refused to discuss her sessions at the gym. Crestfallen, Ethel bolted from the room and fled to her car. Her departure shocked the doctor into remorse over his insensitive manner. Ethel never saw her physician again until hospitalized for her final days. Had she stood her ground that day about discussing Jazzercise, she might have received more palliative care to comfort her last months of life.

Why identify the type of relationship that you already have? Why try to mold a different relationship with your physician? Because you may have a nagging feeling of discontent and not understand the source of it. You may unconsciously be troubled by the style of communication that you and your doctor pursue. With this chapter's framework in mind, it's also easier to recognize that no one role relationship—distant, technical, personal, or complete—is ideal for each and every patient. Encounters change over time. Many patients who begin by focusing only on the medical side of their condition later let down the barriers to disclose other needs. Roles fit situations as well as people, and moralizing about the poverty of a distant or technical relationship may fly in the face of a patient's wishes or welfare at any particular time.

Leon, for example, *wanted* a fairly distant relationship with his doctor. A more personal relationship costs time and emotion and requires disclosures that may exceed the investment a patient is willing to make. Not everyone is determined to like his or her doctor as a person.

Nor should one leap to conclusions about which type of role relationship sustains the best quality of medical care. Settling that question

requires information about the patient's psychological and physiological condition, and what a particular physician is talented enough to provide. When people are handled humanely, sensitively, and informatively,
the full range of patient role relationships opens to them.

## OPENING NEW LINES OF COMMUNICATION

Where should you start to seize your share of control over communication with doctors? The asking of questions plays the most central
part in medical consultations. At first, this seems simple enough. One
might innocently assume that questions are asked mainly in order to
elicit information. They are, of course, but questions also assert the
speaker's self and the speaker's claim to a measure of conversational
dominance. Questions set the agenda, enabling the speaker to announce:
"Here is what is on my mind, and please adjust to that in what you say
or do next." Like a conductor's baton, questions direct each cycle of
exchange during the medical visit.

One study draws a vivid picture of question asking in typical
exchanges between doctors and patients in family medical practices
(West 1983). Patients ranged widely in age, occupation, and race, and
included men and women. Encounters varied in length. Amid this
diversity, one feature beamed through clearly: Doctors ask questions and
patients do not; physicians project their selves forward in the conversational flow and patients react. The asymmetry between physicians
and patients in their behavior is profound. In the majority of cases,
physicians asked 90 percent of the questions and patients asked 10 percent. Half of the exchanges included two or fewer questions initiated
by patients.

Timidity among patients rules many consultation rooms. When
one can muster the courage or curiosity, questions often come out in
a stammer. In fact, researchers eavesdropping on exam-room conversations hear many more stutters and other "speech disturbances" when
patients are asking questions than when answering them. It is as if
patients themselves treat their self-assertions as problematic.

The case to be made against dependency is strong. Being verbally
active and injecting one's own agenda into the medical consultation
promote biological health. Experiments have been conducted to train
patients to be more effective participants in their office visits (Kaplan,
Greenfield, and Ware 1989a,b). In one of these projects, clinic assistants
spent approximately twenty minutes with each patient before consul-

tations, reviewing the last visit and helping clarify the principal medical decisions and options for both diagnostic decisions and disease management. The assistants coached patients to ask questions and negotiate medical decisions. Those who feared embarrassment were encouraged to rehearse questions or discuss points out loud, and to focus on being as objective and as detailed as possible.

Results were profound, for both the consultation and for physical health. First of all, patients' involvement shot upward. They seized more conversational control with interruptions, suggestions, assertions, and questions, even though their office visits took no longer than usual. Physicians responded by offering two to three times the amount of factual information. Doctors opened up to express their own anger or anxiety. Tape recordings of talk preserved signs of impatience, humor, anxiety, nervous laughter, praise, misgivings, frustration, and tension. The emergence of these positive and negative emotions showed greater interpersonal engagement and care by physicians. With encouragement and training, patients' inhibitions to enter into a dialogue with their doctors melted, and the amount of facts and emotions per minute swelled as a result of a modest investment of time in skilled preparation.

Second, the ultimate payoff in better health was striking. Several categories of illness have been studied, including diabetes, ulcers, high blood pressure, and breast cancer. Weeks later, patients who received training in communicating with doctors were much better off than those whom the investigators designated as a control group. The trained people were more active physically. Diabetes patients enjoyed lower blood-sugar levels. People with hypertension got their blood pressure under control. Patients with other conditions scored better in biological status, too.

These findings carry the whiff of revolutionary gunsmoke. Thanks to short visits with a clinic assistant, a diverse array of patients learned a lot about effective negotiation with physicians: volunteering information, asking for clarification, allowing their feelings to show. Doctors responded with their own emotions and involvement. The participants created a human transaction that is seldom seen in examining rooms, and they did this *without prolonging* the length of consultations. Health status shot upward.

Another study reveals part of the reason why a humane and wide-ranging relationship between doctors and patients strengthens physical health (Burish, Snyder, and Jenkins 1991). Feeling in control during medical encounters bolsters immunological processes that protect against disease and help heal tissues. The project involved people undergoing chemotherapy, whose immune systems commonly take a nose dive *before* scheduled treatment sessions. This probably results from the association of clinic visits with nausea and anticipatory fears.

One clinic experimented by preparing patients and companions, covering the psychological as well as physiological dimensions of the disease being treated and various side effects of treatment. A patient model on videotape was shown coping with treatment—first showing some distress but then becoming more comfortable. A question-and-answer session followed the video, and booklets were also distributed. Such care achieved wide benefits for the educated patients, compared to those who didn't receive this attention. Experimental cases experienced less depression and anxiety and resumed their daily lives more quickly. They had less nausea and vomiting before and after treatments.

The advantages of open communication went beyond making clients happier. Their immune functions also remained strong, and their recovery rates were better than patients who got little in the way of psychological attention.

Patients with arthritis, to offer another example, can be helped to learn about their disease and encouraged to do their part in managing it. Among the benefits from such attention are that patients' need to visit the doctor tapers off, by as much as one-half, and their physical condition stabilizes or even improves.

Additional studies have demonstrated that patients can quickly learn how to ask questions and take a measure of control in the consultation (Anderson, DeVellis, and DeVellis 1987). Brief videotapes showing other patients being politely assertive are enough to stimulate appropriate imitation. Even giving a short leaflet to patients urging that they raise questions can empower them in ways that improve the encounter. The lesson is clear: Many people jump at the chance for greater involvement in determining their medical care, if they are shown the way. The rewards include better health, more successful coping with chronic conditions, and swifter recovery.

## THE PAYOFF FROM ASKING GOOD QUESTIONS

We have seen that patients may visit doctors for several reasons and experience widely varying outcomes. But a "technical" or "complete" relationship with medical professionals usually implies an unspoken contract: The patient will expend effort before the next visit. In these relationships, the patient acknowledges that regaining health is the goal, and that depends on compliance with instructions. Taking prescription medications in a proper way matters. Other advice—such as resting, keeping track of physical sensations, changing one's eating habits, exercising, or drinking fluids—should not be ignored.

Despite this common sense, failure to comply with medical instructions is rampant. And no wonder. From one-third to two-thirds of the important information imparted during clinical visits goes in one ear and out the other (Grover, Berkowitz, and Lewis 1994; McConaughy, Toevs, and Lukken 1995). As a result, many of the 1.5 billion prescriptions filled each year for pills, ointments, and other pharmaceuticals go unswallowed or unapplied, or are used in ways that seriously weaken their effectiveness. Only a tiny fraction of doctors' pleas that patients exercise, stop smoking, or change their diet are heeded. The rate of forgetting about medical advice is high, even when we discount those doctor-patient consultations that concentrate on personal experiences, where little information has been imparted about biological issues or about following a treatment regimen.

The literature that many of today's doctors read in medical school placed much of the blame for forgetting and other causes of noncompliance on patients. They are inattentive, it was often alleged, or suspicious that the available remedies probably would not work. Patients are poorly motivated, often failing to take their share of responsibility for getting well. Or their emotional turmoil over being ill leads to escapist styles of coping. Or they see the treatments being urged as more painful and inconvenient than illnesses, some of which don't have troubling symptoms anyway.

Recent research, however, has begun to uncover other roots of not remembering the consultation and of not complying with advice. Some of patients' apparent refusal to cooperate results from doctors failing to share crucial information. Shockingly, the most fundamental barrier to effective communication is plain and simple: Doctors often omit clinically significant facts during the consultation. In many cases, for example, physicians don't tell patients how long their therapy is likely to take. They fail to discuss dosages for drugs, or mention side effects, or interactions between drug treatments and food or other substances that patients may be taking. Doctors often do not explore whether their treatments may interfere with safe driving or hazardous activities at work. They neglect to cover the adverse events that are serious enough to warrant calling them for help. Obvious topics like a treatment's name, purpose, and effects may go unmentioned.

We saw a concrete case of this in Harold, whom we met in our study of office visits by cancer patients. He was chuckling then but had been terrified a week earlier following his infusion of chemotherapy. Hours after that treatment, he had begun urinating red fluid. He thought his bladder was hemorrhaging. An emergency call to the nurse disclosed that a common side effect of the drug was a change in the color of the urine; he was not bleeding and he need not worry. But what a pointless episode of acute anxiety.

The scale of such enforced ignorance is staggering, as the example of drug therapy illustrates. Keep in mind that prescribed medications are involved in two-thirds of the services given in physicians' offices. Put another way, about one-quarter of the adult U.S. population takes a prescription drug during a typical twenty-four-hour period. Yet, as many as one-third of patients to whom drugs are prescribed do not receive counseling at either their physician's office or the pharmacy unless they ask for information—and the vast majority do not. Such lack of counseling has been found even where prescriptions are being written for medications that patients have not used before and for drugs that have the potential for toxic reactions.

The causes behind patients' confusion can be even more frightening—and avoidable, especially when chronic medical conditions require complex sets of drugs and treatments. A study of people afflicted with rheumatoid arthritis or hypertension showed that records in the pharmacy routinely disagreed with notations that physicians had entered in patients' medical charts—about which drugs had been dispensed, their dosage form, strength, and directions for use. Duplicate prescriptions were common, as well. Errors in prescribing medications and patients' misunderstanding of their use lead to adverse reactions, longer hospital stays, and even death, and are an increasing concern in health care (Classen et al. 1997; Lesar, Briceland, and Stein 1997). These are signs that the medical system often keeps unreliable records. No wonder patients find it hard to keep matters straight.

Furthermore, experiments show that when the medical system makes the effort to get its records in order, patients' compliance with treatment improves dramatically. Their physical health gains ground, too; people with hypertension, for example, get their blood pressure under control.

The lesson is clear. When a patient wants the facts about a proposed treatment, pharmaceutical or otherwise, he or she should enter the consultation room armed with a list of questions (about timing, duration of treatment, side effects, and interaction with other prescriptions). When a patient is determined to leave behind a correct medical record, he or she should ask the doctor to "tell me the treatment or prescription again, just like you're putting it down in my chart." Prompted repetition encourages accuracy. Do not leave the consultation unless you feel you understand what the physician is recommending and why.

Of course, patients' memory for the details of medical consultations can falter, even when physicians share clinically significant information. Often the trouble lies with the way that information is conveyed. Consider, first, a general rule about memory. People recall best the first statements or ideas in a series of thoughts and the very last or most recent—tending, by comparison, to forget the middle ones. This is the well-known primacy/recency effect, observed in animal as well as human learning.

How does this apply to a medical consultation? Think of whatever a doctor says after examining the patient as a serial list of statements, stretching from first to middle to last. The first items will be well remembered because they are easily committed to long-term memory in the absence of other statements that could compete for attention and importance. By appearing early in the doctor's exploration, first statements are assumed by patients to be the most important things to remember; subsequent comments or instructions must be very dramatic in order to compete against this presumed weighting and mobilize powers to remember. Or the doctor has to provide his or her own emphasis ("Now here's something that is very important").

So much for the primacy effect. The recency effect concerns those issues discussed at the end of the consultation. We know from studies that this advantage comes from the quick access people have to their working memory (as distinguished from long-term memory). Hence, the edge for recency quickly evaporates with time and the interference of other activities. Therefore, over the long haul, patients recall the early part of consultations better than any other part.

This helps explain why people's recollections are so spotty about

the treatments that have been prescribed, including what they are supposed to do on their own to get better. Physicians usually deliver these
ideas and instructions late in office visits. The physician's earlier comments are usually about the diagnosis, and that is what sticks.

There are ways to combat this bias in human memory and get a
firm grasp on important features of a medical consultation. We share
these later in the chapter.

## READING BODY LANGUAGE AND OTHER NONVERBAL SIGNS

Words alone seldom make a communication experience valuable. A
sense of psychological "presence" is needed, too. Some physicians show
that they are alert to subtle cues that patients may exhibit, and other
doctors seem miles away, even though they are across the desk. Presence
is easy to detect, even by watching videotapes of medical consultations.

Studies have shown that groups of doctors can view tapes of consultations, say between general practitioners and patients suffering from
high blood pressure, and quickly separate their colleagues who give a
high quality of care and counseling from those who miss important
aspects of their cases (Verhaak 1986). Above all else, skillful doctors
make greater eye contact with patients than the less skillful. They also
use conversational continuers—invitations to the patient to keep talking like "Mmmm," "Hmmm," and "Ah."

These basics of an inviting nonverbal style are just a part of presence during consultations. Three other clusters of activity and furnishings contribute, as well. The doctor controls many of these. With
an understanding, however, you can know immediately why an office
visit turns sour. Often, you can take steps to improve the situation.

1. *The Use of Interpersonal Space and Distance.* By and large, presence
   grows where people arrange themselves closely rather than distantly,
   in keeping with the space available in, say, an examining room. Too
   much closeness can, of course, be oppressive, which is why a caring
   physician steps back from inspecting your throat before resuming
   conversation. But normally, presence flourishes when:

   - patient and physician face each other without a barrier of furniture;
   - parties seat themselves at the corner of the table, instead of across from
     one another in an "authority" position;
   - they occupy the same elevation when reviewing important points,

instead of different levels (as when doctor stands and patient perches on the examining table);

- they lean slightly toward one another.

2. *The Use of Bodily Motion.* For the most part, smiles promote presence, especially where they are reciprocated. Head nods encourage warmth and openness. Presence gains from the use of gestures and bodily relaxation, where doctors and patients keep hands, wrists, and arms available to punctuate the conversation, instead of folding them, digging fists into pockets, or clutching a chart or purse. Presence suffers when a doctor shows haste with abrupt movement or by entering and leaving the room often.

   The eyes can promote presence, as when the pupils dilate, which indicates interest and usually warmth. Eye contact by a speaker is more complex. Speakers alternate their gaze between the listener and vacant space to the listener's side, even when seeking presence. Speakers must "shut down" their intake from time to time in order to compose their next expressions. But a listener's wandering eyes signal distraction, a wish to be elsewhere or doing other things.

   People in a consultation do not crave constant eye contact, of course; occasions arise when both parties tacitly agree not to gaze directly at each other. Such routine avoidances often occur during the expression of physical pain and involve a subtle irony. When you seek advice for suffering that has persisted or become acute, you enter into a pair of conflicting duties. On the one hand, you feel obliged to express reasonable grounds for having sought professional help, by speaking vividly about the pain ("I've had this stabbing headache"), or wincing, or demonstrating restricted movement. On the other hand, you also agree to take an objective stance toward difficulties and cooperate with the diagnostic search for their cause. You agree to suppress the extremes of subjective accounts that might easily be shared with friends or family.

   The physician feels free to pummel, poke, bend, or massage until you complain. You curtail outcries in the interests of more clinical comments. You may say with tight lips, "That's where it hurts, Doc," or through gritted teeth, "It feels tender when you touch there." Seldom does a howl of misery escape the lips. The physician, in turn, resists extending sympathy; instead, your report brings additional inquiries and more manipulation within an entirely analytic, impersonal stance.

Importantly, the doctor averts his or her face, displaying a continuing commitment to the physical examination, while you stare into middle distance, grimaces or tears unnoticed. Both parties collaborate in this management of emotions, with the understanding that intense and spontaneous communication would interfere with the diagnostic task at hand.

Tests have been devised for measuring a doctor's ability to read nonverbal cues presented through brief video and audio clips. Physicians—like most—vary widely in how accurately they decode faces, voice intonations, and pacing (when words have been obscured electronically), and bodily postures. What's important for patients to realize is that doctors' actual sensitivity to other people's nonverbal communication is completely unrelated to how empathic or alert to these signs they think they are. Doctors often misperceive their own abilities: Some exaggerate their awareness and others underrate their skills of understanding. Patients should expect to encounter some doctors who think they are adept at noticing subtle cues, but who really don't "get it."

A tip-off that doctors, like many other people, can also be completely unaware of their own nonverbal communication comes from the account by humorist Marjorie Gross about her experiences with ovarian cancer. She's sitting in her physician's office, waiting to get the word: "What really happens is the doctor walks in and gives you the sympathetic head tilt that right away tells you, 'Don't buy in bulk.' The degree of tilt corresponds directly with the level of bad news. You know, a little tilt: 'We've caught it in time'; sixty-degree angle: 'Spread to the lymph nodes'; forty-five-degree angle: 'Spread to your clothes'" (Gross 1996, 54).

Studies don't confirm that this particular bodily posture conveys the signal that Gross read in it, but we all get the point. Some doctors have a very shaky grasp on the value of posture and other parts of humankind's second language. They turn out to be the physicians whose patients adhere to treatment poorly and who fail to keep scheduled appointments. These are the physicians whose case loads include many disgruntled customers, often unclear about precisely why they are so unhappy.

3. *Office Decor.* Also important is the structure of the waiting room, the way the physical layout of the doctor's office reinforces the patient's

position in the medical hierarchy. Here is Jean Craig, who visited many doctors during her husband's illness:

> Doctor More's office was like a zillion other doctors' offices in a zillion other medical buildings. A cookie-cutter decor ordered, it looked to me, from a 1940s Sears catalogue. The waiting room was very small and cramped. The receptionist was behind the sliding-glass window, as usual. The sliding-glass window in doctors' offices has become an important piece of symbolism to me. Not only is it unfriendly, it also says "them" and "us." It makes a separation between the medical staff and the patients. It makes a boundary that says what any boundary says: "Stay out. Don't bother us. Speak when spoken to." If I could wave a magic wand over the medical profession, the first thing I would do is rip out all those glass windows and make those receptionists sit out there with the people and answer the phone in front of them.                (Craig 1991, 139–140)

Decor and interior design can create a moatlike barrier between patients and staff, which might explain the limited communication that typically occurs between occupants on either side of the partition. An authoritarian waiting room for patients may set the stage for guarded encounters with doctors later on.


## A GAME PLAN FOR BETTER COMMUNICATION

Consultations with physicians will stay in the same rut, unless *you* take the first steps. You can nudge communication into new channels of mutual discovery, but don't expect doctors to take the lead. Here are some practical strategies to get you started.


### DESCRIBE THE CHALLENGE

You may be searching for a diagnosis or already under treatment. Or, perhaps, you just feel unwell and anxious. Whatever the situation, the first step toward gaining control is to put your thoughts about the problem into a concrete form, where you can examine them coolly. You should find a quiet corner, away from interruptions. If home or work sites are too distracting, a public library or a church or synagogue, or even a coffee shop will do. You should get comfortable, and be prepared to write nonstop for at least thirty minutes on these questions.

- What is the problem, minor or serious, that is bothering you? When did the problem begin, and how has it evolved since?

- Describe your symptoms, as completely as you can. Are there other symptoms or side effects that you have been led to expect—from physicians or from common knowledge, from the media, or from acquaintances?
- What distresses you about this problem?
- Does the problem have a bright side you've overlooked?
- Do others suspect you have this problem? What troubles you about their reactions? Is there anything positive about the way others react to the problem?
- What caused the problem, as best you can tell?
- Have your decisions to continue or refrain from doing certain things magnified the problem?
- What direction will this problem take if you do nothing about it?
- What options do you have for dealing with the problem?

When you've written everything that comes to mind about the situation, you should snap your notebook shut and put it away for a few days. With the passage of some time, you'll do better at distinguishing enduring thoughts from passing sentiments. When you do pick up your notes again, you'll have one purpose uppermost in mind: deciding which of these ideas to share with others and which to keep to yourself. Those you decide to share provide leverage for boosting your sense of control.

You must also decide what to divulge to medical professionals and what you would prefer to share with a minister, rabbi, priest, or counselor. What should you discuss with work associates, family members, or close friends?

In preparing to see doctors or others, you should keep in mind that most people organize their thoughts about illness using a timeline to narrate the condition. People tend to package experiences so that sensations—dizziness, swelling, pain, watery eyes, and the like—get connected to perceived causes and consequences. Often, symptoms fit into a stereotype developed for common conditions, such as the flu, allergic reactions, or a heart attack. Patients develop models of a condition as acute, cyclical, or chronic; they self-diagnose. The more unhappy, upset, or distressed you are, the more symptoms you are likely to jot down, and the more intensely they will be felt. Humans construct images of illness by mixing personal feelings with medical facts.

## IMPROVE THE QUALITY OF TALK

Before leaving for a consultation, write down the questions you want to ask and comments you want to make. Naturally, other inquiries or statements will arise spontaneously, but studies confirm that prior planning boosts the number of contributions you make and their value to both patient and physician.

Organize your list so that you cover all the ground you want. Try to document symptoms and time sequences as carefully as possible. Consider aspects of your personal values, feelings, and experiences that you would like to clarify. Review issues about your medical situation about which you are unsure. Coping with a condition or treatment usually improves when you frame two lines of questioning.

In many kinds of office visits, your first inquiries should ask for *procedural information:* Step-by-step, what is going to happen during diagnostic and treatment programs? The second questions should seek *sensory information:* What are the tastes, feelings, sounds, or smells that the test or treatment and its side effects bring? When you know about each of these ahead of time, you can anticipate and rehearse what is going to happen. Understanding one's own reactions reduces both anxiety and the sense of physical discomfort. You get back to normal more quickly and require fewer medications.

Suppose, for example, that your physician suspects you have polyps in your colon. He or she might prescribe a barium enema; this involves inserting barium, a chalky liquid resistant to X rays, into the large intestine, making it clearly visible on the film and permitting the doctor to see any defects, masses, or obstructions. Your understanding of the procedure starts your process of coping with it.

*Procedural information* forecasts exactly how the examination takes place. You'll want to ask about how you should prepare ahead of time. (You will eat no solids for twenty-four hours nor fluids for eight hours, and will take laxatives and a regular enema the night before.) Next question: What happens during the procedure? (You will undress and lie on a hard table on your side; a lubricated nozzle will be eased into your rectum; barium will slowly be injected and its progress up the colon monitored.) Who will do all this? (A trained medical technician, not your doctor.) Where? (At a lab specializing in this work or at a hospital.) What happens next? (The technician will continue pumping barium until all the loops of your colon are filled. Finally, several X rays will be taken.) How long will this take? (Probably thirty to forty-five minutes.)

By this point, you would probably benefit from some *sensory information*—all the things you will feel, taste, smell, and hear. Find out before the procedure, so you're not startled by something that's perfectly normal.

Easy-to-understand handbooks about common medical procedures are also available. One such handbook prepares readers for the barium enema with this description:

> With enemas it is usual to have a cramping feeling, fullness, and an overwhelming desire to defecate. A small balloon-type device on the tube helps you retain the barium. If you expel some of the liquid, don't be embarrassed. Doctors and technicians are used to it. Retaining your dignity and sense of humor can be as difficult as retaining the barium. Once the X-rays are taken you are permitted to go to the bathroom and expel the barium, which will relieve much of the discomfort immediately. After the procedure you will probably be encouraged to drink lots of water to ease the constipation that often follows a barium enema. . . . Don't be alarmed if your stool is white for 24 to 72 hours.                    (Wurman 1985, 81)

Armed with facts, you know what to expect before, during, and after the examination. Be alert to asking about unexpected sensations. Abrupt or unusual noises can be disconcerting. Tastes stimulated by drugs can be mistaken for the onset of nausea. A wealth of research confirms that patients who understand what's going to happen to them feel more confident, experience less pain, and recover more speedily than people who remain in the dark.

The power of sensory information to quell anxieties emerges in this case recalled by Erma Bombeck. She tells of a mother whose three-year-old daughter was diagnosed with a brain-stem tumor. How could one prepare the tot for the strange noises and menacing apparatus of radiation therapy? "At night we'd wrap Darlene in a white sheet and lay her on the kitchen table. Then we'd turn on the microwave for sound, turn off the lights so it would be dark, and put the portable sewing machine lid over her head and thump it with our fingers. We set the timer for thirty seconds at first and if she didn't move, then each time we did this we'd do it a little longer" (Bombeck 1989, 10).

Why does concrete and objective information about impending medical events reassure more often that it unsettles? Because a mental picture composed of accurate and unambiguous descriptions of things to come displaces a map that focuses on the unpleasantness or anticipated pain. People worry more about what *could* happen when they are unprepared for what *will* happen. Diverting attention away from emotional dimensions helps to manage your body and to understand the reactions you feel as each new step of a medical procedure unfolds. You understand what is happening, even if you don't enjoy it. Even the toddler Darlene lost some of her fears of the unknown, from learning sounds and sensations that mimicked her upcoming treatment.

## REHEARSE

Practice may not make perfect, but it does make for increased confidence. Now that you have questions and comments in mind, there's one more vital step. Just going over plans in your mind is not enough. It takes *practice* (which builds courage) for many people to speak up during their consultations. Because you don't have a videotape showing how others react during visits to the doctor, you'll have to create your own demonstration. Fortunately, you already own an interactive technology that really helps—a large mirror.

You need to practice saying things out loud, and a mirror helps you observe your own body language. Do your posture and gestures convey feelings and punctuate ideas, the way you wish to be seen? Prop the mirror in a position where the doctor will likely sit, relative to the spot that you'll occupy.

Speaking into a tape recorder can also help. How well do voice inflection and pacing support what you're trying to get across? Are there words and gestures you could substitute that would be more effective?

Mirror and tape machine can boost self-awareness. Studies show that building self-awareness this way reduces the chance of misleading the doctor. And the physician will refrain from asserting dominance, when that's unproductive. Practice with a mirror and tape recorder contributes to genuine rather than faked communication. Fifteen minutes spent on these private rehearsals can make a world of difference in the richness and coherence of the stories you tell.

Watching and listening to yourself ahead of time also strengthens your persistence during the consultation itself. You're less likely to let conversational sidetracks divert you from getting what you want from the visit. You'll be less likely to let a physician's appearance or idiosyn crasies interfere with the exchange. Your motivation to tell the doctor what's really on your mind grows, and you'll show your feelings more clearly, whatever they are. All this will help the doctor make an accurate diagnosis and offer the most appropriate choice of treatments.

## USE NONVERBAL STRATEGIES TO HIGHLIGHT NEEDS

Many patients feel like Sidney, age sixty-three. He suffers from serious heart disease, and had this to say about appointments with his doctor: "He's miles away on the other side of that desk, and the whole time we're talking he's got his eyes glued to my chart, scribbling away. Sometimes I feel like grabbing the thing and yelling, 'Would you please just *look at me?*'"

What strategies can you use to draw the doctor's attention away from reading your chart and get him or her to face you directly? *Refraining from speaking* always captures the needed audience; usually a gap of three to five seconds is sufficient. An *extended pause* such as "Well . . ." in the middle of a sentence can achieve the same effect. A switch from coherent to *perturbed and hesitant speech* ("Errr, ahh, I don't know . . . cough . . . maybe . . . you know") also brings eye contact.

Similar results follow from *sudden movements*. You may lean forward into the doctor's field of vision, or stretch out in a chair, clasping your hands behind your head, or simply gesture with one or both hands to punctuate what you are saying. With these actions, you project a body part toward the doctor, perhaps even into his or her personal space. Faced with activities like these, few doctors will fail to look up from their chart reading or writing. Even more dramatic *shifts in posture* can command the stage—such as rising from a chair, or stepping to a window and turning back to face the doctor. These flamboyant quests for attention are best reserved for crucial utterances. Otherwise they risk focusing attention on themselves rather than on what you have to say.

You can put insights about nonverbal communication to work, seizing control of the consultation when you want it. But sensitivity to nonverbal events also improves your understanding of how the doctor is interpreting the meaning of the time you spend together.

## BE ALERT TO YOUR OWN DECEPTIONS

In the examining room, patients often harbor a hidden agenda, as well as stated purposes for the visit. The announced condition may mask something that the patient feels is unacceptable or hard to report. In primary-care settings, the underlying motivation for visiting a physician matches the announced complaint in only half of the encounters. Sometimes, though, the reasons behind faulty or misguided treatment rest on patients' style of communicating.

More often than some would admit, for example, people give their doctor an idealized picture of physical or psychological conditions. Or they cloud over important topics, failing to report symptoms or underplaying a lifestyle that contributes to illness. It's not fair to brand this behavior bald-faced lying. Many times such patients are completely unaware of the motivations that contribute to their repressed or biased accounts.

Denial comes in two flavors. In one, people engage in self-deception, actually believing in an exaggerated, flattering image of themselves. When responding to questionnaires that measure self-deception, these people may insist that they have never, ever thought that their parents hated them, or ever doubted their own sexual adequacy, or worried over possible misfortunes. With these deep-seated questions about self-image, some people refuse to acknowledge that "terrible" thoughts have crossed their minds.

In the second kind of deception, people try to manage the impressions others form of them by covering lapses in behavior that could be embarrassing. These impression managers fudge their image in socially desirable ways—insisting, for example, that they are always courteous, even to disagreeable people, or that they always tell the truth, or are never irritated at people who ask favors, or never vote for candidates they know little about.

Patients who practice either of these styles, the extremes of self-deception or of impression management, also underreport physical symptoms to the doctor. Pains that may be forerunners of angina go unmentioned, for example, or gastrointestinal upsets or blood in stool are ignored. Such patients' reporting of psychological symptoms is even more biased—silence about anxieties or depression or sexual dysfunction. If the physician doesn't catch onto these omissions and distortions, he or she can overlook or mistreat a condition. Even the doctor's sympathetic manner and guarantee of confidentiality may not insure candor from a patient when unconscious tendencies toward self-deception are in play.

In another kind of miscommunication, patients disgorge symptoms, descriptions of physical pain, or other sensations for which repeated examinations fail to find organic causes. Doctors refer to such patients as "somatisizers." Sometimes these patients' sensations change in elusive and subtle ways, to be followed by a new trail of laboratory tests in an attempt to pin them down. Often, doctors continue to order tests in order to protect themselves against charges of malpractice. And sometimes their persistence actually uncovers a pathological condition that needs attention.

## LEARN SUBTLE CLUES TO WHAT THE OTHER FEELS

Thoughtful patients recognize that unarticulated reasons may stand behind their wish to see a physician. Expressed complaints may serve as thin excuses, opening the door to revealing more urgent concerns, usually of a psychological order. For example, a patient feels tired or has a persistent cough, but the visit's more pressing agenda is really an unwanted pregnancy, marital strife, job insecurity, or the death of a close friend. Will the physician move beyond ruses and throw open the appropriate channels of communication? Not easily, in a rushed or interrupted office environment, or without the doctor's attention to how you look or sound.

When you shrink from putting underlying concerns into words, sometimes you unwittingly let slip, or "leak," what is really on your mind. A patient's self-touching is one powerful nonverbal sign. Scratching, grooming, ear-touching, facial stroking, and adjustments of clothing often reveal a generalized anxiety about the consultation itself. As Freud observed of a patient: "If his lips are silent, he chatters with his fingertips; betrayal oozes out of him at every pore" (Freud 1964, 78).

Importantly, turnabout is fair play in reading nonverbal messages. Patients unconsciously interpret their doctors' cloaked communications. Studies show how physicians as well as ordinary people project their expectations about others through the contours of voice intonation, speed, and rhythm, irrespective of words. Most patients have learned to follow these nonverbal communications by physicians for signals about how fully the doctor expects a recovery. The messages patients receive often have a powerful effect on healing.

Researchers tape-recorded psychologists, psychiatrists, and other counselors during interviews with patients (Rosenthal, Blanck, and Vannicelli 1984). These same counselors also were asked to talk privately about each of their patients for three to five minutes. Thus, the study gathered two samples of professionals' talk—direct talk *to* patients and indirect talk *about* the same patients. This talk was subjected to electronic filtering that removes the high frequencies on which word recognition depends but preserves cues relating to tone of voice and pacing of speech. Independent panels of judges rated these fragments of speech for characteristics like warmth, dominance, empathy, competence, optimism, and professionalism.

Even though the judges were working with snippets of conversation and were deprived of the actual words being spoken, they were able to agree about the emotions and feelings that the different voices expressed. Not only that, the emotions that the clinicians conveyed when talking confidentially *about* patients matched closely with what they conveyed when talking directly *to* their patients. For example, a staff member's cold and domineering manner when reflecting privately about a patient also showed up in that counselor's voice when talking with the patient face-to-face.

Furthermore, staff voices were judged more "competent," more "professional," and more "optimistic" when they were talking to patients they expected to get better than when speaking to those they expected to get worse. Results underscore that even trained clinicians telegraph their assumptions about recovery to patients, setting the stage for self-fulfilling outcomes. No wonder some people have come to believe that patients can be "talked into" a deeper illness than they actually suffer.

What are the implications of all this for the doctor-patient relationship? Both partners need to pay attention to body and vocal signals—modulation, tone, pauses, and the like—in addition to the words being spoken. Both partners should also be aware that facial expressions can easily mislead, even though this is the most conspicuous channel of nonverbal exchange.

Because nonverbal communication carries so much weight in the examining room, it is not surprising that misunderstandings often arise between cultural communities. Most of us are more adept at reading nonverbal cues that originate within our own subcultural group than ones from other ethnic groups or backgrounds. Middle-class whites and inner-city African-Americans bring different norms to their "reading" of a New York Jewish pediatrician, for example.

## IMPROVE YOUR MEMORY FOR CLINICALLY IMPORTANT FACTS

Most physicians are blissfully unaware of the dynamics of memory. So, again, a patient who wants to remember the consultation must take the lead, with two crucial steps. Step one is for the patient to create an occasion for "summing up," when he or she has planned ahead of time to pay close attention to everything being said and, crucially, to ask for an organized capsule of main points.

After all the conversational back-and-forth, seek the bottom line. Say, for example, "Now that we're near the end of my visit, I want to make certain that I understand seven things clearly and simply: What is wrong with me? What tests are we going to carry out (if relevant)? What will happen to me (procedural and sensory facts)? What treatments do I need? What do I need to do to help myself? How long will it take for me to feel better? When should I plan to see you again?" Studies show that patients' memory strengthens when doctors cast information into this explicit structure. Facts align in a coherent pattern and statements that jump erratically from topic to topic tend to disappear.

This summing up defeats another oversight by physicians that weakens memory. Throughout a consultation, doctors often neglect to separate the most important information from nonessential items. They fail to accent or emphasize vital material. Asking for the bottom line overcomes this lapse.

Memory also improves when medical ideas are expressed in specifics rather than general or vague terms ("Lose three pounds before your next visit" versus "You should lose some weight," or "Take the medications with your three main meals during the day" versus "Let's try some medication and see what happens"). Asking for a structured bottom line encourages such concrete instructions. Memory gets better when a few key points are made rather than many; a structured summarization leads toward simplification, too.

Step two toward improved memory requires repetition or rehearsal of information. Ask the doctor to repeat important points during the "summing up." Say them *aloud* yourself, getting his or her confirmation. This helps transfer ideas from working to long-term memory, where you can later retrieve them.

The aim of this effort goes beyond simple recall. You want to interpret correctly what the physician has concluded. Why are you having your trouble? Why is a certain treatment advised: Will it make your condition more tolerable, or cure it, or help investigate it further, or prevent it from recurring? Knowing these things avoids later disappointments and a sense of futility that things haven't panned out as expected.

A determined patient should take notes during this summing up, or, even preferably, bring along a friend to do so. If you do, write the headings down ahead of time to organize ideas—what's wrong, tests, what will happen, treatment, your duties in the healing process—so you can easily fill in the blanks. Again, your goal is to prompt an organized and concise explanation, not just to elicit lots of information. You may prefer to bring a small tape recorder, in order to review the consultation later. If so, still take along your agenda of questions; you need these to shape the conversation.

## COMPOSE A SATISFYING STORY TO EXPLAIN YOUR ILLNESS

Systematic, orderly questions from a patient boost memory for details that help one stick to treatment. But patients who are suffering from a chronic and serious condition may want their office visits to be more than informing. They may be searching for a higher understanding. They may want to compose an explanation about their illness that addresses why this is happening to them. In short, why me?

Most urgently, the need to endure excruciating, horrendous pain demands an explanation that can rationalize distress. People need to find *meaning* in such experience, and three kinds of narratives can come to the rescue. Sometimes people construct their story around motifs of punishment. They see themselves as just or unjust victims of a force. Reparations must be paid to this force (a deity, simple luck, or misfortune) for one's failings, or to appease the fickle power that has brought one to his or her knees. If it's too late in life for atonement, these patients' stories may rationalize suffering without providing a means to keep it at bay.

Other people's stories hinge on a military theme. Pain and disability result from an invasion by hostile elements, externally or internally, stealing valuable parts of life. Under attack, the patient scrambles to find allies (friends, family, a supportive doctor, spiritual aid). When the patient fails to build troop strength, he or she may succumb to an overwhelming enemy.

In the third imagery some people use, the idea of challenge commands center stage. Illness presents obstacles, just like other situations in life. Disease imposes demands and tasks to be mastered by any means available. Diligence and determination to succeed must spring from personal strength ("No one can fight this but me"; "I've got a lot to live for"), even though encouragement from others can help. These stories picture pain as a personal adversary, sometimes even an ennobling one.

Evidence shows that people who weave a story of challenge around their illness feel less subjective pain, marshal more coping strategies, and are less depressed than patients who embrace other explanations. But these can be secondary benefits to people whose lives have twisted out of shape from chronic disease. Having *any* framework for understanding trauma is preferable to none at all. Being able to convey a story about illness to others allows one to feel heard and acknowledged.

Office visits to the doctor provide, in theory at least, an opportunity to elaborate the story behind illness, pain, and frustration. Physicians can embellish a patient's figurative depiction of disease by contributing metaphors, analogies, anecdotes, allegories, and other elements that inspire interpretive meaning. Metaphors are expressions about one thing in terms of another, throwing new light on the character of what is being described. For example, "diabetes is a dictator," unforgiving and making endless demands, only neutralized by shrewd and relentless opposition. Analogies compare things that are usually seen as dissimilar. For example, "Your mood right now is like the sailor who has heard the order to abandon ship, but can't find his way to a lifeboat." Anecdotes are short tales about other people's experiences, or they draw on autobiographical episodes. Allegories capture essential truths about the human condition (courage, devotion to God, humility) in the actions of symbolic fictional characters.

When doctors use such figurative language, in addition to straightforward and literal talk, they help patients construct their own story around the serious illness that besets them. They help patients visualize their life's current objectives—such things as "being a positive model for their children to emulate," "appearing physically attractive," "ending jealousies or anger directed at others," "becoming recognized for excellence at work," and, of course, "eliminating pain or bringing it under control."

When an individual's story about illness clarifies strivings and objectives, these elements can be integrated into a larger framework for self-understanding. The individual can gauge whether goals stand in harmonious relationship (the things required to pursue each goal also help one attain other goals, or at least don't interfere). Or the person can discover that goals lie in conflict (efforts required to attain one goal work against securing others). Once these roots of trouble have been uncovered, options become available. The individual may forsake a goal or find new ways to achieve it that don't imperil other goals. Even more significant, the individual can now talk about the dilemma.

Storytelling and story listening (or reading) fulfill basic human needs. The writer Bill Buford expressed it this way, when accounting for the outpouring of novels and other tales that have swept onto our cultural scene:

> But stories also protect us from chaos, and maybe that's what we, unblinkered at the end of the twentieth century, find ourselves craving. Implicit in the extraordinary revival of storytelling is the possibility that we need stories—that they are a fundamental unit of knowledge, the foundation of memory, essential to the way we make sense of our lives . . . We have returned to narratives—in many fields of knowledge—because it is impossible to live without them.
>
> (Buford 1996, 12)

Ideally, talking with physicians has much to offer, as patients struggle to make coherent the strivings that play a part in their narratives about pain. But patients who are not getting much help from their medical doctors in storytelling and goals clarification may want to seek assistance elsewhere. Psychological counselors offer one resource. Therapists may differ widely in the clinical methods they practice, but most are gifted at sharing apt stories and expressive ideas that enrich illness narratives.

The patient who seeks such help in storytelling, however, needs to be aware of the therapist's agenda. That counselor may cling to biases toward the "best" kind of story for the patient to craft. The therapist may be eager to dispose of "dysfunctional" or "inaccurate" narratives, instead of allowing the patient to find his or her own voice.

Joining a support group can also promote storytelling. The patient may see fragments of his or her own experience in another's tale. Or the patient is startled to find coherence in his or her illness, only by relating it to the group.

One fact remains firm, however. Treatment for disease requires images for the heart and mind, as well as medicine. The seriously ill seek both kinds of relief.

## OTHER STEPS THAT BRING A MORE REWARDING CONSULTATION

Simple, humble tips can work wonders for a patient's confidence. You should remain clothed whenever possible, for example. You'll feel more comfortable in street clothes than in those awkward paper gowns, especially with a new doctor. Tell the physician that you want to get dressed before talking over the consultation's important points. Your composure and memory will improve.

Patients should take stock of their consultations afterward. A diary composed of notes following each session allows you to record details from the talk and the nonverbal feelings you experienced. What topics failed to emerge that, in hindsight, you wish had come up? Did the doctor ask broad, free-ranging questions, or did the inquiries seem confined to yes–no alternatives? Did the doctor solicit your point of view? Were the doctor's postures, movement, and voice inviting, or preoccupied and self-centered?

What about your own contributions? Did you bring up the questions you had in mind? A candid record of the information you think you provided in words—and more covertly in intonations, posture, and gestures—improves the next visit. If you find yourself struggling to imagine the messages you conveyed, consider how vague you might have appeared to your doctor.

Patients should consider *taking someone along* to appointments. The companion can keep notes or remind you of questions that you intended to ask, or simply give you a fresh opinion about how well you got your points across. No matter how well prepared you are for a medical examination, as the object of scrutiny, your ability to process information accurately and compose coherent questions will not be in top form.

Keeping your dignity and asserting what's on your mind improve physical well-being. With feelings of control, the human immune system grows stronger and promotes faster healing. Hiding your real feelings about illness under a blanket of false cheerfulness or feigned indifference might be helpful to people around you in the short run, but you risk impaired health and peace of mind down the road.

## IN THE HOSPITAL

Most of the advice we've shared deals with outpatient situations, the major setting for patient-physician contacts. Should you find yourself in the hospital, though, you need to be especially vigilant. You probably wouldn't think of the most vital protections, but they can spare you agony. For example, write your name prominently on a stiff piece of paper and tape it above your bed (to avoid treatments intended for someone else). To be doubly safe, always ask the nurse to check the name and dosage of any medication he or she is about to give you.

Outline the area of your body to be operated on with a felt-tip marker. Tell the anesthesiologist if you are on any type of medication. You can discover the wisdom behind many more ideas like these from a physician writing from his own experience as a cardiac patient in his own hospital (Blau and Shimberg 1997).

### IT'S JUST NOT WORKING

Suppose you're armed with questions, you've rehearsed, and you've consulted notes from past visits, but you still feel ignored after seeing the doctor? You have tried in vain to capture his or her concern with verbal prompts: "Doctor, I need to talk about this test," or "Doctor, I'd like to review my condition." You may have used gestures or silence to command notice, but failed. You remain confused about the course your care is taking.

Trust your misgivings. Recognize that patients switch doctors for many reasons. "Doctor shopping" has gained an ugly reputation because many assume that patients who change physicians must be grasping for a comforting diagnosis or looking for someone to rubber-stamp their own choice of drugs or other therapies. Fickle or immature or petulant people are not the only ones who change doctors. Some thoughtful, intelligent patients also make changes for a better quality of relationship. Believe in your right to control your life and in the vital part that good communication plays in biological health. Change doctors, and don't allow yourself to feel guilty about taking that step.

### THE CHANGING WORLD OF MEDICINE: HOW TO GET YOUR INSURER TO PAY ATTENTION

The tidal wave of managed care now covering more than sixty million people has raised the public's sensitivity about quality. And, no wonder: Insurance plans differ widely. Take the case of drugs called beta-blockers; given after a heart attack, this medicine can reduce chances of another attack by 25 percent and death by 10 percent. The average Health Maintenance Organization (HMO) provides such medications to six of ten patients who need them, but plans across the United States range from a low of one of seven appropriate cases getting the drugs to a high of every patient getting them (National Committee for Quality Assurance 1997). Clearly this leaves much room for improvement and an incentive for each patient to press hard for attentive care.

Quality-of-care statistics make tricky reading, though. Traditional insurance and fee-for-service payment often score even lower than the average HMO on use of beta-blockers, prenatal care, eye exams for people with diabetes, and other clinical measures. Developing an overall report card for care under different methods of reimbursement is arduous and time-consuming, and rating one HMO over another can prove equally frustrating.

## EXAMINING MANAGED CARE

Health Maintenance Organizations (HMOs) are the oldest form of managed care, starting in the United States on a small scale as early as 1929. HMOs offer members a range of health benefits for a set monthly fee. Several kinds of HMOs have sprouted over the years. A staff or group model HMO means that doctors are employees of the plan, and patients visit them at central offices. Other HMOs contract with physician groups or individual doctors with private offices. These are called individual practice associations (IPAs) or networks. Some HMOs require a co-payment by patients (or for some services). Others do not.

Some HMOs offer an option closer to traditional insurance, known as a Point-of-Service (POS) plan. In this system, the primary-care doctors usually make referrals to other providers in the plan, but members can also refer themselves outside the plan and still get some coverage. If the plan's doctor makes a referral, all or most of the bill is covered. In self-referrals outside the network, patients pay coinsurance.

A Preferred Provider Organization (PPO) is even more like an insurance plan. A PPO arranges with doctors, hospitals, and other providers who agree to accept lower fees from the insurer for their services. As a result, the patient's share of costs is lower than going outside the network. Patients seeing a PPO doctor are charged a co-payment. If they choose to go outside the network, they must meet the deductible and pay coinsurance based on higher charges. In addition, they may have to pay the difference between what the provider charges and what the PPO will pay.

Fee-for-service (FFS) medicine rests on three relatively independent legs: an insurance plan, the patient who signs with the plan (usually through an employer) to get a menu of coverage, and physicians and hospitals that the plan reimburses on demand. For the patient, this means an open choice of physicians, some yearly deductible, and some co-payment.

This thicket of care choices grows even more tangled. Plans within all these alphabet soups change their offerings from year to year. Organizations within a reimbursement system (HMOs, for example) differ in the conditions they handle well and ones where they cut corners. Some consumers know the chronic condition for which they need help, such as adult-onset diabetes, and can shop for coverage with this in mind. Other consumers can barely imagine the conditions for which they may one day need urgent, high-quality, and affordable attention.

Consumers also differ in what they want most when choosing a plan. Some patients prefer bottom-line measures that go to the biological roots of medicine: Do people under one system or plan get care that professionals rate as superior to the attention that people under other systems receive? Do they enjoy greater rates of survival from various procedures? Do they stay healthier and live longer? Other consumers also want to weigh plans for the degree of personal satisfaction they produce, how contented patients are with doctors' friendliness and an absence of bureaucracy. Physiological outcomes offer a different yardstick than contentment with care.

Of one fact we can be certain. Each system of care delivery in use today has its liabilities. The "gold standard" of fee-for-service (FFS) medicine encourages overuse of procedures, especially costly ones, and underattention to preventive care. FFS also imposes rationing of treatment according to patients' ability to pay. The well-off and the well-insured get the pick of the best physicians, procedures, and drugs. The poor and uninsured must resort to low-cost neighborhood clinics, if they are available. Or they crowd into busy emergency rooms for attention to subacute conditions.

Managed care contains its own biases. Simply put, managed systems limit choices by patients and the clinical autonomy of physicians. A patient's preference among primary-care doctors may be frustrated. Furthermore, a patient may not gain access to specialists or additional consultations unless approval is granted. Doctors, on their part, often find corporate bookkeepers second-guessing them. These functionaries search for excuses to deny a procedure whenever they can brand it as "experimental" or "nonstandard," even when no standard treatment exists.

Doctors in many managed-care plans are discouraged from talking with a patient about proposed treatments until the options are authorized. A doctor's own income may suffer if he or she recommends too many referrals or tests. The doctor's contract with the managed-care provider may push him or her to see as many appointments during a day as humanly possible. And these physicians' contracts are usually subject to ninety-day cancellations, without stated cause. Such conditions undermine top-quality medicine.

## KEEPING YOUR DOCTOR AS AN ALLY IN MANAGED CARE

Among the many stumbling blocks in the world of managed care, one seems to rankle patients most: getting approval for a medical procedure or obtaining authorization for a drug or medical device. Patients and their families can overcome the obstacles, but they must be prepared to nag the system—persistently and, especially important, deftly. Two cases from managed care illustrate steps the determined consumer must often take.

Jill, a thirty-six-year-old mother, has had insulin-dependent diabetes since infancy. When we first became acquainted several years ago, neuropathy had begun to damage the nerves in her feet, making them susceptible to cuts, bruises, and blisters. She had been referred to a podiatrist for regular care, and he prescribed custom shoes.

The doctor's office submitted forms asking Jill's HMO to authorize the shoes. Two weeks went by with no response. The doctor's assistant called and was told that there was no record that the request had been received. Another form went into the mail. And then, amid the paperwork of other patients, the podiatrist's office lost track of Jill's case until her next checkup months later.

Jill steamed into the office, fuming over the delay in getting her shoes. The podiatrist was perplexed to hear that she hadn't received the go-ahead. Over the next weeks, a barrage of phone calls and faxes to the HMO finally extracted a reluctant approval. Jill was able to purchase her shoes 254 days after having them prescribed, enduring needless pain across many months.

This opening chapter in Jill's HMO torment resembles many patients' experiences. HMOs often stonewall. They "lose" paperwork, buck callers to other offices where action on the request is supposedly stuck, or simply take an unfathomable length of time to reach a decision. Other times, the HMO will reply by asking the doctor for additional clinical details or other justification; the doctor may or may not have time to answer. Individual cases sink from sight under a burden of paperwork or forgetfulness. That is the intent some HMOs practice: Keep enough physicians and their patients on the defensive so that a share of their requests for enhanced services, or even routine approvals, falls through the cracks.

There is more to Jill's story, however. We reconnected with her three years later. By then, she had suffered a serious and festering wound on the bottom of her right foot, a common progression in the ravages that diabetes can bring, often resulting in gangrene. Her primary-care physician suggested referral to an orthopedic surgeon, who recommended amputation. Although surgery and recovery would cost tens of thousands of dollars, Jill's HMO would probably approve the procedure. Medical directors at most HMOs recognize amputation as a definitive resolution for lower-limb infections.

Jill, however, had read in publications by the American Diabetes Association that amputation curtails people's mobility and plunges many into depression. Statistically speaking, amputation below the knee often hastens a patient's decline and death. So Jill sought another solution, based again on her reading of stacks of materials. She was again determined to seek a referral to a podiatrist. He, in turn, took time to tell her about long-term wound care. This new treatment protocol uses state-of-the-art drugs and procedures: debridement (or surgical removal) of infection and dead tissue from her foot, taking a culture to identify appropriate antibiotics, and two to three months of moist dressings and casts to keep pressure off the wounds.

Jill chose this over amputation. Although long-term care is less expensive than amputation, perhaps one-sixth the cost, Jill's troubles with her HMO resumed. Long-term wound care is innovative and unfamiliar to the bureaucrats who pass on authorizations. Their answer was "no." She might have simply wrung her hands in despair, but Jill kept her sense of humor, telling us that her HMO's response reminded her of Robert De Niro's line in *Night and the City,* screaming "No can do! No can do! What's that? A Chinese appetizer?"

This time, Jill was prepared to play the skilled medical consumer. Here are the steps that won her authorization for wound care and that can achieve the same kind of results for others.

- Start by making certain that your physician's request for authorization has actually been sent to the HMO. If your appointment was in the late afternoon, for example, call the nurse or other staff next day and remind them of what needs to be done.

- Make friends with nurses and staff. Know them by name. They will serve you well, as savvy insiders who know how to work the system. Acknowledge their help with token gifts and thank you notes (better than spoken words).

- Understand that you must secure your physician as an ally. In all communications with the HMO, depict the doctor as your partner and not the butt of your complaint. You want to present a seamless unity, even where that stretches the truth, to escape being pigeonholed as a crank.

- Realize that few doctors or their staffs have the time to follow up on your request; they don't scroll through a computer every morning, for instance, searching for overdue authorizations.

- If nothing has happened within a week, start a series of telephone calls at regular intervals to the appropriate targets at your HMO or insurance company—it may be the medical director's office, customer relations department, claims office, pharmacy manager, or others. Calmly and simply state your purpose; have notes in front of you so that you are accurate about dates of appointments and other details. Ask whether the decision has been made, and announce that you will call again in three days to follow up. If the HMO objects to this schedule, ask for a recommended date and hour to telephone. When the time comes, call again.

- When making follow-up calls, ask for the person you last reached. When someone confesses that they can't solve your problem or don't know how, ask for a supervisor, working your way up the HMO's ladder. Get the names and direct-dial numbers of any representatives with whom you talk.

- When an HMO stalls or denies a worthwhile request, plan your campaign with care. Begin with a letter to the HMO's medical director that focuses on the *delay* that is taking place in medically appropriate care. Write "I'm extremely concerned about my condition. . . . My physician assures me that (drug, procedure) is the most effective care for my situation. . . . He (or she) has been attentive and skilled in providing treatment. . . . I have been waiting for (span of time) for your decision. . . . Please expedite your action on this request (or please reconsider your denial of this request) in light of the urgent clinical situation I am facing."

In cases like Jill's, vascular deterioration can be rapid. Wherever you can include medical reasons behind asking for prompt action, do so. Send this letter by certified mail. That won't gain it any priority within the HMO, but you will have an undeniable record of transmittal for later use.

- When your appeal involves a drug or a costly medical device, ask your doctor for the maker's name. Some firms maintain hotlines staffed by reimbursement specialists who can help deal with insurance difficulties. Call the company's public affairs department to ask.

- Following a stubborn delay, write a second letter to the HMO and place another call. Calmly announce that you intend to write your employer's benefits office (contractor for HMO coverage) and your state legislator about the HMO's processes, asking them to intervene. You will also correspond with the local chapter of a national health-care association, describing the clinical facts and complaining about the HMO. Ask for a decision (or reconsideration) by a certain date before launching this salvo.

  When you have been handed a denial, ask immediately about the insurer's internal appeals process. Activate that with a letter and follow-up calls.

- Finally, pursue formal avenues of complaint that we describe below in Stage 2 in the section on shopping for managed care.

Another successful example seems humble enough, but, again, it shows how persistence and preparation paid off for a mother whose child has asthma and allergies. After months of severe nighttime coughing, postnasal drip, and shallow breathing, Karen's eight-month-old daughter was diagnosed and was prescribed liquid medications and an inhaler. At the pharmacy, Karen was told that she was "denied" on the aerochamber, a device that allows a small child to inhale the medication properly. Desperate to begin the treatment program, Karen bought the aerochamber and began a seven-week battle for reimbursement. She finally did receive her check to cover the cost of the aerochamber, but it took four phone calls (starting with a customer representative at the end of an 800 number) and a formal letter.

These are the realities of dealing with medical insurers. Jill strengthened her hand by becoming knowledgeable about her condition and various therapies. That allowed her to write convincingly and speak on the phone with confidence. Karen, wisely, understood that she must pay out of her pocket for a device that would allow her to administer the recommended medication to her daughter. Her story also ended successfully, but not without effort in communicating with her HMO. When patients cannot shoulder such tasks, other family members or friends must step in to help. With managed care, each patient is a lonely soldier.

### SHOPPING FOR MANAGED CARE

There are a million stories like Jill's and Karen's, leading some people to despair that managed systems are simply "cash box care." This is not the place to enter this debate. We can, however, side with readers who must choose among systems in order to get affordable treatment. Our suggestions for shopping fall into two areas of homework. First, there are basic questions that most prudent consumers want to ask. Second, you must take steps to make a refined choice between providers, or to wring top-quality care from the system under urgent circumstances.

*Stage 1.* Start, naturally, by learning about a managed provider's or insurance plan's rules and preapproval for existing conditions before enrolling. What will the plan pay if you require services outside the network of providers? What limitations on coverage apply—such as visits to a chiropractor (or other "alternative care" service that interests you), mental health specialists, vision and dental services, or infertility treatment? Are there lifetime caps? What about medical attention when traveling outside the geographic coverage area? Would you need prior authorization for emergency treatment?

Does the published list of doctors include a choice of specialists you are likely to need? Are they nearby? Commuting grows into a painful disadvantage when repeated visits are necessary.

If you have a chronic problem, are you permitted to use a specialist as your primary-care doctor, or will you always have to see another doctor first before visiting a specialist? Which of your needs for this ongoing condition does the plan cover?

Some HMOs are starting to accredit nurse practitioners as providers of primary services that were formerly reserved for doctors. The nurses help patients deal with chronic conditions like asthma and diabetes, treat common complaints, prescribe drugs, and refer complicated cases to a doctor. State laws differ about how independently these nurse practitioners can work. Inquire into a plan's use of nurse practitioners.

Some patients see their increasing involvement as a blessed gift in access to nurturing care; others fear that nurses are being used as a cheap substitute for superior treatment.

The informed patient also considers the potential pitfalls in choosing a particular HMO simply because it includes a familiar doctor or presents a fat roster of physicians from which to choose. Such choice does not always lead to superior care. Among HMOs, for example, the ones with central clinics and medical staffs on salary almost always offer better care, according to clinical measures the health industry uses for quality. They have lower rates for cesarean sections, for example, more cancer screenings, and better mental health follow-ups. Their doctors practice medicine under just one set of rules, the employing HMO. They collaborate with colleagues in the same firm. This type of managed-care plan can quickly capture evidence about successes and failures with its patients, and use these data to improve services.

By contrast, physicians reimbursed through networks of HMOs that are IPAs or PPOs (see above) typically work under the shelter of a half-dozen or more separate plans in order to broaden their competitive access to patients. As a consequence, the physicians' reporting and accountability are divided. Information about patients gets shared among doctors at arm's length, if at all.

A handful of managed-care providers have joined with consumer groups (such as the American Association of Retired Persons, or AARP) to propose a patient's "bill of rights." Compare the providers you must choose among against these standards:

- Which, if any, offer a range of health-care options? (More than half of employer-insured consumers have no choice of plans, and they are stuck with what's offered.)
- Will you have access to round-the-clock care seven days a week?
- Do women have direct access to obstetricians and gynecologists as their primary doctor?
- Do the plans pay for emergency care in any situation that "a prudent lay person" would regard as an emergency? HMOs sometimes refuse, for example, when chest pains result from indigestion rather than a heart attack. Would you need prior authorization for emergency treatment?
- Do the plans have an ombudsman, a review process within the organization, to investigate complaints and help patients appeal a denial of coverage or services?

*Stage 2.* All these worthy points made, many people's situations call for
more information and advice than can be offered here. You will find
savvy reports about managed care in columns by Ellyn E. Spragins
that appear frequently in *Newsweek*. You can locate articles that interest you by using a local library's electronic tools for bibliographic
searches in leading magazines (ask for help at the reference desk). You
can also find hard-headed advice from a physician about contending
with the quirks of managed care (Steinberg 1997).

In addition, there are at least five other ways to dig out information about individual providers:

- Your employer's benefits office should have copies of reports by the
accrediting agency for managed plans, the National Committee for
Quality Assurance in Washington, D.C. (NCQA). The organization's
"Quality Compass 1997" shows how 329 HMOs compare on many
indicators of clinical performance and on their patients' satisfaction.
Ask your benefits representatives to help you interpret the ratings. If you
want written information about how these ratings were collected, call
NCQA at 202-955-3500.

- The Center for the Study of Services in Washington, D.C., publishes
an annual guide covering some 300 HMOs; call 202-347-7283.

- You can order a report on any of approximately one hundred plans
from CareData, a firm that conducts independent surveys of people's
satisfaction with managed providers; call 212-583-9350 or consult your
employer's benefits office.

- *U.S. News and World Report* has published its rankings of HMOs nation-
wide; see the October 13, 1997 issue.

- In many states, the major daily newspaper has published its own guide
to health-care planning. It may have included ratings of managed plans
available to you. Call the newspaper's community relations department
or use an electronic search tool at your library.

Here are some other guidelines, which clarify the benefits that
patients can demand and the risks they bear under managed care.

Do you have access to a computer and modem, and an on-line account
to use in searching the Internet for information about the condition you
suffer? If not, a young relative with access at school and experience surfing the Web may come to your rescue, or a local library can assist.

Searching the Internet will uncover information about the range
of therapies for your situation, which you can use when questioning

nurses and doctors. Start at the National Library of Medicine Web site, or look in other directions suggested by an up-to-date guide to medical resources on the Internet (Ferguson 1996; Ryer 1997).

Use your new information to inquire about care options. That way, you will learn about the drugs and other treatments that your provider prefers and those it discourages. Ask why some are off-limits. Then, pay for an independent consultation with a specialist, asking about the same medical regimens. You can unearth a lot about the economic and subjective biases in care this way.

Some state governments have procedures by which seriously ill patients can appeal their managed-care provider's decision about treatment to an independent panel of physicians or another arbitrator with no financial stake in the decision. Does your state offer this service? If so, how long do such appeals take to be settled? What would happen if you were denied care that was urgently needed? Does your state have an 800 number where complaints against HMOs can be lodged? Your state medical society can tell you about this process.

Each state has a Medicare peer-review organization that receives complaints against providers when reimbursed through this coverage. Your state medical society can tell you how to contact this organization, and you can ask for its standards and procedures.

What is the status of your state's consumers' rights laws affecting access to health care within a managed plan? How about policies that limit how managed-care organizations may curtail their physicians' decisions? Contact your representative to the state legislature and ask him or her to query the National Conference of State Legislatures Health Policy Tracking Service by calling 202-624-3567.

Does your managed-care provider allow subscribers to participate in clinical trials approved by the National Institutes of Health or the Food and Drug Administration? These are often the last best hope in acute cases, including exotic cancers. When providers say "never" or "rarely" to such care, you are forewarned about possible anguish in a critical and unusual situation.

Does the company where you work monitor the quality of care provided by plans it offers to employees? Some large firms send undercover sleuths to hospitals and clinics to learn firsthand, and independently, just how providers handle cases. Some hire doctors as consultants to review records, looking for mistakes that have impaired care: primary-care doctors who didn't recognize crucial symptoms; specialists not consulted in time; and other debacles. Ask your benefits office about this. When such checking takes place, the quality of employer-approved plans is likely to be above average.

Finally, it's important to retain a sense of perspective about surviving modern medicine, doomsayers to the contrary. You will seldom—perhaps never—feel driven to take all the steps we've described; just one crisis, however, will make our menu for action worth reviewing. Remember, too, that another principle has not shifted with the advent of managed care. Informed and inquisitive patients, aided by their family or friends, tend to get superior medical treatment, regardless of the means by which physicians are paid. Today's daunting plans for coverage are just a fresh inning in medicine, not a whole new ballgame.

---

## CHAPTER 2

# Making the Best Medical Decisions

TODAY'S PRACTICE of medicine delivers bewildering options and calculated risks for almost every patient. Should you take prescription drugs or surgically implant a device in order to correct a heart arrhythmia? What about surgery or radiation or hormones or cryoablation for prostate cancer? How to choose a form of birth control that's effective as well as compatible with your lifestyle? Every procedure has pluses and minuses.

This chapter's story begins with your own style of making choices and rationalizing the outcomes, because certain lifelong habits of thinking set the stage for falling ill in the first place. Second, we warn you about potholes along the road to medical decision making—flaws in judgments by your doctor or by you that commonly lead to clinical mistakes. For example, what bumps in care result when you and the doctor interpret the "remote" chance of side effects differently? Are cheerful doctors better at reaching decisions than those who are anxious or grim, and how can you lighten the physician's feelings?

Third, we dig deeply into habits of thinking that lead any sort of decision making off course, medical or otherwise. What happens to the calculus of choice when deadlines are rushed? Is feeling regret over past mistakes a waste of time, or can you turn these sentiments into better plans for the future? Fourth, we sketch ways to sharpen your consumer skills in choosing medical care, getting the type of practitioner you really want. Finally, we share simple steps to help you clarify a confusing situation in any diagnosis or treatment.

No single chapter can offer a pathway through all the decisions that illnesses or accidents bring. But people will take wiser steps when they stay alert to subtle tricks of the mind that can warp choices, and where they develop an orderly way to sort through medical options.

## LITTLE DECISIONS ADD UP TO BIG HEALTH OUTCOMES

Most of the insights that follow help readers overcome difficulties in reaching a specific decision. It's worth pausing, however, to learn how mental habits of daily living accumulate steadily over the years, shaping people's very survival. The manner in which individuals explain events can actually affect their overall health. These explanatory styles also influence judgments about specific questions, such as which treatment (if any) to follow. People who act confidently enjoy greater well-being than those who fear that matters are spinning out of control, that fate or blind luck rules the course of events.

When people feel in control, they are convinced that they have options. They experience a boost in their self-worth. Compared to those who feel powerless, they can even resist physical pain from medical procedures. Chronic pessimism, on the other hand, should carry a warning label: This style of thinking can be injurious to health.

Psychologists gained an early appreciation for this in a landmark study of undergraduate men at Harvard (Peterson, Seligman, and Vaillant 1988). Researchers screened many students to identify a group who had superior physical and psychological health and who were academic achievers. Each subject took an extensive battery of physical and psychological tests, some of which focused on how the students explained events that occurred in their lives. Participants were asked about difficult situations they had encountered and why they had succeeded or failed.

The optimists in the group told stories full of confidence. They were responsible for their successes; and where they might have failed, they believed circumstances or other people were accountable. They predicted that good things would keep happening, whereas bad things were only temporary. They felt that one good experience spawned many other happy ones, but that a failure was just an isolated event.

Of course, not all the students explained their experiences with this rosy glow. The gloomier individuals in the group ranged all the way down the scale to abject pessimists. According to these people, good things occurred by accident, and bad things grew out of their own limitations. Successes were fleeting and isolated; failures endured and were woven tightly into a barrier against achievement.

It is important to note that these explanations—both optimistic and pessimistic—were personal constructions or theories about life. Many of the students' explanatory stories did not correspond to reality. Like all of us, these young people had individual styles of interpreting events that had become the foundation upon which they acted, regardless of the facts of the matter that may have appeared very different to onlookers.

As you might expect, the investigators were interested in whether the optimists and pessimists differed in physical health, down the line. For thirty years following graduation, the men filled out annual questionnaires about employment, family, health, and more. They also provided details of periodic physical exams by their own doctors. Indeed, the health consequences from these graduates' styles of thinking were profound: The rates for irreversible chronic illnesses, disabilities, and death were much higher among the pessimists than the optimists.

These research subjects launched their adulthood in a privileged and enviable position—male graduates of America's leading university, favored by social class and circumstance. Optimistic and pessimistic styles of thought led them to very different ends in life, however. Other studies confirm that pessimists report more sickness and cope more poorly with illness than do optimists. Pessimists take poorer care of themselves in many ways.

Biological processes help account for some of these results. When a person no longer feels in control, stress floods the central nervous system and weakens tissues. For example, a sense of helplessness can lead to abrupt and undischarged arousal of the cardiovascular system and, over time, to hypertension. Moreover, feeling out of control suppresses neurohormones that prompt vital processes such as appetite, sexual stimulation, regular cycles of sleep, and clear thinking. Powerlessness attacks the body's resistance to bacterial and inflammatory threats. The immune system weakens, as measured by natural-killer (NK) cell and lymphocyte (white blood cell) activity. People lose resistance to diseases such as respiratory disorders.

When people do not learn how to cope with stress, it can weaken the endocrine system, making them more susceptible to such pathologies as rheumatoid arthritis, an autoimmune disease in which the body's immune system launches an attack against its own tissues. Laboratory studies of mammals show that the growth of malignant tumors accelerates where animals have been taught that there is nothing they can do to relieve a mild torment, such as irritation from an electrical charge (Visintainer, Volpicelli, and Seligman 1982). These experiments offer a chilling prototype for much of human experience among pessimists and those who suffer from depression.

Therefore, on average, a serene confidence in one's abilities and health brings its rewards. People who dismiss minor aches and pains are busily maintaining their sense of control over life and reaping benefits from doing so. Large surveys of self-evaluated health and mortality rates actually show that death comes more quickly to people who think they are in "bad" or "poor" health, regardless of what their physical exams indicate.

Perhaps the cartoonist had all this in mind when he sketched a patient perched on the end of an examination table facing his physician. "Blood pressure is fine," the doctor says. "Now let me just check your pessimism."

Emotional tone in specific situations often crimps human judgment, too. A spirited outlook makes for sounder decisions, other things being equal. Feeling glum or stressed impairs anyone's quality of thinking. When a person's medical condition weighs heavily on emotions, as it naturally can, it's time to recruit others who feel less burdened into the picture. People alone and in a funk habitually make bad choices about their care.

From such contemporary findings as these, it's easy to see why evolutionary survival by the human species over countless generations has tilted the bulk of people toward optimism. That style of "sense making" favors problem solving and success. A corollary, however, deserves some vigilance: Most individuals vastly underestimate the risks they face throughout life. Surveys have been conducted asking adults to predict the chances that they will suffer a heart attack, be diagnosed with cancer, be injured in a car accident, have a nervous breakdown, develop a drinking problem, and be stricken by a wide range of other unfortunate conditions. Most think themselves relatively immune compared to actual statistics that describe their peers in age and gender. People don't reflect much on the factors that contribute to personal risk or the circumstances that shield them from danger (Weiner 1985).

Thus, when physical symptoms do appear, many ignore them, especially the most optimistic people. Signs such as swelling or mild pain usually resolve by themselves, anyway. On occasion, continuing to dismiss the hints of illness can lead to a delay in diagnosis and treatment, undermining the potential for a cure. In many cancers, for example, survival rates and quality of life depend on how far the disease has progressed when doctors detect the abnormality. Early screening spells the difference between recovery and death.

A familiar pattern of events describes many people's discovery of illness. First, a few symptoms crop up that are easily neglected, sometimes unwisely. Continued or growing distress (pain, discharge, coughing, bruising, diarrhea, loss of energy, restricted movement, frequent urination), however, starts to raise anxieties. People consider making the effort to visit a doctor. Most flatter themselves by thinking they are accomplished at tracking ailments and identifying the real source of trouble; they usually do a poor job at this. Hence, they form convincing but wrong assumptions.

Finally, after some delay, they decide to seek medical attention. The simple phone call escalates speculation and worry to a new level. That is why patients become so annoyed when they have trouble arranging an early appointment. By the time they walk into the doctor's waiting room, they are teeming with grim possibilities and convinced of the worst. Even people with optimistic spirits slump into a doleful mood between telephone call and office visit.

The pages that follow pick up the story at this point. We carry you through the most frequent kinds of judgments that you will need to master when faced with the possibility of a routine or serious medical condition.

## POTHOLES ON THE ROAD TO MEDICAL DECISION MAKING

Between consultations with your doctors, skim through this section to review the missteps that choice can take, usually without either you or your physician realizing it. Take notes and open your next office visit with questions that focus on the issues in decision making you have spotted.

## THE NUMBING INFLUENCE OF NUMBERS

Physicians may consult research studies to assess the risks and benefits for various treatment protocols. However, the results of scientific research in medical journals are less easily applied than you might imagine. Sometimes these reports categorize patients according to stages of disease, age, gender, or general health, allowing an easier match to your case. Other times, though, ratios describing treatment successes and failures have been averaged across all types of patients. The location of your individual situation among this crowd of statistics may not be easy to pin down. Don't be surprised, therefore, if the doctor seems imprecise about guidance from the medical literature.

Another problem with numbers often rears its head. Primary-care physicians and specialists may receive your diagnostic test results embedded in a swarm of data and obscure markings, shorn of interpretive aids. A doctor's chart literacy can be shaky, particularly when he or she needs to decipher results from unfamiliar readings. Understand that your physician farms out most testing to separate diagnostic laboratories, each with its own protocols for reporting results.

In documenting his fight against prostate cancer, Michael Korda learned only too well how difficult it could be to sort through the numbers with a doctor. As he describes it:

> The radiologist even had charts and papers to give us for further reading. He stabbed at the statistics with a blunt finger. Even if the cancer has spread, he told us, radiology offered far better odds for survival than surgery—it was all there in black and white, for us to study at our leisure. A survival rate of five to seven years, even with sky-high PSAs [Prostate Specific Antigen test]—go find a surgeon who could show you those kinds of results!
>
> I could see that Margaret [Korda's wife] was taking in only the numbers, assuming that the radiologist was telling us that *my* "survival rate" was five to seven, whereas he was, in fact, outlining an aggressive case for radiology and talking averages. Still, I thought it best to head him off at the pass and turn the consultation more firmly toward my case specifically, before Margaret broke down altogether.
>
> Did he think my case lent itself to radiation? I asked. I had been given the impression that it did not. Was that a mistake?
>
> (Korda 1996, 80–81)

In "talking averages" with patients, doctors may present survival and death rates, such as number of cases per thousand, or per hundred treated. This can be helpful, but patients need to be sure that

TABLE 2.1
### WOULD YOU CHOOSE
### TREATMENT A OR B?

CHART 1

| | NUMBER OF PATIENTS OUT OF 100 | |
| --- | --- | --- |
| Time elapsed | Treatment A | Treatment B |
| 1 month | 90 alive;  10 dead | 100 alive;   0 dead |
| 1 year | 68 alive;  32 dead | 77 alive; 23 dead |
| 5 years | 34 alive;  66 dead | 22 alive; 78 dead |

CHART 2

| | | |
| --- | --- | --- |
| 1 month | 90 alive;  10 dead | 100 alive;   0 dead |
| 1 year | 68 alive;  32 dead | 77 alive; 23 dead |
| 2 years | 51 alive;  49 dead | 48 alive; 52 dead |
| 3 years | 40 alive;  60 dead | 28 alive; 72 dead |
| 4 years | 35 alive;  65 dead | 23 alive; 77 dead |
| 5 years | 34 alive;  66 dead | 22 alive; 78 dead |

their doctors consider the fit between the averages and their specific case.

Another distortion can come in interpreting statistics. The amount of information presented—and the way it is sliced—make a big difference, even where both pros and cons are included. Here is an example (Mazur and Hickam 1990b). The two charts are identical in representing the results of two treatments across five years. Or are they?

Chart 2 in table 2.1 shows survival and mortality figures for more points in time than the first. In this expansion of the information field, the second chart adds three time periods where treatment A reports greater medium- and long-term survival than treatment B. But treatment A offers less attractive outcomes at one month and one year. The enlarged information field draws people's attention to the longer-term figures. In a research study that presented the shorter version of the chart, half of the subjects preferred Treatment A. When participants were given the fuller chart, a much greater number (eight of ten) preferred treatment A.

It's not only patients who are influenced by the field of information presented. The same study asked a group of experienced physicians to look at the abbreviated chart and choose between the two treatment options, whereas a second group worked with the full array of data. Physicians were as swayed by the longer version as were patients.

What is happening here? The field-of-information principle is actually quite straightforward. When the information given to us is more vivid, or simply more available for mental processing, we tend to favor that information. This is the case even though objective odds favoring medical procedures stay the same. Choices are sensitive to the volume of information leaning toward one option, regardless of the hard-nosed chances of correcting a medical condition or surviving a procedure.

Which version of the chart gives patients the best shot at making a wise choice: a condensed account of survival and mortality, or a longer and more complete comparison between treatments? More information is better, by and large. But completeness helps only where patients truly take advantage of it.

If you are faced with treatment options that present different possibilities for survival and mortality over time, ask your doctor to draw survival curves for the competing procedures, using several points in time. That way, you'll be able to see whether or not there's a wide gap in survival, favoring one procedure over the other in the middle range—perhaps followed by a crossover that gives the second procedure a slight edge in long-term life expectancy. In your case, it may be rational to choose a course of action that is dramatically more successful for two or three years, even though it is inferior in the long run. An older patient, for instance, might be especially interested in early- to mid-range results like these. In any event, counteract your own selective bias to rely on just the beginning and end points in data displays. Get the full range.

The human tendency to fasten on information that is vividly presented crops up in other ways. For example, a physician might talk at length about one procedure and give cursory attention to others. Because the procedure that was given lengthy discussion is more vivid in your mind, your judgment tugs in that direction. How can you resist this slant? Get the issue out on the table. Ask directly: "Are you really recommending procedure A? That seems to be the one we're talking about most." Getting a second opinion (see later in this chapter) is another excellent way to correct this tendency and receive a more balanced array of information.

Likewise, patients' own preferences among treatment options can lean toward the procedures that friends have followed. Such experiences and stories come promptly to mind. Nevertheless, these interventions may not always be the best choice for the next case in line—yours.

News frenzies in the media can be another misleading source of cues about the best health practices, as the controversy over silicone breast implants, a medical procedure in use since 1962, vividly illustrates. In the early 1990s, television, magazines, and newspapers flocked to anecdotal accounts of adverse side effects that seemed to be surfacing after implants for reconstructive (post-mastectomy) or cosmetic reasons. The apparent consequences ranged from hardening of breast tissues to diagnoses of cancer and rheumatological disorders.

The media often dramatized the issue as a horror story—a bewildered and defenseless woman suffering medical complications, while her wealthy plastic surgeon raced indifferently on to the next victims (Vanderford, Smith, and Olive 1995). Importantly, scientific evidence at the time did not challenge the use of these implants. Nonetheless, highly publicized lawsuits ensued against both clinicians and the chief manufacturer of implants, and a small army of lawyers reaped large fees from litigation. Still today, the evidence is not clear about any adverse reactions (Angell 1996).

The case highlights three kinds of questions that contribute to judgments about medical causation. First, are doctors observing that patients with a certain disease were also exposed to a possible cause, in this case the implants? Second, do scientists consistently observe a significant increase in the disease among large samples of people exposed to the possible cause, compared to people unexposed—an association that can't be explained on other grounds? Third, do controlled experiments (using animals or human subjects) reveal a biological explanation for how the disease results from its conjectured cause? (Lamm 1995)

Media that reach the general public leap on stories, when spurred on by the first level of evidence, anecdotal reports. By contrast, stories grounded on the second and third levels seldom make splashy headlines. The patient's best defense is to recognize that confidence in a medical procedure rises dramatically between levels one and two. Confidence increases again between levels two and three. Ask your doctor to explain the reasoning behind his or her recommendations in ordinary language. Are the arguments for a treatment, or assurances that there are

few side effects, based on a few clinical cases, on large-scale comparisons of ill and healthy people, or on trials buttressed by a biological explanation?

Be alert to the other ways that statistics or emphasis, this chapter's
lessons, can bias your decision making and possibly your physician's.

## THE EQUIVOCAL LANGUAGE OF RISK

Doctor-patient talk about medical interventions may never refer to
statistics such as survival rates. Instead, the clinician's statements can
rely exclusively on words. A side effect may be "common," for example.
A benefit can be "usual"; a risk is "rare" or "remote." A symptom may
be "normal," but nonetheless worrisome. The lexicon includes "may
occur," "occasionally," "possible," "small chance," "frequently," and similar terms.

Psychologists have presented these words to patients and health
professionals, asking what the words mean in a numerical sense (Brun
and Teigen 1988; Mazur and Merz 1994). What, for example, does
"occasionally" indicate in the context of side effects for chemotherapy?
Does it mean half of the cases, a quarter of them, or some other number? What does "rarely" mean when referring to risks of recurrent heart
attack? Does that mean a third of the patients, one of ten, or fewer than
that? These studies paint a sobering picture, finding that people differ
widely in their interpretation. There's little consensus and ample room
for misunderstanding between doctors and their patients.

We saw such a communication gap in the case of a young couple,
Rachel and Jon, whose infant son developed a blockage in one tear
duct. Tearing and infection were evident in the first weeks after birth.
Following their pediatrician's instructions, the parents applied antibi-
otic drops and wiped the affected area clean in an attempt to stem the
condition. Despite these efforts, the tearing continued and green pus
discharged intermittently over the next several months. The condition
refused to clear up.

They were referred to a specialist, who presented these options:
(1) the blockage and associated infection might resolve by itself; (2) if
it didn't, a pediatric ophthalmologist could place the infant under general anesthesia and surgically clear the tear duct; (3) it would be wise
to resort to surgery (if needed) relatively early in the child's development, because cartilage and other structures toughen, complicating the
procedure; (4) on the other hand, surgeons were reluctant to submit

infants to anesthesia until they are as mature as possible. In a nutshell, there were arguments for waiting and reasons for scheduling the operation.

What to do? Consistent with today's philosophy of patient autonomy, doctors left decision making in Rachel and Jon's hands. The couple flopped back and forth between waiting and arranging for the surgery. They continued to worry that they would miss the window of opportunity for this procedure, and they struggled with unanswerable questions such as, "Will my child be less traumatized by general anesthesia at six months or a year old?"

Without realizing it, Jon and Rachel misunderstood key terms. Doctors kept referring to blocked tear ducts as "common" in newborns, and said that "a large percentage" of these cases resolve on their own by six months or clear up with simple medication and cleansing. The couple inferred that this meant that half of all children experience the condition in their first year, a very comforting assumption, and that all but a handful of blockages open on their own, again reassuring. The parents concluded that doctors were implicitly urging patience.

In fact, studies show that only 5 to 6 percent of newborns experience this problem, far fewer than the 50 percent that Rachel and Jon imagined. About seven of ten of these infections spontaneously resolve, leaving more than just a "handful" of stubborn cases. Furthermore, after one year of age, the failure rate of the relatively simple probe would climb sharply (to approximately 10 percent), necessitating a second operation with general anesthesia and a more difficult procedure.

As the weeks rolled by, doctors increasingly felt they were nudging the parents toward surgery. But Rachel and Jon held back. Neither the medical team nor parents discovered the contradictions between their perspectives until the infant was fourteen months old and still experiencing periodic eye infections. Finally, the operation took place (successfully). But the couple had gone through months of wrenching uncertainty, using a different equation to determine their child's care than doctors thought they had been suggesting.

People interpret the meanings of words based on their own experiences, and the experiences of people trying to communicate can be drastically different. In this case, Rachel and Jon's specialist, merely by virtue of her job, saw many pediatric eye infections in her practice. She had implied that a duct blockage was more "common" than it truly is. To her, the infection *was* common. In the general population of infants, however, it is not.

Here is a word to the wise about words: If you are determined to estimate risks and benefits for yourself or loved ones, ask for the intended meaning behind the language that is used. Terms indicating the likelihood of events are sprinkled throughout documents such as consent forms and bandied about in presurgical consultations and other kinds of medical communication. Press for numbers. Make sure that you and your doctors share an understanding. It is within your rights as a health-care consumer to ask for these details, and essential if you are to make careful decisions.

Understand, too, that the risk of failure or of side effects may be expressed as a range instead of an average. "Generally, between one of five and one of ten patients experiences severe cramping with this medication," for example. You shouldn't infer from such a presentation that the doctor is being evasive or just doesn't know vital facts. Quite the contrary, he or she is honestly confiding one of medicine's inherent uncertainties.

Another snag when talking about risks deserves attention. People tend to confuse risks with benefits, and assume that uncertain treatments have few merits to recommend them. To the contrary, however, risky treatments can produce profound improvements, just as safe procedures may bring few gains.

Don't allow the realistic odds of different treatment outcomes to sour your views about their advantages. Try to establish a separate list for each procedure's risk of failure and unwelcome side effects, apart from the list of its potential benefits in fighting your condition. Accept or reject a treatment, keeping both these features distinctly in mind.

## SPECIALISTS' DEVOTION TO THEIR SPECIALTY

Specialists often cling to a particular procedure or diagnostic screening, even though other techniques might be just as valid. Coronary conditions offer a case in point. Despite the decline of arterial disease in the United States, there has been a relentless increase in the number of people undergoing bypass surgery. Reliance on this operation was expected to diminish with the advent of angioplasty; in fact, the use of both procedures has grown in tandem.

There appears to be an ever-lowering threshold for carrying out both bypass surgery and angioplasty. At first, these interventions were recommended for severe or intractable cases; now, even asymptomatic patients are not exempt. Indiscriminate use of a diagnostic procedure tilts doctors and their patients toward invasive action: Many heart specialists can't resist advising their patients to have coronary angiography to measure the degree of arterial blockage. Once patients are informed of the magnitude of obstruction, they see only disaster from not "cleaning the plumbing," by one means or another.

In fact, there are better indicators of coronary health than vascular anatomy. Studies show the advantages of diagnostic results from exercise stress testing, a far less invasive step than angiography, and one whose findings don't drive patients automatically into surgery. In one second-opinion follow-up of patients recommended for angiography, nine of ten were found not to need this diagnostic procedure (Grayboys et al. 1992). Most followed the advice to cancel their angiogram, and their health four years later was not poorer because of it. Precise estimates vary, but a knee-jerk reliance on angiography shunts tens of thousands of people every year into bypass grafts or angioplasty—where these procedures are ineffective or place patients in needless peril from anesthesia or medical mishaps.

Michael Korda's experience with an enlarged prostate (well before his cancer diagnosis) provides an echo. For months, Korda dealt with symptoms that seesawed between frequent urination and an inability to urinate. His sex life suffered. Finally consulting a urologist, he found himself in the grip of a specialist devoted to one type of treatment over alternatives:

> Surgery was one option. Surgery, he went on, was the best solution, the "gold standard" against which all other therapies were measured. What *kind* of surgery, I asked. He was more cheerful now that we were on the subject of surgery. Urology is a surgical specialty. Urologists are therefore all surgeons, men of action, true believers in their own skill and the technology at their command; the prospect of solving the patient's problems with a scalpel generally appeals to them a lot more than sitting around talking to the patient. There were several approaches, he said, warming to the subject, all of which involved removing enough tissue to free the pressure on the urethra and open up a strong, steady flow of urine.
>
> I asked if there were possible after effects. He thought about it. Not really, he said. Some men experience—he paused—"erectile dysfunction." Others, temporary incontinence.
>
> Oh boy, I thought. Impotence and incontinence. We sat in silence as he tapped his fingers impatiently on the blotter. Were there any nonsurgical treatments? I asked.

He sighed. There were a number of new and relatively untested drugs, he suggested rather unwillingly—his heart was clearly in the surgery as an answer to my problem.          (Korda 1996, 25–26)

Korda probed for the possible side effects of drug treatments and decided that "all things considered, either drug seemed a better alternative than surgery, and I left the office with samples of both. The urologist looked disappointed."

This patient managed to see past his doctor's personal leanings and assess which treatment was best for him. Other patients, however, are less assertive. They don't want to offend; they're already thrown off kilter because of illness and nervous before their white-coated physician.

Be alert to the fact that a physician's preferences may be personal, professional, financial, or shaped by a host of other influences. As you consider the doctor's manner of presentation, ponder whether he or she dismisses procedures without reason. Get a guide to your disease at your local library or bookstore and pepper your medical team with questions about options for diagnosis and care. Go on-line, searching the Internet (see suggestions in chapter 1). Try to budget funds for second and third opinions if your health insurance or HMO will not approve and pay for these. And, like Korda, be suspicious of "gold standards."

## THE POWER OF PRESENTATION

The very phrases that doctors use to express treatments affect which course their patients choose. The method of presentation influences which alternative looks best, and you will reach more informed decisions if you understand how language shapes decisions. Psychologists call these *framing* effects.

One of the most powerful examples of framing can be found in a seemingly trivial distinction. The threat of a *loss* usually has a greater impact on decisions than the possibility of an equivalent *gain*. We can see an ordinary example of this instinct in people's common reluctance to accept a fair bet on a coin toss in which the odds are fifty-fifty. The thought of losing a sum of money is stronger than the idea of winning the same amount. The hesitation to take on this bet is not "rational," in the strict sense of the word, but it is normal.

This human quirk, departing from objectivity, explains the failure of many efforts on behalf of preventive care. They're often couched in words of gain, which fail to motivate. The superiority of *loss-framing* over *gains-framing* has been well documented in such areas as drug counseling, smoking cessation, and the care of people with AIDS. For example, look at these two appeals to women to perform breast self-examination (BSE).

Imagine that Jean's physician urges monthly self-examination, which brings the risk of finding a dreaded lump, with these gains statements: "By doing BSE now, you can learn what your normal, healthy breasts feel like so that you will be better prepared to notice any small, abnormal changes that might occur as you get older. Studies show that women who do BSE have an increased chance of finding a tumor in the early, more treatable stage of the disease."

Wanda's doctor, on the other hand, uses a nearly identical script but with a subtle variation, emphasizing the losses or the negative side: "By not doing BSE now, you will not learn what your normal, healthy breasts feel like so that you will be ill-prepared to notice any small, abnormal changes that might occur as you get older. Studies show that women who do not do BSE have a decreased chance of finding a tumor in the early, more treatable stage of the disease" (Meyerowitz and Chaiken 1987, 504).

Research on these presentations shows that Wanda and other patients visiting her physician, who presents the issue in loss terms, are twice as likely as Jean to perform self-examinations, and to keep doing so in future months. In fact, patients who are given the positive or gains-oriented approach are no more likely to follow through than women who get no urging to self-exam at all. The effect of loss-framing is that strong.

Realizing these effects of framing, some doctors try to persuade a patient to undertake a chancy medical intervention by focusing on the potential losses that the patient will suffer if he or she doesn't take action. Wise consumers of medical care, though, will recognize that the language in which recommendations and alternatives are presented affects their choices. Especially when these decisions are life-threatening, it is essential to note which frame—loss or gain—is being emphasized.

People's instinctive avoidance of losses also helps explain the popularity of some elective surgeries, which studies of medical utilization show are often unnecessary. It's not uncommon for a physician to urge a hysterectomy to provide immediate and permanent protection against possible future cancer of reproductive organs. The operation often impresses patients as better than having to face possible medical treatments with less certain outcomes in case cancer develops later on.

How can you protect yourself against the influences of gains and loss frames and make wise choices between treatments without simply bending to the power of presentation? The solution is straightforward: Frame the decision both ways. Ask your physician to express treatment choices using two vocabularies: "What will happen to me if I follow this course, versus what will happen if I don't? How do treatments A and B compare on the plus side, and how do they stack up on the minus side of the ledger?"

If the medical problem is serious enough, write down the options so you can inspect them carefully. Then, pick the solution that makes most sense to you. Ask about quality of life in addition to survival. Your sexual functioning, mobility, cognitive abilities, and emotional strength after treatment can be as important as life itself (see chapter 5).

Of course, it can be satisfying and comforting to rely on the single perspective that the doctor or the "facts" seem to favor spontaneously. However, patients should understand that their decision can be warped by the physician's choice of arguments and the language used—aside from medical facts about the situation.

## THE UNDERTOW OF EMOTIONAL MOOD

Feelings regulate the capacity to think creatively—for the professional as surely as the layperson; for the doctor as surely as the patient. The hidden costs to quality care often escape notice, but they are real.

Our friend David had a persistent cough and occasionally spat flecks of blood. He had lost ten pounds over the previous six months. Finally, David phoned his physician to arrange an appointment, and the doctor scheduled chest X rays even before the consultation. David was sitting in an examining room waiting his turn. Here's what happened next.

His doctor pushed open the door and apologized for the delay. David saw right away that something was wrong; the doctor looked as if the weight of the world had fallen on his shoulders. David kept quiet, but his doctor explained anyway: "I was just tied up, arguing over the phone with the new administrator at Memorial Hospital. The jerk is turning everything upside down and completely ignoring those of us who started the place." Then the doctor forced a grin in place of his frown. "Let's look at your chart and see what's cooking here."

And that's what they did. But should David have worried about his doctor's emotional state that morning, and even done something about it? Does any patient have legitimate reason to be interested in the physician's feelings, what's happening in his or her own life as diagnoses are taking place and treatments being launched? Does the doctor's emotional state influence his or her approach to diagnosis and care?

Evidence from studies of human judgment say loudly, "yes." Emotional states profoundly influence the quality of decision making, even among professionals like medical clinicians. Feelings, even when provoked by unrelated matters, can shape the precision and thoroughness of care.

An experiment with third-year medical students shows how (Isen, Rosenzweig, and Young 1991). The students were given files describing six patients and asked to identify the one who probably had lung cancer. Reassuringly, all the budding doctors arrived at correct answers. But they differed in important ways on their styles of judgment, matters that affect the type of care offered to patients, and feelings influenced these judgments.

At an earlier stage of the study, the medical students had been shown a series of difficult anagrams, five-letter scrambled words. Half the subjects were asked to solve the anagrams, and told they had done very well. This success at a word game boosted their positive feelings. The other medical students were asked just to judge the difficulty of the word game and not to solve it, leaving them relatively neutral.

The medical students with positive feelings made more efficient use of their time in reaching clinical judgments about lung cancer. They studied all the cases more thoroughly, and were more clear-headed about their decisions. They incorporated a greater mix of information from each patient's chart before deciding whether or not that person had cancer. In short, positive feelings triggered by an experience that was *completely unrelated to medicine* influenced the thoroughness and enthusiasm with which the clinicians tackled their professional assignment.

Why is this the case? Two psychological explanations are at work here. Of course, when people feel positive they take greater pleasure in the tasks at hand, which means they are more likely to give their best effort. A second, less obvious contribution to the quality of decisions comes into play, too. Experiences are stored in memory according to their emotional charge as well as their content. Ideas and information of similar emotional tone tend to be linked. A positive value attaches to most of the things that doctors have learned about medicine; these things have been judged "useful" and have been stored that way.

When any of us—including a doctor—feels good, our memory rummages through its inventory of positively charged items more efficiently than when we feel neutral or, even worse, out of sorts. If we feel positive, our decision processes quickly match positive items in memory to see if they contribute to each other in some beneficial way.

Positive feelings lead people to more creative solutions in several ways. First, positive feelings make it easier to see connections among ideas and to visualize things in a more inclusive manner. Doctors in a positive frame of mind consider the possibility that symptoms normally indicating one condition might actually provide clues to another. They resist an assembly-line approach, in which each new patient's illness is seen as just another case like those who have gone before. Positive-feeling doctors also remain open to novel strategies when choosing among treatments. Patients benefit because they and their condition are less likely to be swiftly typecast.

Furthermore, when decision makers are feeling good, the possibility of making a mistake torments them; consequently, they remain determined, thoughtful, and careful to do their best. Feeling good can even slash the time necessary for reaching decisions, if that is important. Finally, doctors in a positive frame of mind are more willing to cut loose from failing diagnoses and treatments without fear that this would damage their self-esteem.

What does all of this mean for you as a patient and consumer of medical care? It takes only small pleasures to perk up the quality of decisions. Better judgments result when people have been praised for their capabilities or success, given token gifts like a greeting card, flowers, or a book or—especially powerful—told a joke or funny experience.

Decisions also improve when feelings have been boosted by chance, such as finding money on the pavement, being offered a snack, or unexpectedly tuning in to a stand-up comedy routine on television. The emotional tone of surroundings matters, too. Pleasant work spaces bring better decisions than cluttered or run-down quarters, even when obvious factors like level of illumination, distracting noise, and oxygen content are held constant.

David may have gotten less from his harried doctor that morning than the complexity of his case deserved and needed. The same possibility faces you when undergoing a medical exam, unless you go armed with a retaliatory strike against gloomy moods and emotional fatigue. Recall a previous experience with the physician with gratitude, or bring a token gift. Share a cartoon that pokes fun at yourself or at a target that the doctor and you both disdain.

## WHEN THE PRICE TAG BIASES CHOICE

Patients and physicians reach decisions within the limits of what seems possible financially as well as medically. Insurance coverage brings a harsh reality to their decision making: By wide margins, physicians and patients favor procedures that are reimbursed over those that must be paid for out-of-pocket. Lack of insurance altogether is even more serious. Among nonelderly people well above the poverty line, one of nine adults plus their children have no health coverage whatsoever and must rely on their own financial resources, forgo care, or misuse emergency facilities (U.S. Bureau of the Census March 1990–94; Swartz, Marcotte, and McBride 1993).

Even when insurance cushions the sticker shock, doctors increasingly struggle with reimbursers over standards of care (see the discussion of managed care in chapter 1). As you examine the provisions of health plans available to you, consider their limitations and what those might mean to your decision about treatments. Two illustrations—psychological services and hospice care—drive this point home.

*Psychological Services.* A wide range of conditions lead people to seek out or be urged into psychological care. Among such problems are general anxiety, depression, feelings of panic, phobias (e.g., fear of public places, height), eating problems, substance abuse (alcohol, drugs), sexual dysfunction, and stress. Sources for therapy include psychiatrists, psychologists, social workers, support groups, marriage counselors, physicians, and others. These providers practice many different techniques, depending on the therapist's training and the nature of the client's problem. Length of time for treatment varies widely, too.

Interviews with users of psychological therapy suggest that most feel they have gained dramatic improvements (Seligman 1995). A large majority of those feeling "very poor" when they began say they are feeling much better at the time of the survey. Problems that led them to seek care had lessened, and general functioning had also improved:

productivity at work, interpersonal relations, insight, and personal growth. In short, therapy had helped.

Importantly, improvement doesn't seem to depend greatly on which methods the therapists had used. Champions of one school of counseling over others dispute this furiously, but research evidence that backs a single, best approach is hard to find.

Other major influences on effectiveness do emerge, and these hinge on reimbursement limitations by insurance plans. A patient's length of time in care is apparently related to his or her improvement. Patients getting psychological services for just a few months, for example, claim dramatically less improvement than people who have been in care for more than two years.

Unfortunately, though, more than four of ten persons who obtain some form of therapy report that their insurance plan limited its coverage in some way. The insurer had disallowed access to a type of therapist, curtailed how often the patient could get counseling, or shortened the length of care. When this happened, improvement fell far below the experience of patients who got help until they felt better, from the care provider they thought best for treating their condition.

Of course, many needy people are discouraged from seeking psychological services at all, because their health plans offer little or no coverage. Other needy people resort to subterfuge. They see a family doctor for conditions better treated by mental health specialists, knowing that he or she can disguise services to make them reimbursable. Unfortunately, patients may pay a price for this practice. Many people with psychological problems who consult regular physicians get better only in their first six months or so, but stay at that level thereafter. By contrast, people who consult mental health professionals continue to improve with longer treatment, on average.

Insurance companies argue that liberalized benefits for psychotherapy would unleash public demand; patients would convert into therapy junkies, bankrupting the system. Or the therapy industry would ratchet its recommended length of treatments upward to fit just beneath more liberal ceilings. These are plausible fears, given that many mental conditions lack good clinical protocols for evaluating when therapy is no longer needed.

Some hard evidence, however, argues in the opposite direction (Landerman et al. 1994). It has been shown that limiting the insurance of people with pronounced psychiatric disorders curtails their care as hurtfully as limitations placed on people with less severe problems, but who would nonetheless like to see a therapist. This evidence suggests that insurers' stinginess harms people with uncontestable but unreimbursed needs, not just groups of patients that may include a few malingerers.

Regardless of debates over justifiable or frivolous services, the lesson is clear: Availability of insurance coverage makes a serious difference in people's quality of psychological care and in the options they can exercise among treatments.

*Hospice Care.* End-of-life choices offer another illustration of how economic constraints force patients into surrender. The hospice approach for terminally ill people has received growing support, with patient loads increasing at an annual rate of 10 to 20 percent. Hospice care emphasizes the relief of physical, emotional, and spiritual pain, rather than treatment of underlying diseases. Compared to traditional hospital-based terminal care, home-based hospice plans provide better pain relief and encourage patients' self-determination in their last days.

The availability of insurance often controls whether patients can make this choice, however. In the vast majority of cases, enrollment in a hospice means that the patient remains at home and is cared for by a family member. Professional hospice staff visit, bringing their skills in home nursing, spiritual counseling, treatment for pain, and other forms of palliative care. Insurance programs and Medicare make the hospice staff visits possible by paying an average daily rate of ninety dollars. Were it not for special hospice coverage, many of these noncurative medical and support services would not be reimbursed.

To qualify for such aid, though, a patient *signs away* all rights for reimbursement of medical treatments aimed at underlying causes of disease. The patient's doctor also certifies that death is likely to occur within six months. The physician's statement is not trivial; the government actually penalizes hospice plans that register high rates of survival past the requisite six-month cutoff through retroactive denials of payment.

As a consequence, hospices have become favored ways to seek terminal care for some conditions but not others. From the insurer's financial standpoint, the most desirable candidate is someone with a relatively predictable, brief final course of illness who needs intensive management of symptoms. Many cancers fit this profile. In 1994, not surprisingly, 80 percent of the approximately 340,000 dying persons taking part in hospice care had cancer.

Unfortunately, however, more Americans die from other causes: heart disease, stroke, lung disease, and other types of chronic organ failure. Even when patients are desperately ill, the timing of their death is unpredictable and may not occur within the six months. Therefore, these patients become unwelcome prospects for hospice treatment.

Regulatory and cost pressures on hospices limit them even more severely. Half the enrollees die within five weeks, many in the first week or so. The tragedy of these late referrals is that they leave far too little time for many supportive services that hospices have pioneered. Furthermore, patients should be able to benefit from hospice care while still mentally alert. Alas for their eligibility, people who retain their faculties survive a wide range of terminal illnesses longer than the incompetent or comatose.

A dark and unintended side to hospice care emerges. Few except cancer patients can be offered this option. The rules of reimbursement impose their own cruel rationing of dignity in life's final chapter. The decision about whether or not to have hospice care results more from reimbursement policies than personal choice.

The list of distortions in U.S. health care runs much longer than this. Many critics have decried insurers' inattention to preventive measures such as nutrition and their skepticism about alternative medicine, even recognized methods such as chiropractic techniques. Insurance plans vary too widely, however, for any advice here to help—except one very practical step. Seek a benefits counselor where you work to help explain provisions of care available to you and your family, and don't be surprised if this person has disappointing news to pass along.

## HABITS OF THE MIND THAT CLOUD DECISION MAKING

People settle into ways of dealing with choices. Sometimes the gravitational pull of these habits leads people to defer decision making or default to shortcuts, economies in thinking that clear the mind but can bring unwelcome consequences.

### THE POWERFUL PULL OF THE PAST

People are generally unaware of it, but they implicitly renew their decision to continue a course of treatment every day, in contrast to trying something different. Ideally, each day's decision should reflect a refreshed estimate of the therapy's prospects for success, regardless of the investments in the course of action thus far. To their regret, though, many people have a habit of overlooking this principle.

In the field of accounting, this is called the bias of *sunk costs.* Sunk costs occur whenever people have invested substantial resources (time, pain, reputation, money) that cannot be retrieved and are still waiting to get commensurate benefits. It is not that benefits do not or will not occur; rather, they have *not yet occurred,* although costs have. Faced with a decision to quit with certain loss or to continue with the *possibility* of a gain, people resolve to continue. The inertia of the past glues them to their course of action.

We're all familiar with how people can be fond of throwing good money after bad. Consider the man who paid thousands of dollars to join an exclusive tennis club. Several weeks later, he developed tennis elbow. Routine ground strokes brought excruciating pain; serving was even worse. Nonetheless, he continued his weekly appointments on the courts, plunging his arm into a pail of ice after every match. Why this obstinate and agonizing behavior? He had paid too much for his membership to quit playing.

Similar stories flood the business and governmental worlds. Failing ventures continue to suck capital from firms and appropriations from legislative bodies, because it would be "shameful to stop now when we have put so much into this project already."

Women during childbirth show how medical decision making can be influenced by sunk costs—not actual money, in this case, but pain that has already been endured. Many who originally decided to deliver without anesthesia stick with that commitment even after long periods of painful labor. These mothers-to-be tend to delay getting relief even though they come to feel that anesthesia is preferable to delivering naturally. Their sunk costs in pain warp their decision-making preferences.

Other medical applications come easily to mind. Therapies that have already begun tend to be continued, even in the face of disappointing results. The more costly or difficult treatments are, the more doggedly doctors and patients may cling to them.

Another wrinkle of sunk costs involves setting deadlines. Ironically, this can strengthen people's value on investments already made. Take the case of Ted, a fifty-two-year-old assembler in the aerospace industry.

He suffered sharp pain down his arm and deadened nerves in his hand. His doctor diagnosed a pinched nerve, complicated by whiplash from a rear-end car collision. The doctor prescribed an anti-inflammatory drug to relieve the discomfort, a strong medication that often brings intestinal upset. Like many patients, Ted was eager to know when he would feel improvement. The doctor offered his best bet. In due course, the predicted time for improvement arrived, but Ted's arm continued to ache.

Paradoxically, however, Ted kept thinking that positive results from the anti-inflammatory would show up "any time now." His sunk costs in therapy included a modified diet that he and his wife went to some trouble to organize, in order to avoid the medicine's side effects. With each passing day and its specially prepared meals, he became more tolerant of the stomach aches and diarrhea and more willing to stick with the medications, instead of less so. In this, he acted true to form in response to the combination of mounting sunk costs and a passed deadline.

Many times, of course, patience with therapy pays dividends. Other times, however, persistence proves fruitless, as it did with Ted. He stuck with the anti-inflammatory medication and bland meals for six weeks beyond the time when results should have appeared. He resisted exploring other therapies.

What can you do to eliminate the sunk-cost influence on medical decisions? Patients and their doctors can periodically review the course of medical action, tallying up the costs and benefits of a procedure during each week or month, from start to the present. Are costs mounting, with absolutely no sign of offsetting rewards? Have some benefits appeared, and then vanished? Establish a mental timeline to track these.

Write down even subjective opinions; these are preferable to marching blindly ahead. What are the medical alternatives, with their predicted advantages and disadvantages? Does sticking with the chosen procedure bring health risks, as well as inconvenience or annoyance? The wise patient is willing to jettison a choice that's just not panning out.

## THE COSTS OF IMPULSIVENESS

People are a restless and impetuous lot, anxious for closure and results. Unfortunately, carrying out a medical treatment program or undergoing a procedure usually involves a stretch of time and gnawing ambiguity. Patients decide on a treatment today, but the benefits (or failures) may take some time to appear. Impatience for these results can bias expectations, which in turn can lead to bad decision making.

Have you ever noticed how people get relatively more upset when their hopes aren't met, than happy when an unexpected reward comes their way? Researchers have called this tendency the "delay-speedup asymmetry" (Svenson and Maule 1993). Picture an airport scene. The loudspeaker announces that a flight will not depart on time. Travelers waiting in the lounge groan loudly and their shoulders slump. They're upset. But how about the people running down the corridor who would have been late for their flight but now are able to make it? Strangely, there's little sign of joy from these ticket holders. They're simply, and usually undemonstratively, relieved.

In other words, once people have set their heart on an outcome, being prevented from reaching it irritates them a lot more sharply than unanticipated, early results might please them. Your point of view about improvements in health can follow the same course. Say that you have undergone a vasectomy. Intercourse without risk of conception can't take place until your semen is cleared of live sperm, which can take fifteen to twenty ejaculations following the operation. Your urologist wants to collect a sample to confirm that it's safe for you to have sex without protection. You're looking forward to the go-ahead. If you don't get the green light when you expect it, you'll feel upset at postponing intercourse; your frustration will exceed any pleasure (several times over) you could have taken from an early announcement that all was safe. Furthermore, your resentment may spread to the doctor and his or her medical advice on other matters, needlessly poisoning future relationships and discrediting good ideas.

In such ways, impatience for immediate results often distorts people's attitudes about the quality of their care. The demand for "results, now" even leads patients into premature actions—driving an automobile before incision from a bypass operation has properly healed, for example. Or, with a vasectomy, it could lead to resuming sex while sperm are still ready to do their biological duty.

The human fascination with immediate gains shows its hand in other ways. Under the spell of short-term thinking, patients often ignore the magnitude of different benefits and commonly decide in ways that are contrary to their genuine but unrecognized interests.

Imagine that a medicine to alleviate the symptoms of flu promises quick but limited relief. A different course of treatment—say, bed rest and drinking fluids—takes days, but brings complete results. Facing such choice, many feverish and aching people swallow the nostrums and keep up their busy schedule. They fall for the immediate but partial solution within twenty-four to thirty-six hours, in preference to the delayed and thorough one.

A simple mind experiment would readjust these people's priorities. Suppose they imagined that nostrums would start to relieve some of their flu symptoms in one week (instead of just hours). Suppose also, by comparison, bed rest and fluids would bring complete relief in ten days. Faced with this time-shifted choice—superficial help in seven days versus thorough help in ten—almost everybody chooses to hit the sack and drink hot tea instead of trusting over-the-counter potions.

What's happening here? It's true that people lunge for the quick fix, but they do a flip-flop if they imagine a delayed span of action. Near-term, an immediate but small benefit looks better than a greater one postponed slightly. By contrast, greater rewards reveal their attractions over lesser ones when all are cast in the future by even a few days.

Unreasonable preferences for immediate over delayed results sometimes get expressed in a slightly different way: People overvalue outcomes that are considered certain, compared to ones that are merely probable. When this happens, a patient may opt for the treatment that's sure to produce small gains instead of taking a chance on another procedure that might bring much larger improvement.

Shrewd physicians and savvy patients blunt the distortions from short-term fixes: They make time seem to go faster. They identify intermediate stages of medical improvement, which breaks a large ambition for improved health into a number of smaller and swifter achievements. Patient and physician can work together to keep customary interests like hobbies alive as treatment progresses; these distract from a tedious progress toward recovery. Patients with nothing to do except get well are the most zealous for speedy results. Children and others who do not recognize their impulse toward immediacy and certainty are especially vulnerable. Sometimes the greatest gift a parental caregiver can make is persuading the child to divide recovery into manageable stages: first "let's get well enough to enjoy your favorite food," then "let's feel like playing a board game together," and finally "let's be able to ride your bike a couple times around the block."

## LOOSENING THE VISE OF DEADLINES

No one would mistake medical decision making as one of life's leisurely pastimes. Time pressures hasten many choices. Patients are asked to make up their minds about a therapy now, while in the doctor's office. If they need an operation, the surgical team and facilities must be booked soon, before others schedule them. Life-threatening conditions obviously require swift action. Even with less pressing problems, however, a clock may be ticking—physical strength dribbling away, tumors growing, infection looming, or some other biological marker announcing that your narrow window of choice has arrived and may not reappear.

How does the human decision maker perform under intense time pressures? Badly, many times, and certainly less successfully than when there's an opportunity to weigh options. A dangerous cycle gains hold: (1) when hedged by a deadline, a decision is more difficult and tiring to make than under other conditions; (2) this leads the decision maker to fixate on how hard things are, wasting scarce time; thus (3) difficulty ratchets up another notch, exhausting the decision maker even more. When caught in this cycle, the besieged patient often cuts himself or herself off from others. Regrettably, the loss of time-consuming social contact sacrifices information and opinions that others could provide, further depleting the opportunity for sound judgment.

There are a number of systematic ways that people slip into unsatisfying decisions when haste rules. They embrace shortcuts that they wouldn't tolerate in themselves under other circumstances. An approaching deadline encourages them to filter information and criteria, paring things down to what appears essential (Keren and Roelofsma 1995; Roelofsma and Keren 1995). People omit considerations. And, unfortunately without realizing it, they delete evidence selectively. As a consequence, individuals commonly reach diametrically opposed results, depending on whether they are rushed or are given a more leisurely pace to make choices.

Hurried people tend to edit away the positive and appealing characteristics of options, concentrating instead on negative and adverse criteria for making their decision. Choice A may have more advantages than B, but A may also present more risks or disadvantages, too. People in a rush opt for B, focusing all their attention on the disadvantages of A and ignoring the greater benefits from A. In a calmer frame of mind, many would give the nod to A.

In such stealthy ways, time pressure crimps the aperture through which people view their decision: A particular option becomes relatively acceptable just because it could prevent the worst from happening. Under these circumstances, the possibility of maximizing benefits often vanishes from consideration.

Small wonder that tight time constraints often lead decision makers to throw up their hands, growing discouraged and less and less attracted to any of the options they face. And once a decision is reached under pressure, the chooser often shows little satisfaction with the result, no matter how well things may turn out. The seeds of regret are sown (see the next section).

People who are alert to the handicaps from time constraints are better prepared to counteract them. Two strategies can aid the harried and hurried decision maker. If at all possible, try not to make urgent medical decisions alone. Keep a calm and cool friend by your side, one who will be less rattled than you by the approaching deadline. Continue asking this ally: "What am I overlooking here? Am I balancing this information correctly?"

In addition, challenge the ground rules. Health-care providers may have laid these down to suit their own convenience. Ask "Is there a genuine, biological reason why I must make up my mind as quickly as you say?" The insistence on speed may simply help the medical bureaucracy: another day in the hospital costs money; the surgeon will be on vacation next week; putting off a procedure requires scheduling another office visit. Meditate on whether you really do need to rush, or would prefer to take a breather. Of course, give yourself time for a second opinion, if appropriate.

In some medical crises, the clock can't be slowed. Just the same, recognize that you might be unhappier with the outcome than if you had been given time for thoughtful choice. Clem, seventy-two years old and a retired menswear salesman, went into life-threatening respiratory failure while hospitalized with pneumonia. He was conscious but severely distressed; his blood gases were abnormal; his acute condition was rapidly getting worse. Physicians asked Clem to choose between surgical intubation—sedation and insertion of a pipe into the larynx to aid breathing—or noninvasive ventilation using a mechanical pump and external mask. He had only moments to choose and opted for the less invasive procedure.

Happily, normal breathing and blood readings returned within forty-five minutes. But Clem became irritated anyway, complaining that the face mask was painful and that he found it difficult to breathe, despite objective signs to the contrary.

Clem, like others, interpreted a pressured choice as a denial of freedom of choice. Such circumstances, even when unavoidable, leave a residue of unhappiness. Embrace this lesson: In routine medical situations it's best to avoid needless rush. Greater satisfaction with results and happier doctor-patient relationships are just two rewards.

## REACTING TO MEDICAL DISAPPOINTMENT

One of life's most familiar experiences is regret (Landman 1993). People examine what's become of them and compare that against some standard or expectation of what could have been. They conclude that another outcome was possible. Their thoughts turn quickly to what might have happened (1) if only they had done something earlier that they failed to do, or (2) if only they could take back or reverse an earlier decision or action. They wish to undo reality. Regret can torment people. Replaying events leading up to a spinal cord injury or a child's death from Sudden Infant Death Syndrome (SIDS), for example, can infect people with guilt that they should not bear.

Encouragingly, though, regret can also become a catalyst for helping people take new action. Sometimes, upon reflection, people can ease (if not fully correct) the consequences of their earlier behavior. Other times, ruminating on past deeds and missed opportunities can help make better choices next time around. "Backward thinking" frees people to imagine brighter and more satisfying futures. Trying to undo an event by thinking of ways one could have acted differently offers a means for taking personal responsibility. Regret, in other words, need not always paralyze, be a melancholy enterprise, or lack benefits.

Even world champions, such as Olympic athletes, feel regret and toy in their minds with what might have been as a means of doing better next time. Surprisingly, silver medalists feel more regret after their competitions than do bronze medalists. Athletes who earn the silver think about what they almost accomplished: "If only I had won the gold." Athletes who receive the bronze are in the same shoes as silvers, having missed the top prize with its singular rewards, but they enjoy knowing that they have risen above the rest of the pack to reach the medal stand.

Psychologists have surveyed Olympic athletes in the weeks that followed the Games (Medvec, Madey, and Gilovich 1995). Just like other people who feel they didn't perform at their best, the second- and third-place finishers ruminate about how they would have performed better if they had only done things differently before the Olympics ("started their comeback sooner," or "had more scientific training," or "competed in the Pan Am Games the year before").

Medical encounters are full of regrets when abnormal outcomes take place or when you just don't regain as much health as expected. Nonetheless, you can turn your natural human response of regret into a valuable, constructive experience by understanding the dynamics of rearview thinking. In order to make better health-care choices and improve well-being, you must focus on re-creating the past in a way that illuminates future decisions. That way you can consciously consider scenarios that don't pop quickly to mind.

Notice, first, the distinction between *adding* imagined things to the past as opposed to *subtracting* them. With additions, people imagine extra acts that could have improved the outcomes; there's usually a great variety of these. With subtractions, people think about deleting something they already did; the range of options here is obviously more limited.

Interestingly, when people grapple with failure or disappointment, they think much more naturally about additions than subtractions; what they could have done instead of what they did wrong. In fact, additions spring to mind two to three times more easily than subtractions. Moreover, if a disappointing condition persists or gets worse, people dwell on imagined additions even more fervently, five to six times more often than subtractions.

In some medical situations, thinking about additions may be a sensible way to reassert control. However, additions without considering subtractions may not always lead to more creative decision making, even though they come more easily to the imagination.

Consider the case of Samuel, a sixty-three-year-old construction foreman with adult-onset diabetes. His endocrinologist was concerned because Samuel's blood-sugar readings were all too often high and fluctuated widely. Samuel kept showing up for his appointments with the same results, and he grew increasingly concerned and regretful himself. He began to imagine additional changes he might make that could stabilize his situation. He should eat more fresh vegetables and fat-free foods. He should exercise. He should test his blood sugar regularly. He should take his oral medications more faithfully. All were medically sound ideas, and Samuel even began to carry through on them, although fitfully.

Samuel neglected to consider subtractions with the same determination, and in his case, there was a big one that begged attention. Samuel put away a couple of hard drinks and two or three glasses of wine with nearly every dinner. Eliminating that custom would have brought more immediate control over glucose levels than adding the other sound habits Samuel thought of embracing. In this instance, a search for behaviors to *subtract*—as unaccustomed and challenging as that can be—would have allowed him to profit more from his regret over disappointing results in controlling his disease.

Psychologists who study decision making have not come up with prescriptions for how one learns best from a differently imagined past— when to try adding elements and when to try deleting them. The alert patient or doctor, though, recognizes the human bias that favors grasping at new straws.

Other factors besides a preference for adding to the past, instead of subtracting from it, can distort people's decisions about medical care. When people revise the past in order to imagine a happier outcome, they alter some parts of history more readily than others. For example, people tend to rewrite events that occurred *recently,* more than events in the *deeper past.* Carl, a fifty-six-year-old real estate salesman, complained of angina, intense and suffocating pains in his chest. He blamed his recent job change, which made him responsible for the sales performance of eighteen other agents and created extraordinary stress at work. "I should have stayed with the old firm," he moaned. Carl never considered the role that his thirty-year, two-pack-a-day cigarette habit played in his current predicament.

This search for recent causes of regret can also lead to blaming the last person in a chain of action. Anne, a high-strung marketing executive of thirty-seven, had been dashing from one doctor to another with complaints of abdominal pain. None diagnosed the ulcer that finally erupted in a hemorrhage, sending her to the emergency room one night. She held the last physician she had seen at greater fault than the others. Our check of her medical charts at the three doctors she visited actually revealed that the last clinician had come closest in his reading of her symptoms and test results. Nonetheless, Anne acted like the basketball fan who faults the player who misses a last-second, desper-

ation shot instead of other team members who fluffed a greater number of plays during easier periods of the game.

Moreover, people are fonder of rewriting their past *actions* than
their *inactions*. A bit of medical detective work often shows, however,
that actions may be no more at fault for one's bad health than missed
opportunities. Jennifer, a nineteen-year-old college student, returned from
a trip to Bali and a remote area of Celebes with a case of infectious hepati-
tis. Jennifer's first regret was to have included the jungle village in
Celebes on her itinerary. Probing questions by her doctor back home
uncovered a more likely cause: She forgot a crucial vaccination before
traveling.

It's common for people to see causes for their distress in *exceptional*
situations rather than in *familiar* or mundane conditions. Georgina, a forty-
three-year-old housewife, developed an allergic irritation in her nasal
passages. Her life hadn't deviated much from her routine of late, except
for the trip she took to Italy, her first time outside the United States.
She was flooded with regret when the allergy developed, blaming
her decision to go abroad and feeling annoyed at her sister for pres-
suring her into this vacation. Actually, Georgina's allergic reaction was
caused by construction in her neighborhood; a builder had mowed
nearby fields choked with ragweed and mustard to make way for his
development.

In these examples, the most natural ways in which people rewrote
their past helped ease their regret and frustration, but these habits also
turned out to be inaccurate assessments and poor guides for the future.
Reimagining the most recent events prior to distress did not spotlight
real causes. Focusing on actions instead of inactions missed the real
point. Exceptional life experiences were not to blame. In these cases,
and perhaps in yours too, people needed to swim against their natural
currents of thinking in order to profit from regret.

The point is to urge you to consider many replays. Rewriting past
events to account for present medical agonies or disappointments is
normal and even helpful. You will draw more positive results from
ruminations where you are willing to experiment, testing the usefulness of alternative drafts of your story.

Finally, refashioning the past, natural though it is, carries a threat
that deserves your notice. An unreasonable sense of guilt may lie in
wait. To some people, moral or other personal weakness seems inescapably
to blame when trying to account for serious illness or devastating acci-

dent. These unfortunates flail themselves for tragedies that were clearly beyond expectation: crime victimization, brain tumors, multiple sclerosis, and more. Their ruminations dissolve into shame and self-loathing. Acute depression lurks closely behind. Such individuals get into a rut and won't let go of mulling over their past. People whose self-esteem is already shaky are especially prone to endless self-reproach.

Thus, undoing the past in your mind could carry a double dose of bad feeling: preoccupation with current distress, plus guilt over the belief that the distress needn't have happened except for your own negligence. It takes a hardy person to try rewriting the past without falling prey to the process.

## A BIOLOGICAL AMBUSH SHADOWING DECISIONS

Elusive forces govern physical and emotional vigor, silently upsetting many people's decisions about medical care. Patients submit to diagnosis, choose a therapy, and wait for results, but no improvement is seen, or matters actually get worse. What's wrong? Sometimes, the trouble lies in ignoring rhythms of biology, many of which lie beyond people's notice.

Cycles that we only dimly perceive regulate well-being and even our capabilities of thinking clearly (Rosenthal and Blehar 1989; Hrushesky, Langer, and Theeuwes 1991). The mind works more swiftly and surely at some times of day than others. Drugs administered at certain times of day have better ratios of effectiveness versus toxicity than when taken at other times. Women are more susceptible to asthmatic attacks just prior to and during their menstrual cycle than at other times of the month. Research has observed (but not yet fully understood) biological rhythms through which our bodies gather strength for resisting or dealing with illness. If people acknowledged these ebbs and flows, they would be able to deal with illness in a more thoughtful and calculating manner.

The field of "chronobiology" focuses on the mechanisms by which cells, tissues, and organisms sequence activities across time. For example, heart attacks strike in a circadian rhythm, a daily cycle. Other medical conditions are keyed to a seven-day cycle; still others to the menstrual cycle. Few of today's medical practitioners were exposed to the therapeutic consequences of these facts during their training. Few adapt their treatment of patients to biological rhythms. But these systematic ups and downs affect the sensitivity and results of screening tests, such as mammograms with pre-menstrual women, the measurement of urinary peptides as a marker for ovarian cancer, and blood analyses. Interventions may succeed or largely fail according to their timing during the day, as with the potency and side effects of drugs to fight colorectal cancer and other solid tumors.

The most documented case of biological timing involves the circadian cycle of circulatory conditions. Heart attacks and strokes, "the malaria of the developed world," commandeer the largest share of the West's health-care and research budgets. These emergencies occur with clockwork regularity. The hours from waking to noon are the peak period, four times greater than other times, leading to the chorus of sirens as ambulances rush through morning traffic. The circadian pattern holds for sufferers of both mild and severe coronary artery disease, men and women, younger and older people.

Several factors contribute to this cycle: a morning increase in blood platelet aggregation, a regular increase in arterial blood pressure, and cycles of hormonal secretion. Further research is needed in order to distinguish these physiological processes from intervals of rest and activity in the typical day, to which they are related.

Menstrual cycles are also recognized demonstrations of chronobiology. Nonetheless, clinicians have blithely ignored them in the treatment of many illnesses. Recent studies of women with breast cancer underscore spectacular opportunities that such attention could bring (Hrushesky 1996). Several years ago, laboratory studies with mice began indicating a connection between the timing of the breast surgery in relationship to menstrual cycle and future metastases (the spreading of cancer). Evidence suggested a much better prognosis when the surgery was performed during ovulation; recurrence of disease occurred more often when the operation was timed during menstruation. Researchers believe that the immune system's functioning explains this phenomenon. Natural-killer (NK) cell activity fluctuates during the menstrual cycle, peaking around the time of ovulation and falling to its lowest point during menstruation. NK cells play a critical part in the rejection of tumors, hence the suppression of metastases.

Could such a simple, bureaucratic consideration as the timing of their operation affect the fate of tens of thousands of women who undergo breast cancer surgery every year? Just asking this catches one's breath. Fortunately, some oncologists have kept menstrual history in the charts of their breast cancer patients. Results from just one report show the amount of difference (Hrushesky et al. 1989).

Among women whose surgery had taken place during menstrual intervals, 37 percent had a recurrence seven to fourteen years later. Among women who were ovulating during surgery, only 14 percent had a recurrence. In this time period, nearly one-third of the first group had died, compared to 5 percent of the ovulatory patients. None of the usual clinical indicators could explain the large gap in outcomes. Current research is refining the window of surgical opportunity even more closely, so premenopausal breast cancer patients should ask their physicians to consult the latest journals before scheduling surgery.

If chronicity affects bodies, does it also affect minds? Yes, it does. Rhythmic cycles show up in the way people think. Motivations and capacities to process information follow circadian (daily) patterns. Research confirms that there really are "morning people" and "night people," hours of the day when individuals are at their prime. Naturally, performance declines steadily with sleep deprivation; most people can sense that growing tiredness saps their thinking skills. But circadian rhythms are processes distinct from fatigue itself.

Because of circadian rhythms, skill and insight for problem solving fluctuate (Bodenhausen 1990). "Morning people" are sharper early in the day rather than in the evening. By the same token, "night people" perform their best in the evening. During off times, people are more likely to fall back on deeply rooted ("automatic") ways of thinking instead of carefully weighing the pertinent facts; individuals go for the easiest explanation rather than work for the more complex and possibly accurate one. Changes also take place throughout the day in the efficiency of people's working memory. Differences in flexibility of problem solving are often quite large, even within a single day. Circadian variations can be as great as one-third the average level of performance on a particular task. Daily oscillations among these primary functions affect safety at many jobs, general achievement, and of course, medical decision making.

Daily peaks and valleys in problem solving are only one source of short-term variability. Studies of mood swings have also considered weekday, compared to weekend influences. Headway is being made in tracking cycles in brain functioning across longer time spans, too.

What use can the ordinary patient make of these insights, other than finding them intriguing? For starters, you can add these questions to the list you prepare before seeing your physician:

- Is the onset or severity of my condition related to daily cycles or other systematic biological rhythms?
- Is there any best time of the day to take medications, so that they have maximum effect and minimum toxicity? Any best time for another intervention you are recommending? What about the timing of the tests that you've ordered for me?
- For women who are still menstruating: Is there any best time of the month to schedule drug or other therapy?

Finally, acknowledge your own mental limitations during off periods. Refrain from making critical decisions about health care, if you can, until you have reviewed options during your peak time, depending on whether you are a morning person or a night person. Refuse to become alarmed or defensive if you see that your own performance varies by day of the week and time of year. You're simply responding to nature.

### SHARPENING YOUR CONSUMER SKILLS IN CHOOSING MEDICAL CARE

In light of all the things that can go wrong during medical decisions, the patient's pick of which doctor to see ranks high in importance. Statistics confirm that physicians differ dramatically among themselves in how they reach decisions and in their prescriptions for care. Regional differences in medical costs, adjusted for local cost-of-living, provide some of the groundwork. Per-person medical expenditures in some states are twice the level found in other states, a dizzying swing in health care (Weil 1996). The rates-of-use for specific treatments fluctuate, too, such as surgery for breast or prostate cancer; these choices depend heavily on the region where patients get care. For example, when treating women with the same kinds of tumors, some areas' doctors favor radical mastectomies over simpler breast-saving lumpectomies, while doctors in other places lean in the opposite direction.

Rates differ state-by-state, and even city-by-city, on other procedures as well: the use of bypass surgery versus medications for heart disease; the decision to operate on those with chronic back pain, rather than prescribing rest, weight loss, and exercise. In another example, the number of procedures doctors order per Medicare patient varies enormously; this index of intensity of care is often simply related to where patients receive their health services.

There is little evidence that people are healthier or live longer in areas where costly medicine is practiced. There is plenty of evidence, instead, that an oversupply of doctors and a surplus of hospital beds fuel higher costs and a reliance on aggressive procedures and increase the number of treatments prescribed. In the Humpty Dumpty world of health economics, supply of services drives "demand."

Quality of doctors' training varies and adds its own uncertainties to care. The stethoscope dangling around the neck symbolizes everyone's image of medicine. Yet when listening to sounds, many general practitioners miss four of five of the most commonly encountered and important indicators of heart or lung disease. Many doctors on whom people rely for regular checkups are ill-prepared to pick up clues to deadly cardiac abnormalities like the murmur of aortic stenosis (Mangione and Nieman 1997).

An even closer peek inside doctors' examining rooms confirms how differently physicians interpret the same case. Researchers have presented doctors with videotapes of a patient being examined for chest pain, a common complaint that sometimes foretells health calamity (McKinlay 1996). Although carefully trained actors played the roles of patient and physician, these enactments were based on actual cases. Workup sheets summarizing each patient's basic physiological measures accompanied the videos. The physicians in the study rendered their diagnoses and treatment recommendations in their own offices as if the patient were one of their own.

Four of ten doctors thought the condition was primarily psychological in origin. Another four of ten blamed cardiac abnormalities. Still other doctors thought gastrointestinal causes were at work. A quarter of the doctors prescribed a cardiac drug; about the same number urged a change in lifestyle. Just three of ten suggested quitting smoking (a habit included in the patient's workup). One of five prescribed an over-the-counter antacid or pain medication.

Doctors were more likely to see cardiac abnormalities with older patients' complaints than with the younger patients with exactly the same clinical signs and dialogue during examination. These older patients were even more often seen to be suffering from heart problems if they had insurance than if they did not. Many doctors dismissed complaints of the uninsured as psychological in origin.

The subjective face of medical decision making showed in other ways, too. HMO-based doctors were half as likely to make a primary cardiac diagnosis that requires complex and costly steps to confirm, compared to their fee-for-service colleagues. Thus, reimbursement policies for medical treatments cast a magnetic pull on diagnoses.

Such facts remind us that the myths inspired by Dr. Kildare and Marcus Welby, M.D., should have faded with those television series. It is dangerous to think of the doctor as a parental figure, weighing evidence within a uniform scientific formula, and delivering precise alternatives. Instead, medical choices often hinge on highly subjective and often intuitive judgments, unconscious factors operating on the physician as well as the patient.

But how do you get to the best doctor? The patient is David and the health-care system is Goliath when finding a physician. First, managed care may have narrowed your options. Beyond that, much of any physician's technical abilities and motivations can lie beneath a camouflage of starched lab coat, framed diplomas, erect bearing, and authoritative voice. You can't easily tell, for example, how up-to-date he or she stays with the medical literature. It's hard to judge how thoroughly a doctor examines you, until you have comparative experiences with several who probe and pummel and test for the condition you are suspected of having. It would be worth knowing how many times the doctor has performed a surgery or other procedure you need, but this carries little meaning unless you also know the norm for specialists in your area. Gauging a doctor's instincts—is he or she a dedicated helper or in it mainly for other reasons—strains the intuitive powers of many patients.

You may want to get advice about how to compare providers from an inside source, an informed doctor attentive to the quality of professional care (McCall 1995). Another, general strategy also helps narrow your search, when you want to find the best oncologists in your city, the most respected orthopedic surgeons, talented allergists, cardiologists, or whatever. Ask your general practitioner: "Who would you send your family to?" Ask doctors you know socially or at church or synagogue the same question. Ask friends to ask their doctors and physician friends. Ask specialists of one type, say obstetricians, who they would recommend in another specialty—plastic surgery or ear-nose-and-throat, for example. Continue until you find some convergence.

This works when you are in search of a second opinion or are willing to pay for care outside coverage by a managed plan. Be aware that doctors offering their advice may not know what plans other physicians have joined. If you are determined to stay within your HMO, you'll need to cross-check recommendations against the HMO's list of approved providers. Inside a staff-based HMO (see chapter 1), your quest for recommendations from others' doctors will probably center on coworkers; ask them to query their primary-care physician, if they have grown to trust his or her judgment.

Often, people's choice of doctors reaches beyond the circle of conventional practice, to what have usually been called *alternative* therapies. Actually, the term *alternative* is a misnomer; *unconventional* would be better. Each year people pay more visits to providers of chiropractic, acupuncture, massage, homeopathy, mind-body interventions, osteopathic medicine, and other forms of treatment not taught in mainline schools of medicine than they do to general practitioners of conventional medicine. Reliance on these other treatments is hardly alternative. In many cases, people see both kinds of practitioners concurrently, the conventional and unconventional (Eisenberg et al. 1993).

Patients usually turn to unconventional care when they have chronic ailments, such as musculoskeletal problems, allergies, anxiety and depression, or gynecological or viral diseases. Referrals by satisfied friends, coworkers, and family members figure strongly in this choice. Generally, people pay out of pocket, although a small but growing number of insurers include unconventional therapies within their plans, especially acupuncture, chiropractic, massage, naturopathy, and herbal medicine.

Some patients are confident that their chosen means of unconventional treatment helps control or cure the condition they suffer. They subscribe to a holistic view of connections among physical, mental, and spiritual well-being; the therapy elevates the importance of these connections, instead of depending on aggressive interventions. Often these patients continue seeing a mainstream doctor for physical treatment, adding unconventional providers in order to resolve emotional needs, gaining a sense of control over their illness.

Other patients feel driven to their unconventional treatment out of desperation, because "nothing else has helped." Literary mileage has been gotten from the cancer patient who flees to Mexican clinics practicing exotic remedies. Nonetheless, few cases of desperation involve people with acute or lethal conditions; among cancer patients, to illustrate, less than 10 percent rely on unconventional care.

A final reason for seeking unconventional care deserves special comment. Many users of such treatments find their providers to be more caring and interested in them than orthodox doctors. The use of auxiliary therapies provides patients longer and more rewarding office visits than they would otherwise enjoy. In the words of chapter 1, they achieve a *complete* relationship with health care through a division of labor—one provider giving *technical* care and another providing *personal* treatment.

## WHY SECOND OPINIONS MATTER

The range of care options, conventional and unconventional, and the wild swings in quality of health care convince many people that they need a second opinion for almost any serious condition that resists early care. Merciless, even insidious practices by the care bureaucracy also put patients on guard. The contractual arrangement between doctors and some managed-care plans discourage the medical team's candor with patients. One HMO's contract reminds physicians that: "Physician shall take no action nor make any communication which undermines or could undermine the confidence of enrollees, potential enrollees, their employers, plan sponsors or the public in [name of HMO], or in the quality of care which [name of HMO] enrollees receive" (Pear 1996, E7).

Corporate working conditions like this split doctors and their patients into adversaries, instead of uniting their interests. But there's an added reason for seeking a second opinion, as a check against hasty and narrowed recommendations by the initial care provider. More doctors than ever before chafe against bureaucrats over allowable treatments and reimbursements. As these contests wear on, doctors feel a valued part of their professional autonomy slip away. Faceless accountants now join them in the clinical driver's seat. Studies show that when doctors feel themselves hedged in this way, they grow less participatory in their manner with patients (Kaplan et al. 1996). They deliver their opinions more abruptly, leaving less room for discussion or challenge. They tend to discourage patients' input about care choices and underplay patients' responsibility for helping manage their own treatment. In short, the doctors' battle with insurers leaves them edgy and damages the quality of care by shortchanging involvement with patients over decisions.

Often, the second opinion serves as the best safeguard against such impoverished care. With it, you can compare two medical voices before plunging into a program that costs time, inflicts pain and inconvenience, poses risks, and raises your expectations.

Some patients are nervous about taking the step of seeking another opinion. It often requires asking your original physician to send records and test results to a professional competitor. Some doctors subtly discourage second opinions by frowning at their mention or by stalling. The doctor may discount the need for such advice, saying, "Your situation is pretty straightforward."

Even so, a second opinion can have value, as one of our subjects shows. Margo had asked her father's cardiologist for a recommendation, following his diagnosis. The physician snapped: "You'll just waste your money and another doctor's time." She invested her money and time, anyway, with satisfying results. The second physician confirmed the first, and Margo gained peace of mind that she considered well worth the effort.

Some patients, of course, fear that their doctor will be disappointed in them, or angry, if they seek a second opinion. Don't worry about offending your physician; it's your right to become as deeply informed as you can.

Seeking a second opinion offers you the chance to compose questions you probably didn't think about when talking to the diagnosing physician. Always ask about alternatives. Jocilyn, forty-seven, was bleeding from fibroid tumors, benign growths in her uterus. She was told that surgery would be a quick and conclusive solution, but she wondered whether it was the best choice for her. In seeking a second opinion, she learned that medication might slow bleeding and shrink the tumors, and it would be less invasive. She chose that route.

You may also want to seek a second opinion for a lingering problem that does not seem to resolve, or whenever options are presented that you feel you cannot untangle. For six months, Carolyn, a thirty-two-year-old advertising salesperson, went through periods when she lost her voice. Her doctor suggested speech therapy so that she would use her diaphragm more in speaking, relying less on straining her vocal cords. However, speech therapy was time-consuming and expensive, and Carolyn's busy schedule interfered. The quick-fix option upon which Carolyn had been relying, to take cortisone regularly to shrink the vocal cords, was dangerous over the long term.

Carolyn sought another opinion and discovered a completely different course of treatment: eliminating orange juice and other high-acid foods from her diet. The doctor suspected that Carolyn's high consumption of these foods had been literally "burning" her vocal cords through acid indigestion and reflux. She was advised of other measures, too: Take an antacid medicine at night, and use a firmer pillow when sleeping to prop her head higher. When she tried these approaches, the vocal cord problem began to clear up.

When it comes time to visit the physician for your second opinion (self-referred or within an HMO), come prepared with a list of topics to cover. First, you want to brief the physician about your previous and current medical condition. You'll want to bring your medical records and ask the first physician's office to forward copies of his or her diagnosis and other documentation, such as X rays and written results from pathology labs. These are essential for the second doctor to assess your medical history and compose an informed diagnosis.

To decide among your options, you'll want to inquire how various treatment options:

- will affect your day-to-day activities;
- compare on amount and type of discomfort, and length of convalescence;
- depend on results of further diagnostic tests;
- differ in the percentage of patients who experience complications (and what are they?);
- differ in the percentage of people who attain the best possible outcome (and what are the best results, treatment-by-treatment option?).

Many procedures have grown so common that videos and visual aids are available. Ask to see these. Inquire about current books and articles prepared for lay readers. Consult Internet sources (see suggestions in chapter 1 under "The Changing World of Medicine"). Don't be timid about asking for estimates of the costs, and break them down: surgery, drugs, hospital, continued consultations with doctors, home care. What kind of costs are incurred immediately, and how much is spread over future months? What share of this will your insurance cover?

It's best to get a second opinion from doctors who are not associated with your regular physician. In a smaller community or with an uncommon condition, you may need to travel to another place to find an independent point of view. All this costs money.

As in Margo's case, over half the time a second opinion serves to reassure you in the original recommendation, not to contradict it. But be prepared to find disagreements. A second opinion may advise completely different treatments (including a different surgical procedure), delay instead of haste, or more tests. Resolve your course of action by asking questions and weighing responses according to your own priorities. Along the way, you will need to learn a bit of medical terminology to understand your condition, and, in some cases, you might need to solicit a third opinion.

Wide-ranging advice can be your best defense against falling into one of medicine's most common snares. In recent years, the growth in number of surgical operations has more than doubled the rate of growth in population. The United States is increasingly a cutting and probing culture. Your situation may be unclear and not as urgent as made to appear; if so, hang back from joining the ranks of patients recuperating from surgery until you have carefully considered other options.

Understand that if you must struggle to get a second look, persevering against reluctant doctors and even paying for the consultation yourself, it's natural to exaggerate the second opinion's worth. People value difficult accomplishments. Give yourself a few days, if possible, to sort through all the advice you get and weigh it calmly.

## HOW TO MAKE CLEARER AND LESS AGONIZING DECISIONS

In facing the uncertainties surrounding medical choice, perhaps you feel like the character Trudy, in Lily Tomlin's one-person comedy routine. "I made some studies," Trudy drawls, "and reality is the leading cause of stress amongst those in touch with it. I can take it in small doses, but as a lifestyle I found it too confining. It was just too needful; it expected me to be there for it *all* the time, and with all I have to do—I had to let something go" (Wagner 1986, 18). The attractions of daydreaming and other vacations from life may seem irresistible. That's when an uplifting plan for coping needs to swing into action. To help, we've assembled a set of tools called CUT: Control Uncertainty Training. Only half in jest, we offer CUT as a way to slice discouragement and self-blame out of your path, as you make your way through the thicket that obscures a health-care decision.

To practice CUT, you must first begin by separating three kinds of uncertainty that may confront decision makers (Yates and Zukowski 1976). There is *ignorance,* in which information that contributes to a choice is knowable but unknown to the decision maker (you know that information must exist about the success rate of an upcoming procedure, but you don't yet have that information). Then there is *ambiguity,* in which information about options is inherently unknowable (will surgery distress my six-month-old infant more now or when he is a few months older?). Finally, there is *risk*—what's at stake, the gains and losses that flow from choosing; options with almost equal numbers of costs and benefits create more uncertainty than options with lopsided ledger entries.

Conventional wisdom has given uncertainty a bad reputation by calling it a problem to overcome. It's easy to see why. From childhood onward, our culture weans people from ignorance or even appearing unknowledgeable. The modern worship of science argues that anything important is, in principle, knowable. The aura of mysticism hangs over people who feel that some things lie beyond ordinary human capacities to understand. Our culture also abhors doubt about evenly balanced choices. The human species has cultivated an instinct for seeking the causes behind events so that even difficult options can be discriminated. People harbor the vain hope that judgments will be perfect.

When doubt or uncertainty escalates, many people decline to make choices, or they delegate their decisions to others. They can't handle the thought of being ignorant, facing ambiguous circumstances, or finding themselves in risky situations. These aversions are singularly human.

It's also possible to see uncertainty in a more positive light, as a powerful and beneficial force. Up to a point, feeling uncertain—when matters "could be" or "might be," instead of "are"—can motivate people to pay close attention to their surroundings. People who feel in some doubt favor alertness over mindless habits of thought. They feel more vital and alive. Thinking that we "know" can close off options.

If ignorance challenges you, search for information. Where choice turns on inherently unknowable factors, trust your emotions and instincts. If risk is your nemesis—the appearance of evenly matched alternatives—be especially persistent in searching out reasons why one choice is actually superior to others. Beware of "premature closure," becoming committed to a choice just because the earliest scraps of information you dig up happen to tilt that way. Don't let uncertainty stun you into magnifying the first signs that point to one option over others.

Once you understand the nature of your uncertainty—whether it's ignorance, ambiguity, or risk—you can take positive steps. CUT, Control Uncertainty Training, offers simple techniques. CUT consists of a variety of mental simulations. With these, people can escape the fear and shame of not knowing, or of acknowledging the unknowable. CUT also helps confront equally attractive or equally unpleasant options when they are part of a choice that one eventually must make.

The core of the CUT program is to pose "what if" questions. You ask yourself, "What if I chose option A in this medical situation? How would I feel then? What if option B?" Then you imagine different scenarios about outcomes that might follow from option A and from B, C, and others, including the option of not choosing for awhile. You play at different resolutions and discard the ones that produce the least anticipated satisfaction. You rehearse different reactions to successes and failures from your particular choices. Thinking liberates the imagination and usually requires only a modest investment in mental turbulence.

In the most powerful simulations, the decision maker replays choices with the aid of another person. Often, that way, benefits and pitfalls crop up that the decision maker might not think of, thus enriching the process.

Josh's case shows how this works. He was forty-three, gay, sexually active, and in good health. He had lost ten pounds during the past year, but credited this to his switch to a vegetarian diet. Josh's doctor was unconvinced, though, and wanted to test him for the HIV antibody. Josh felt that he would rather not know.

From his perspective, the pluses and minuses from testing balanced out. If he knew, of course, doctors could monitor his T-cell count and start him on medications in a timely way, but Josh was surrounded by people with AIDS, and he felt obligated to extend them strength and companionship. To do this, he needed to remain known as "well."

Josh was like a lot of people who are equally drawn to and repelled by a medical test—whether for prostate cancer, genetic factors affecting reproduction, or other conditions that present dilemmas. Like many others, Josh grew increasingly anxious.

Josh continued seeing his doctor to learn more about AIDS treatment because he misread the source of his uncertainty as ignorance. Somehow, Josh felt, knowing more about therapies would unravel his dilemma. Josh's doctor helped him see that he was actually frozen by the perceived risk of testing. With the doctor's encouragement, Josh rehearsed his options. First, he imagined continuing to refuse testing, playing out this decision and its consequences. He might be lucky (HIV negative) and continue to be the mainstay among his ill friends. On the other hand, how was the lingering uncertainty about his HIV status already affecting these relationships? He began to wonder. Suppose he was, in fact, HIV positive? His friends might be even more devastated if Josh unexpectedly developed AIDS later on and went into steep decline.

Josh then imagined what would happen if he *were* tested for HIV. He visualized how long it would take to get the results and who he would want with him when he found out. As these thoughts ran through his mind, Josh's pulse quickened, his blood pressure increased, and he began to sweat. He actually experienced the emotions of getting bad news as well as good. He considered what he would tell his circle of friends to soften the blow if he had the antibody. He simulated how this might alter their relationships and dependencies, and how he could minimize that. He also anticipated the results of testing negative—not only being negative, but not having to worry anymore.

Josh's mental rehearsals affected him in several ways. Thinking about testing made that option seem more real, not just the hovering menace it had been. Thinking also allowed Josh to fabricate episodes into an entire scenario—the test and its immediate aftermath, telling others if he was positive and then managing the impact, or learning that he was negative. Imagining the story of his own future allowed Josh to separate himself from dry and fearsome statistics about HIV detection and disease control and see his situation in a more singular way. Josh's simulation of emotions helped bring them under greater control.

Before rehearsing his choices, Josh hadn't considered how his friends would react to the surprise that he had AIDS, too. And Josh had only a skimpy realization of how he might gradually break bad news to his friends and continue to support their coping with illness, even as he developed new needs of his own.

In short, a loathsome option became real, a plan for adapting to it emerged, and emotional turmoil was tamed. After three weeks of playing scenarios, Josh ended his quandary and had the test. His mental preparation proved invaluable when he learned that he, in fact, had the HIV antibody. After a few days of shock and disbelief, he adjusted to the news and remained a rock of support to others. Unlike many who have been stopped in their tracks by such news, Josh didn't sink into denial or lament that "I can't believe this is happening to me."

To ask "what-if" questions and simulate choices stretch some patients beyond their level of tolerance. When the need to face medical decisions collides with wrenching fear aroused by the illness or disability, people are sometimes unready to face uncertainty.

In an achingly honest account, the novelist and poet Reynolds Price describes such a case as he tells of his discovery that he had cancer. A ten-inch-long tumor had grown inside his spinal cord. Despite the highest technical quality in medical facilities and expertise, Price's doctors often handled him brusquely. As details of his diagnosis grew worse, Price reacted as others have before him and since: "After routine pre-dinner visits from my internist and neurologist, I knew nothing more. Inquisitive to a fault though I'd been all my life, some deep-down voice was running me now. Its primal aim was self-preservation. *Don't make them tell you, and it may not happen. Whatever they tell you may be wrong anyhow. Stay quiet. Stay dark.*" And later: "I was only beginning to realize that all my doctors had now entered their laconic 'Tell-him-nothing-he-doesn't-ask-for' mode, but I doubt I asked another question—no fishing for predictions or probabilities. My buried censor was guarding me still against news I couldn't handle at present" (Price 1995, 11, 16). Price had retreated into the dimly lit corridors of information shutdown. Medical events had forced him to surrender a basic principle that nurtures human biological endurance: a sense of having control over your decisions and destiny.

Fortunately, Reynolds Price was eventually able to escape from information avoidance and play an active role in his recovery because he never saw his condition as a personal weakness. Ignorance, ambiguity, and risk became personal adversaries. Price gradually reclaimed parts of his life from their grip. Other sufferers, however, are not as strong-willed, as positively imaginative, or as fortunate.

Draw this lesson for medical decision making. You may feel completely unable to consider options, much less select among them. You may see a paralyzing brew of causes behind your predicament. If so, you are likely to remain out of control and in information shutdown until you rethink the nature of uncertainty that rules your situation.

Ignorance can only dissolve with a determined quest for information. Ambiguities, when properly labeled, remain the province of trust in your emotions. Risks may teeter in balance, prompting a daisy-petal approach to choices; or risks between options may tilt more certainly, pointing to one solution over others. Simulating and rehearsing alternative futures offer your best hope for subduing the fear that uncertainty kindles.

## CHAPTER 3

# Seeking the Right Kind of Social Support

RUTH CONVINCED US that cancer patients struggle to find the social support they need, often against heroic odds. We met her in the driproom of a busy oncology practice, as she settled into a La-z-Boy recliner to receive her regular chemotherapy. A leafy plant by the chair gave her surroundings a homey air, a transplanted scrap of rec room from suburban American housing. But any visitor would need to squint hard to block out the room's true purpose. Bottles of fluids dangled from stainless steel poles. Other patients were lined up in their chairs like passengers on deck at sea. Worn covers on the magazines announced that many distracted people had passed through this space. This was a room for taking medicine—with resignation or grim determination for survival.

Ruth welcomed our questions, preferring a chat to her usual solitary reading. Her cancer was a recurrence, following a tumor removal four years earlier. Most of her hair had fallen out, though a trim wig disguised that fact. She knew that other unpleasant side effects awaited her.

"How has your illness affected your family life?" we asked gently. "The kids are a lot of help. Both Geoffrey, seven, and Melissa, eleven, are real troopers." They did chores around the house, putting on adult airs as they dusted furniture and carried in bags of groceries. She talked with them candidly about the fact that she was ill and that the harsh treatments were necessary steps on the road to recovery.

"And what about your husband?" Ruth's smile faded. Well, Don was another story. He adamantly refused to talk at all about her cancer. He was okay four years ago, but this time he simply clammed up, declaring illness, treatment, and their attendant emotions off-limits for negotiation or sharing.

We sought a way out of this conversational blind alley. "What does Don do for a living?" we scrambled to ask. Ruth answered matter-of-factly: He was the chief pharmacist at a neighboring hospital.

We blanched. Here was a spouse knowledgeable in the ways of medical treatment who could not cope. All other evidence pointed to a loving relationship until now: They shared in PTA events at school, camped on weekends in nearby desert parks, decided together which new car to buy. But spousal communication had suddenly vanished; the nourishment of social support had withered and apparently would not reappear unless someone or some event intervened.

Many others, not just those with cancer, share Ruth's situation. Even where health has not declined, people often lead lives in which social ties are scarce or easily fractured. Current lifestyles tend to magnify personal isolation. Young professionals move from city to city in quest of career advancement, leaving family and friends behind. Children grow up in single-parent or even no-parent households. Elderly persons, whose lifelong friends have died, live in nursing homes remote from familiar neighborhoods and close family. The social ecology of American life presents gaping holes, lacking continuous and varied exchange with others.

A stark irony faces many: Just as medical science is yielding powerful new tools for physical healing, the society's comforting blanket of personal relationships is wearing thin. But new drugs and medical procedures fall short of their potential where social estrangement shadows people's lives. This chapter documents the benefits that social ties bring and the punishing costs from their weakening. Even more important, it shows how you can forge the kinds of social connections that bolster physical health.

## THE PROTECTIVE SHIELD OF COMPANIONSHIP

This chapter's story begins with a blunt truth: Health and life expectancy depend on the quality of social relationships. Scholars at the University of Michigan reviewed a wealth of research on this topic, concluding that the link between social support and wellness rivals the Surgeon General's evidence that established cigarette smoking as a cause of disease (House, Landis, and Umberson 1988). Isolation can be life threatening.

Some of the earliest signs pointing to this fact come from long-range studies that track the social characteristics and health status of large populations. In these investigations, a great deal of information was gathered from surveys—including the presence or absence of chronic illness, history of smoking, regularity of exercise, and other data related to health, such as income. Six to twenty years later, public records for deaths were compared to earlier survey evidence about susceptibility to illness and social ties. These massive epidemiological studies have been carried out with representative samples of thousands of adults residing in different regions of the United States and in European countries.

Results from just two investigations capture the essential lessons from all of them. One, a Swedish study, used an especially thorough measure of social connection (Orth-Gomer and Johnson 1987). Nineteen separate questions probed for contacts with parents, children, siblings, companions from youth, neighbors, friends, and coworkers. Higher death rates followed hand-in-hand with poorer social integration. The most impoverished third in terms of social ties died at 1.3 times the rate of others across the six-year follow-up period, even when other factors contributing to death were considered.

An American study in Alameda County, California, came up with even more impressive differences across a seventeen-year follow-up (Seeman et al. 1987). Socially integrated people had survival rates 1.3 to 2.0 times the rates for more isolated people, after removing the influence of health risks at the beginning of the study period. Being married was the most important factor for those under sixty years at the initial interview. Ties with close friends or relatives assumed greater importance for those over sixty. This is encouraging evidence that one kind of social contact can substitute for loss of another. When a spouse dies or divorce interrupts marriage, friends and relatives can fortify people against illness and decline. The bottom line is clear: Although the content of social support may change across the life cycle, benefits from close contacts with others persist as long as people live.

Crediting emotional support as a potent therapy against illness strikes some as a branch of New Age philosophizing. After all, conventional thinking these days about how to avoid premature death focuses on diet and cholesterol, lack of exercise, exposure to infections—undisputed physical threats to health. How could concerns about social estrangement rank in importance alongside such publicized and authentic roots of disease as these?

The value of emotional sustenance gains credibility, though, from demonstrations of how human warmth even from strangers reduces medical complications and boosts life expectancy. The case of women giving birth confirms this. Physicians in the United States and Guatemala have conducted controlled experiments in hospitals where cramped conditions prevent family from accompanying mothers in labor (Sosa et al. 1980). In some cases, the mothers received support from a lay woman in addition to the usual attentions from medical staff. The lay women chatted with mothers throughout labor and birth, rubbed their backs, held their hands, and simply stood by as a friendly companion. Other women were left without such social support, but received the usual medical care from staff.

Mothers who were given unexpected social support from a stranger experienced half the problems as those who received just the routine care. For example, cesarean sections and injections to aid dilation decreased. Among mothers with uncomplicated deliveries, length of labor from admission until delivery was cut in half by the lay support. Mothers who were provided a companion were more alert after delivery; they stroked, smiled at, and talked to their babies more.

This shows that even temporary, fragile social contacts bring swift and decisive outcomes for health, in this instance for newborns, too. Small wonder that the embrace of kith and kin might shield many from illness.

## QUALITY OF SUPPORT MATTERS

Comfort from strangers notwithstanding, people's natural affiliations provide the greater balm that social support can bring. Instinctively, most people realize that the quality of human relations must count for something. Lessons about these issues come from the experience of people rebounding from a sudden crisis.

Investigators in Australia followed the progress of men who had been hospitalized after a car accident (Porritt 1979). These patients spoke about their situations twelve to sixteen weeks after their injuries occurred, when they were back home trying to get their lives together again. The study used a combination of three outcomes to judge the degree of successful adjustment: any signs of emotional distress; problems in adapting to work; and the men's current enjoyment with their lives.

The men were questioned exhaustively about who had been available to them since their injury. Had parents been present, a spouse, children, friends, siblings, other relatives, the boss at work, strangers, health providers, or others? Even more importantly, the interviews dug deeply into the *quality* of each source's help. Specifically, the accident victim answered questions like these, about each family member, friend, and other contact:

- Were you able to talk with him/her about how you felt? Did he/she seem to understand your feelings and situation?
- Did (the other person) seem to reject you and not accept your feelings? Did the other person accept you and the way you felt? Did (the other person) even challenge you to cope better?
- Did (the other person) seem to be hiding how he or she felt, or pretending in any way? Or did you feel his/her reaction was completely open and sincere?

Details about this study merit close scrutiny because they provide a vivid script for how valued social support takes place. Results were strikingly clear. The sheer number of people available to these men recovering from accidents counted for naught. People rushing to the bedside, making visits at home, or stopping to chat in public places may enlarge the patient's social circle, but the size and diversity of these social ties do not help a person recover emotional balance, reenter the workplace, or look optimistically to the future.

The study underscored that it is the quality rather than the quantity of support that aids in recovery. Improvement after the accident was related to the number of sources who were empathic, conveyed respect, and were constructively open—contributions that tended to go together. In fact, recovery was slowed where there were many sources, but they failed to communicate and act in ways that bolstered emotional strength.

Thus, social contact does not always equal social support. Family members or friends can easily provoke disputes, arouse embarrassment, stimulate guilt, or cause other frictions. They can simply be unaware of how to reach out with unfeigned concern. Therefore, there may be times when someone needs to step in and manage a patient's recovery, posing the following questions: (1) Who should be encouraged to see the patient and who discouraged? (2) Are there ways that visitors can be quickly educated to provide the ill or injured the quality of contact they desperately need? (3) Should someone be delegated to canvass the patient's social network for people who are most understanding and nurturant? (4) Should someone locate a role model, a person who has recovered from a similar crisis? This last option is not necessary, as we make clear below. But sometimes a person who has "been there" can boost the patient's spirits with realistic optimism based on shared experience; and such a helper can assist people around the patient by interpreting what the patient is experiencing and how others can help best.

One hospital in Rhode Island is so determined to get its patients off on the right foot during recovery that it has launched a care-partner system. When people check in they bring a friend who stays the whole time, helping hospital staff with noncritical tasks. Besides cutting the hospital's costs, the partner system raises patient morale.

All the available evidence shows that social support is something like a dance, involving companions locked into complementary steps. How the patient copes stimulates different reactions by caregivers and hence different patterns of interaction. The unrealistic or fantasizing patient may prompt criticism from others; the problem-centered coper may encourage others to rally support. Whatever the case, a web of self-sustaining relationships can result.

## THE WEAR AND TEAR OF CHRONIC ILLNESS

The damage that negative attitudes among family or friends can inflict becomes especially apparent in chronic, deteriorating illnesses. For example, patients with rheumatoid arthritis place special burdens on their partners, who do not always respond with charity and understanding. Researchers at Arizona State University surveyed arthritic women and their spouses (Manne and Zautra 1989). The patients exhibited a wide range of ability. Some had such deformed and painful joints that they needed a wheelchair and were dependent on others for all tasks, including combing their hair or toileting. Others had no limitations and functioned independently.

Across the board, however, wives coped well if their spouses provided positive support. When women felt that the husband was "always around if they needed assistance" and "was right there . . . in the stressful times," they pursued active means of dealing with limitations. They kept up with leisure interests, set goals and worked toward them, and reappraised their lives in the most positive light possible.

Some husbands, however, mixed helpfulness with hurtful attitudes, and some were withdrawn and critical a great deal of the time. The investigators gauged spouses' underlying feelings by interviewing them alone and asking how arthritis had affected their lives. The researchers listened carefully to taped recordings for signs of resentment, criticisms, or disapproval of how a wife had come to grips with illness.

Husbands' negativism in these confidential remarks cropped up in the same cases in which wives were practicing maladaptive habits of coping. These included fantasizing by the women that their condition would somehow go away and blaming themselves for contracting arthritis in the first place. These self-destructive thoughts were often coupled with poor psychological adjustment—anxiety and depression—and submission to illness.

Why might a spouse react harshly to his wife's condition, or why do many husbands do this at least some of the time? Some explanations come quickly to mind: The burdens of long-term care can wear down anyone; some marriages may have been weak prior to illness. Or some wives' defeatist attitude may have caused discontent among their husbands as much as the inconveniences from arthritis itself.

Two other, insidious forces are also at work in these situations. One is a human need to search for justice in life's affairs; bad things happening to good people strikes at one's sense of order and reason. Reliance on a "just world" theory—people get what they deserve and deserve what they get—can color the interpretation of human events. Friends and family of the ill can act in mean-spirited ways out of an unconscious urge to restore logic to an otherwise puzzling situation.

Another explanation stems from the onlooker's own sense of vulnerability, brought to mind whenever adversity strikes close at hand. A spouse with a chronic ailment is a daily reminder that other threats may lurk just outside the household door. Either factor, blaming the victim or fearing for self, can prompt family and friends to raise walls of psychological defense, isolating the person who is ill. These common psychological tendencies appear across a wide spectrum of threatening events, starving ill people of the quality social support they need.

Patients are quick to spot the subtle clues associated with psychological separation: avoidance (a spouse lingers in other parts of the house) and evasive conversations. A forced cheerfulness or a glib assurance that "everything will be all right" impress many patients as ignorant and insincere or as a sign of retreat. When potential sources of social support cannot bear to express what is on their minds, patients would settle for simple quiet affection.

Chronic conditions that people may manage, but seldom vanquish, confirm the benefits of a dynamic partnering between the ill and a friend. A study at Johns Hopkins involved long-term sufferers of hypertension (high blood pressure) and offers a riveting case in point (Morisky et al. 1983). Most patients were knowledgeable about the disease, its treatment, and the possible consequences of skipping medication, but they tended to neglect office visits, to forget taking pills, or to fail to make changes in diet and exercise that are essential to contain this crippling illness.

Researchers tested three strategies to improve blood-pressure control: (1) helping each person grasp the essentials of an individual regimen tailored to his or her health status, using an intensive, one-on-one interview; (2) building the patient's self-confidence in gaining control, through group meetings with other patients; and (3) creating family and social support in behalf of compliance. With some patients, staff tried just one of the three strategies; with others they used two techniques; and some patients received all three.

Results clearly showed that nothing worked in the absence of creating family and social support. To secure involvement, staff would visit the patient at home, talking directly to an adult with whom the patient had the most frequent contact. Staff taught this person how to help the patient stick to treatment and to modify habits of eating and exercise. Twice as many patients had their blood pressure under control five years later whenever such social support had been sought, whether as the only intervention or in combination with other techniques. Among these fortunate subjects, risks of stroke, kidney disease, heart attack, angina, and congestive heart failure dropped dramatically.

Devoted allies make a difference, even when the patient may already appear to have committed to getting well. We saw this in our own studies evaluating the Pritikin Exercise and Nutrition Program (Evans and Clarke 1986). This regimen advocates a diet low in fats, cholesterol, protein, and refined carbohydrates (such as sugars), and high in starches, fruits, and vegetables. Changes in eating are to be accompanied by moderately paced exercise; regular and sustained walking is often enough.

Weight control and general vitality are only the most apparent goals. Benefits are also seen in the cardiovascular system and increased resistance to a variety of degenerative diseases.

Enrolling in Pritikin requires motivation and cash. Our study included people who had paid fees to join classes, investing sizeable chunks of their own money and time toward acquiring new habits. We wondered whether participants would stick to the program six to eighteen months afterward. What factors would separate people with nearly flawless compliance, those adhering unevenly, and those who backslid to their former eating habits and sedentary ways? We tracked people who had signed up for a full-time, twenty-six-day residential program, and others who had joined evening classes that met several times each week for six weeks.

One striking difference divided participants who were faithful to their new regimen from people who lapsed into old habits. The former group had friends or family close at hand who kept watch over their behavior and were not shy with reminders about approved practices. Not every member of a faithful follower's circle needed to reinforce the Pritikin schedule, but *at least one did.*

Some strict adherents faced skeptical or even disparaging comments from others, but a participant's ally helped deflect such doubts and bolster new practices, even when the ally did not subscribe to the Pritikin plan in his or her own behavior. Backsliders lacked this social support, or, if their family and friends had learned about features of the Pritikin lifestyle, they often conveyed mixed signals about appropriate and taboo foods or the significance of exercise.

These results remind us of the cartoon showing a glum couple seated opposite each other at the dining room table. The wife says, "That's right, Phil. A separation will mean—among other things—watching your own cholesterol."

## THE PARADOX OF TOO MUCH SUPPORT

While celebrating empathic support, it's important not to ignore instances of a surplus of conflicting attention. These cases appear in some of our own fieldwork, as Ed illustrates. He was sixty-four, a professional of international renown, who had a herniated disk. He had unexpectedly fallen prey to sharp pain from hip to toe coupled with localized numbness in the calf and foot. He was in agony with every movement—from sitting to standing to walking. An orthopedist advised rest and oral medication; remaining options included physical therapy, traction, injections, and finally surgery.

Ed had expected to be cured within a matter of days. When this did not happen, he grew increasingly frustrated and engrossed by his situation, which he saw as opening the final chapter in his aging process. No friend or casual acquaintance, from colleague to airline reservation clerk, could escape Ed's plaintive chatter about his pain, limited mobility, and sense of vulnerability.

Not surprisingly, Ed was bombarded with conflicting advice, an overflow of information. One person declared that surgery was the only way to go; another assured him that invasive procedures would exacerbate the condition; someone urged acupuncture; another, megadoses of vitamins; others promoted chiropractic treatments; a chorus of people guaranteed that the problem would disappear with rest and time. Many of Ed's advisers joined their opinions with expressions of genuine affection, promises to stay in touch, and tangible aid—handling matters at the office, taking him to appointments, cooking, shopping, laundry, and more.

Ed's quandary arose from a surplus of help. He received too many kinds of help from the same sources—emotional sustenance, information, and tangible aid. How was he to pick and choose among points of view? How could he express gratitude when it would soon become clear that he was not accepting that person's entire prescription? Would he alienate valued friends?

Later in this chapter you will find many practical suggestions for mobilizing social support and for negotiating among the people who may offer it. Ed weighed his options carefully and decided to hold off on surgery. He continued to ask for tangible help from people whose "medical advice" he was rejecting; and in this way, he reaffirmed his need for support and for continued connections with concerned friends.

Ed also confided to us that he would act differently, should he face another medical crisis. He would be more selective with whom he shared details, and he would curtail his requests for lay medical opinions. He had discovered some unexpected conflicts and embarrassing contradictions that careless solicitations of medical advice can bring. Targeted requests for help with tasks at home and office would suit his needs and allow his friends to feel supportive.

Ed's experience warns about a downside to social support. Being overwhelmed by contrary signals can paralyze a patient's decision making as surely as a crabby, insensitive spouse or friend. A shower of out-reach from others can complicate illness.

## SUPPORT-SYSTEM BURNOUT

Sometimes, a network of potential support shreds in the face of a health crisis. This can happen when a patient expects too much from a circle of sociability, forgetting that lots of friendships are low-key and founded on simple camaraderie. Other people may expect joking, story-swapping, shared interests in a hobby—taking pleasure in just being together. Suddenly asking for more, by divulging intimate details about illness or asking for tangible aid, sends these acquaintances running for cover. Evasion sets in.

Burnout also occurs where deep and abiding friendships have been stretched beyond their breaking point. We saw this in the case of Diane, married and fifty, whose mother had died two years earlier. Diane was devoted to Mitzi, her mother's greatest friend. Diane and her husband drove three hours every Sunday to visit with Mitzi, shop for the week's groceries, and keep up with chores around the house. They finished nearly all of these outings with a sit-down meal geared to Mitzi's dietary needs.

Mitzi was in deteriorating health and refused to hire anyone to help with cleaning or cooking. She used an electric scooter to move around town and a wheelchair in her home. Among her other frailties, she had poor vision.

The problem was that Mitzi seemed to have used up all her available support and nurturance, other than Diane and her husband. Mitzi's friends and neighbors no longer wanted to visit, help with errands, or invite her for a meal because she always ended such overtures by asking these accommodating people to do unappealing tasks—cleaning the house, folding laundry, changing bedsheets.

Diane wondered what she could do to help Mitzi reconnect to her friendship network, most of whom were angered by what they considered rude and selfish behavior. We suggested that Diane have a frank conversation with Mitzi about the way she treated people and the demands she placed on them. Diane's obvious devotion to Mitzi would give her leverage to be brutally honest.

We also urged Diane to plan a tea, to which Mitzi would invite the many people who had helped her over the months. This gesture would be an opportunity to thank people for their efforts. In addition, since it would be a gathering of eight to ten people, no one person would fear being asked to perform the usual dirty work that had routinely been part of visiting Mitzi.

The tea turned into a cheerful gathering where Mitzi assured all that she valued their affection. Without having to say it, Mitzi communicated that she wanted to be included and apologized for her insensitive and alienating demands. Afterward, Diane and Mitzi took stock of the tasks that needed attention, assigning unpleasant chores to a paid helper engaged to come each week, and distributing agreeable ones among friends. The two made a plan that followed our two rules for avoiding burnout: (1) think about the depth of friendship you test by the favor you ask; and (2) don't forget to thank others.

## WHEN ILLNESS STIGMATIZES AND SOCIAL SUPPORT WITHERS

Some conditions strike terror in the beholder, undercutting the chances for social support. Cancer offers one poignant example. Friends may offer hollow cheer and then quickly retreat; employers sometimes terminate jobs; romantic partners flee to other relationships. Throughout modern cultures, cancer ignites special fears that often find their outlet in isolating the patient socially.

We have conducted research to evaluate whether videoconferencing between cities can be useful in connecting cancer patients and survivors in social support groups (we describe another of our studies using this conferencing technology more fully below). Support groups offer a means of substituting for social ties fractured by the stigma of illness, allowing patients to voice their most keenly felt needs. One of our experiments brought together young adults from two cities, who shared their adjustments to diagnosis, treatment, and future plans. Listen, for example, to Mike, who had been in remission for two and a half years but was still bitter about others' reactions when he was originally diagnosed:

> When I was nineteen and I came down with cancer, it wasn't the illness that freaked me out or anything. It was something I had to hurry up and get taken care of and you go in for all your surgeries and treatments. It was the after part of knowing that, "Gee you could have died, or you still can. You can still catch it again." I lost my job, I lost all my friends, lost my girlfriend, and I had a school counselor at UCLA who just turned around and said, "Why don't you just quit? It isn't worth it." And I thought, "Who is this bitch to tell me what

I'm gonna do with my life?" Pardon my French, but I got so angry. I think that became a driving force in my life to say, "I'm gonna make it, I'm gonna survive, I'm gonna beat the system." Took me a year to get a new job just because whenever you fill out an application and they'd ask your health and I would be honest, I'd tell them. I think the friends that I chose after that were a different breed of people because first off I would tell them, "This is where I'm at in my life. If you want to be my friend you are going to have to be able to deal with it. Don't waste my time because I don't need to be hurt any more."

Another survivor explained that the large scar left from his surgery continued to dampen his social confidence:

> I'm reminded of the fact that I have cancer every time I look in the mirror. It's not until I get fully dressed that I feel real comfortable with myself. And the thing where it bothers me is before I was diagnosed I was a very active dater. I don't do that any more. It's unfortunate because it's a problem that I have now: How will they accept me?

Many other conditions besides cancer stigmatize the ill, with results that are only marginally less cruel. People reject sufferers as flawed, limited, and undesirable. They direct anger at them, sometimes covertly; they avoid the ill and withhold help. Relationships grow strained, tense, awkward.

Many diseases and types of accidents have acquired distinct images in the popular mind. Two features of these perceptions explain whether or not people stigmatize and reject sufferers: the condition's controllability and its severity.

Controllability means the patient's presumed culpability in falling prey. For example, infections and immune diseases that people think are sexually transmitted become stigmatized. Conditions such as alcoholism, bulimia, obesity, and trauma to the driver from a high-speed car wreck are thought avoidable; they are seen as the consequences of personal choice. Even contagious illnesses can mark their victims, if they did something rash to place themselves at risk. By contrast, few people attribute asthma or juvenile diabetes to the behavioral weaknesses of sufferers.

Ironically, an onlooker's belief in a just world aggravates unrealistic assumptions. When people work from a theory that afflictions are merited, they naturally overestimate a sufferer's responsibility. For instance, some people nod smugly over teenage drug abusers from the wrong part of town, without considering whether a parent's own addiction or a mother's fetal environment is to blame for a poor start in life. Kids from the right part of town, by comparison, get second chances in the court of public opinion whenever people blame indulgent or careless parents for the children's misbehavior.

The second contribution to stigma is severity, a burden that weighs especially hard on many cancer patients. People with a poor prognosis or having a condition that's difficult to treat often face rejection. Symptoms that disrupt social contact (disfigurement, hair loss, deterioration in speech, hearing disorders, loss of motor control, relying on a wheelchair) trouble "normal" people who lack a script for how to behave. They avert their gaze, reduce eye contact, shorten conversations, avoid encounters. Conditions that suddenly worsen (when cancer metastasizes or a second heart attack strikes, for example) sharply reduce social exchange.

Stigmas are highly symbolic. Only rarely are onlookers actually in danger from continuing social contact. People shun harmless though stigmatized persons, the obese for example, as surely as those with typhoid fever.

What can be done to dilute stigmas and reintroduce patients to their social network? It helps to emphasize humanizing details about a person—facts about family upbringing, education, occupation, hobbies and interests, tastes in fashion and popular culture, religious values and beliefs. These humble scraps of information tend to reestablish an ordinary identity and mask physical impairments. They make the patient appear more normal for his or her gender, age, and social class.

Some patients, of course, have "made their own bed and are now sleeping in it." It helps, where possible, to portray the behavior that led to illness or accident as an aberration, a momentary lapse from the straight and narrow. Where justified, stress how hard the person is working to do the right thing now. It also helps if one can concentrate on the medical community's search for a cure to the malady, or on cases of recovery from similar accidents. These stories blunt the image of severity. These are strategies to use in cases where onlookers are simply unable to accept patients for the persons they are.

## THE GENDER GAP IN SOCIAL SUPPORT

Gender plays a role in social support. That rings true. But precisely how, one might ask? A fundamental irony forms part of the answer: To win social support, women must extend themselves more than men to get the same payoff. To appreciate why, one needs to understand how gender shapes people's well-being and whether or not help from others comes easily.

It seems paradoxical, but men die sooner, although women endure higher rates of illness. This is because serious disease and traumatic events are more likely to strike men, or to occur earlier in their life span. On the other hand, nonfatal chronic conditions and psychological distress befall more women.

Men are raised to be adventurous and take risks, which leads to serious accidents. Their focus on achievement and competition can breed tendencies toward a type of hostility that spawns coronary death. Suicides linked to failure at work occur more among men. By contrast, women log more days of restricted activity due to sickness, more days in bed, and greater use of medications and health services in general. An alertness to symptoms and willingness to admit being ill or depressed account for some of women's apparent lack of well-being, compared to men. But women's deficit in day-to-day health also arises from different rates of chronic and burdensome diseases. These can fester for years before raising complications; some are rarely listed as the primary cause of death.

To illustrate, hypertension afflicts more women than men, across the full span of adult years. The same can be said for arthritis, infectious and parasitic diseases, upper respiratory conditions, diseases of the urinary system, and many other dangerous or annoying conditions. Women are more prone to excessive and inconsistent dieting, scrambling to fit into images advertised in popular culture (attempts at weight loss feed a $35 billion per year industry in the United States). Among people over sixty-five, women suffer more than men from diabetes, anemia, and chronic bronchitis, among other frequent illnesses.

Besides such differences in risks, women's relative unhealthiness sometimes flows from how the medical system slights their condition, once disease has struck. Consider heart attacks, which older women suffer almost as commonly as men of the same age (Beery 1995; Bergelson and Tommaso 1995). What happens afterward underscores a gender gap. Women receive less aggressive treatment, even when their cardiac health is similar to men's. They are less likely to be referred for rehabilitation. Not surprisingly, then, women report more serious and persistent symptoms following their attacks—even considering their greater sensitivity to bodily sensations and willingness to express these. Women suffer more related complications, making it harder to return to work or resume other activities.

Studies also show how women sometimes find their diagnostic needs being shortchanged (Franks and Clancy 1993). Women whose primary-care physicians are male get fewer Pap tests and mammograms than women with female doctors. Thus, women often enjoy less access to the highest quality of health services. Across the board, they are less likely to be covered by insurance, as well.

What light do these facts shed on gender differences in social support? First and foremost, women's greater physical and psychological distress throughout life places them in greater need of support—to buffer the body against tension, strengthen the immune system, avoid health risks in the first place, prompt the seeking of medical care, and encourage compliance with care. On this basis alone, they require more of the benefits that companionship brings.

Nature's evolutionary processes of selective survival across thousands of generations might seem to have responded in kind. Whether in Western cultures or other settings, ethnographers agree that women practice communal styles of behaving, compared to men's self-assertiveness. Women, somewhat more than men, concentrate feelings, enjoyment, and ambitions in things outside the self; women make other persons, or even surroundings such as the home, the focus of emotions and accomplishment. Men tend toward more egocentric styles; that is, they make themselves and private pleasures the center of their world.

The availability of social support, at least in modern societies, is not quite so happily matched to gender as one might wish. Precisely because many women lean in a communal direction, they find themselves called upon to *provide* a great deal of social support to others who face anxious circumstances. They must give, as well as get, and often they give much more than they get.

Therefore, we find that marriage reduces the risk of death for men more than it does for women. Furthermore, it takes a companionable marriage for women's health to show an advantage, but any quality of marriage gives men a health edge over other males who are single or separated. Widowhood and divorce weaken men's health more than women's, because, on average, these events bring the loss of one who monitored health and urged corrective steps.

Friendships carry similar outcomes. Men's health improves if they have only a few close attachments, compared to being socially isolated. Significantly, women need a larger network of close friends to gain the same advantages that men enjoy from one ally. Thus, for women, the need threshold is higher for intimate and sharing ties with family, friends, neighbors, and coworkers.

To summarize this fundamental irony about gender: (1) the health needs of women cry out for more social support than men; (2) on average, women are more sociable; but (3) by the same token, it takes more of this resource to provide the protections that women need; and (4) women contribute more than men—in paying attention to others' health and trying to bolster it. In the race to secure social support, women seem to run hard just to stay even.

We saw these dynamics, in exaggerated profile, when interviewing Fred and Martha. Fred, forty-nine and an overweight smoker, had suffered his first heart attack. The doctor urged profound changes in lifestyle, as well as other treatments. Fred, true to a familiar script for men, resented these incursions on his freedom and independence, his opportunity to assert himself. He turned surly. Martha, on the other hand, focused on the threat that coronary disease presented for her relationship. She devoted herself to Fred's needs and urged compliance with diet, exercise, and giving up cigarettes. Fred, in response, interpreted this aid as overprotectiveness. In short, Fred's utter need to shield his coveted ways of self-expression clashed with Martha's communal instincts.

In the weeks shortly after Fred's attack, this conflict between two coping styles plunged Martha into depression, which she tried to hide in order to remain a "responsible and caring wife." Martha became ill herself, with a bronchial infection that just wouldn't disappear. Gradually, however, she reached out for new friends and for deeper, more confiding relationships with old ones. Unconsciously, she tried to attain the advantages women can reap from a greater store of social support than men require. In the process, Martha also learned to hide her new and strengthened ties from Fred. He interpreted her new friendships as a sign of abandonment.

## WHEN TREATMENT ENDS BUT NEEDS CONTINUE

Experiences with a wide range of patients underscore another important lesson. The most intense period of medical treatment may draw to a close, but needs for social support continue. With heart bypass, for example, surgery doesn't end the struggle. A regimen of drugs, changes in diet, and close monitoring for signs of new difficulties stretch well into the future. The shadow of mortal risk lightens slowly, if at all.

Despite patients' continuing needs, however, support from family and friends often slumps—particularly empathic listening, tangible aid, and reassurance. Those around the patient think the crisis is over. Ironically, this withdrawal of extra friendship sometimes affects the outwardly successful copers most, because they give off signs of self-sufficiency. But many of these patients are only pretending. A wide variety of evidence shows that many ill people are reluctant to ask openly for support. They think it gauche or unreasonable to voice even oblique hints to friends and family.

Our own studies of cancer patients and survivors, linked by cross-country videoconferencing (more about this below), have provided poignant cases in which the fears and pain aroused by illness continue long after treatment has been completed. Two women in particular stand out. Like many patients, their final chemotherapy session was simultaneously exhilarating and terrifying: exhilarating because it was a major milestone toward full recovery; terrifying because the women understood that they were now unprotected, again vulnerable to a diagnosis of cancer.

Lily was forty-four years old, married, with three grown daughters and one grandchild. She worked as a receptionist for a cruise line. She underwent a lumpectomy and received both chemotherapy and radiation. Lily was very optimistic during her treatment program, rating her physical progress against cancer at 100 (on a scale of 0 to 100) and her emotional level at 80, but her hardest struggles lay ahead. Three months following the last treatment, Lily's spirits had sunk:

> I finished my treatments (chemo and radiation) in July. I went back to work within the following week—it was one of the hardest weeks I had—by Friday I was totally exhausted and stressed out—my muscles hurt so bad I could hardly walk—I went back on disability—and just within these past two weeks have I felt more like myself, gaining strength and energy. I have been very emotional which I wasn't during treatments—have felt anxious—trouble making decisions, wanting just to stay at home in my safe place—I have made myself go out and usually always feel better. I am on tamoxifen and dealing with hot flashes—and also another area that is really hard for me is my hair—it is growing back, but very slow. I do realize my hair will grow back—I just dislike it.

Many of Lily's friends and family had retreated, assuming that she was well on the road to recovery. During the first interview, she reported five people in her social support network who "listen to concerns, give helpful information, and do errands." In her interview six months later, her close social network had narrowed to only two people.

Rosa was thirty-five years old, in her second marriage, and the mother of a thirteen–year-old son. She had a mastectomy eleven months before the support group began and had begun on chemotherapy. Just prior to the videoconference, she judged her emotional state to be 20 on a scale of 0 to 100. She revealed that she was tense, worn out, unhappy, confused, and very concerned about her ability to conceive another child. She confessed that there are "some topics I'm uncomfortable discussing with my husband—I am afraid of complaining about all my fears. I am afraid of driving him away. Sometimes he does not understand how much of me has been taken away." She listed three people in her close social network.

Immediately following the group sessions, Rosa's emotional state climbed sharply. However, five months after the group sessions had ended, Rosa was very discouraged again. She reported her emotional well-being as zero. Over the course of these few months, she had deteriorated severely. Her own words describe her feelings:

> I recently went into menopause, at thirty-five. The doctors think the chemotherapy may have caused this. My blood pressure has risen. I need to take medication for it. Emotionally I am not confident that this is over. Every little ache starts to concern me. I am having a lot of anxiety. I seem to be walking in fear. I don't know why. I overreact to even the smallest thing. I am also having a problem concentrating. Every little task seems to be a major chore. I feel like a walking time bomb. It seems like a long time since I have been happy. My whole life is different now.

These women's reports are reminders that social support is full of subtleties. The ill may not ask for support, in so many words. Improvements in their apparent condition may seem to signal that support is no longer needed. Other family and friends may return to familiar habits, behaving toward the patient as they did before surgery or treatment. Physicians may become perfunctory during office visits. But supportive others must not be deceived or prematurely comforted by signs of normalcy. The ill still require all the empathy, information, tangible aid, and reassurance that friends are able to give.

## IS CONTACT WITH A "SIMILAR" PATIENT NECESSARY?

Some feel the urge to join support groups, where reciprocity kindles emotions and skills at problem solving. People wrestling with many different kinds of conditions gravitate to these temporary groups. Some organize around diseases or procedures; cancer, heart attack, bypass surgery, infertility, and multiple sclerosis are just a few. Others form around conditions—such as eating disorders, caring for elderly parents, divorce, single-parenting, step-parenting, co-dependency, menopause, grieving, and more. Any day's edition of the newspaper and direct-mail pieces from local hospitals carry notices of meetings, often scheduled weekly. Call-in radio programs (on cancer, for example) add to these opportunities for exchange.

In groups, candor is the coin of the realm. Acceptance by others hinges on self-revelation. Michael Korda decided to attend a support group during recuperation from surgery for prostate cancer. At the first meeting, he was drawn into a frank confession of incontinence and how bothered he was by using a condom catheter. An older regular embraced Korda in the group by replying: "You'll see kid. It'll work out. Hell, if the worst that happens is you piss in your pants a little every once in a while, you're a lucky man" (Korda 1996, 212).

However, many people shy away from support groups, sometimes after an encounter that leaves them confused or disappointed. They had expected that others who have endured their situation would be most able to reach out with care. In other words, people who "haven't felt my pain themselves won't sense my needs nearly as well."

There are reasons, though, why this thinking often leads to frustration. First, people who have shouldered a devastating condition sometimes have had all they can take. They may cringe from being reminded of personal distress—although they would gladly reach out to patients facing a very *different situation*. There's a second body of evidence for why people need not have been there to care, and studies show that men differ from women in this regard.

Among men, similarity of experience does not easily predict empathy. Some men, for example, who have endured a medical experience will then distance themselves from people undergoing the same fate. They like to believe that other patients should be as stoic as they like to imagine they once were themselves. By contrast, other men are moved to help their fellow sufferers. The net result is two opposite kinds of behavior.

Women in our culture, on the other hand, usually grow responsive to signs of another's similar plight. Gender stereotypes generally encourage women to partake in communities of co-sufferers. As a result, similarity in prior experience often brings a surge of empathy from women, above and beyond the level of compassion that seeing others in trouble yields on its own.

The moral of this brief tale: When you are hurting, don't limit a search for support to others who have walked the same path. Having been in your shoes is neither necessary nor sufficient to galvanize others on your behalf.

## HOW SOCIAL SUPPORT WORKS

The pages of medical journals contain scores of studies demonstrating the healthful benefits from social support, which reduces risks or speeds people to recovery—on top of any biological advantages they may enjoy. Coronary bypass patients with supportive companions leave the hospital more quickly, require fewer painkillers, and regain robustness more easily than the socially less fortunate (Kulik and Mahler 1987, 1989a,b). Support for adults undergoing bone-marrow transplants can double their two-year survival rate.

But a nagging question remains: Why and how does support work? One explanation views social support as achieving its benefits through people's visible emotions. This theory suggests that a lack of supportive relationships unleashes negative feelings such as anxiety or depression. In turn, these emotions weaken health by causing people to act in self-destructive ways. For example, anxious people may misinterpret their needs and ignore health care, or they may turn aside the assistance that other people offer, mistrusting attempts by friends to do favors. Depressed people may come to feel helpless in the face of events or may try to escape by isolating themselves or by drinking excessively, for instance.

In this account, weak friendship ties lead to damaging emotions; these impair one's ability to seize advantages or to cope when trouble occurs. Being vulnerable, in turn, makes one less pleasant to be around, curtailing social support even more.

This grim scenario sounds convincing. But an explanation for the value of social connections must also consider the positive effects of unexpectedly receiving social support from strangers, as with the mothers during childbirth. How could the brief lifeline thrown to them have conferred such stunning benefits? Might the warmth of human kindness act, instead, like a powerful drug injected directly into the body's most vital systems?

Ponder the following example from emergency-room care (Lynch 1979). In certain circumstances, trauma victims are completely immobilized with curare, paralyzing every muscle in the body. Patients lose all physical control. They cannot move, speak, open their eyes, or even breathe without artificial respiration, yet the drug leaves them perfectly aware of what is going on. In these terrifying situations, studies have arranged for a nurse to clasp the patient's wrist and offer reassurances that medical staff are doing all that they can. This gesture immediately calms the patient's pulse rate, which is completely beyond voluntary control.

Evidence like this has inspired physiologists to develop a plausible account of how social support acts in a primary way, rather than indirectly through conscious emotional states. The story begins with the brain's genetically programmed ability to determine instantly what internal autonomic and endocrine responses are most appropriate for situations a person faces. Circumstances that suggest danger or even uncertainty increase heart rate and blood pressure, and trigger rising levels of blood glucose. These protective reactions for dealing with shock empower people to fight or flee. Importantly, such stress can help preserve life. Often, however, activation simply wastes energy on symbolic rather than real threats.

Circumstances that signal safety generate different processes, however. Socially supportive situations release hormones that promote cell multiplication and growth throughout the body, strengthening tissues and healing wounds and fractures. Surroundings that are socially supportive activate the assimilation of nutrients into tissues and the elimination of waste.

The importance people place on social ties also affects their immune systems, including the presence of natural-killer (NK) cells in the body. NK cells form an important component of defenses against viruses and abnormal growths, like malignant tumors. To illustrate, researchers at Princeton University measured people's immune functioning and their "need for affiliation" by presenting ambiguous drawings and asking subjects to write or tell stories about what had just happened or might soon take place (Jemmott et al. 1990). People's tendency to see affiliative themes in ambiguous pictures indicates the importance they place on personal, supportive relationships in their own lives. Evidence shows stronger immune-system functioning among people who value human connections than among those who do not. People's long-term susceptibility to disease appears to depend on their use of social cues to interpret behavior.

This helps explain why the number of "frank and confiding" relationships people have correlates strongly with how well their immune systems resist toxic substances, prolonging life. The bond between social support and lymphocyte (white blood cell) activity is especially strong among women, owing perhaps to the greater significance they place on intimate social connections. Investigators have also determined that a *spouse's* immune functioning depends on the quality of social support he or she gets, while being stressed by the *partner's illness.*

In short, getting social support builds physical strength in powerful ways, even though friends cannot observe these biological improvements directly. Social support promotes bodily health directly. People have good reason to hone their techniques for gaining help from others.

## HOW YOU CAN ARRANGE FOR SOCIAL SUPPORT

One of our subjects, Linda, fifty-one, wrote this letter to friends after a lengthy recuperation from back surgery. Her words communicate the rich tapestry of help that can flow during a crisis:

> I have recently stopped to see and smell the roses. With a less hectic schedule, I have had time to enjoy the gift of family and friends. One of the lessons I have learned from you is how to be a good friend. What did you do that was so special? You called, you came to the house, you sent cards. You brought books and magazines, casseroles and soups; you accompanied me to doctors' appointments. Whether it was helping me to make confusing medical decisions, taking me for a walk, driving an extra carpool, meeting me for lunch or carrying on for me at work so I could rest, you've been there. You have listened to me complain, worry, cry, question, and get very confused. And you stayed with me. Your hugs assured me I was no less lovable. Each of you, my family and friends, gave me special loving gifts.

Many of Linda's friends talk about how lucky she was to have received such support. Lucky? Well, sure there was some good luck.

But there was a lot more of planning, pleading, prodding, and prompting on her part. Linda created her own good luck and *you* can also learn how to figure out what you need during times of crisis and stress.

Life's stresses wear many different masks. Thus, it is not surprising that the role of social support in helping cope depends a great deal on the particular problem and on other resources available for meeting it. Social support comes in many different varieties, as does stress itself, and can confer widely different benefits.

Psychologists have made considerable headway toward identifying the different kinds of support that may be helpful (Cutrona and Russell 1990). *Emotional support* is the opportunity to turn to others for comfort and security; it leads you to feel cared for. *Network support* is being part of a group sharing common interests and concerns, such as a hobby. *Esteem support* bolsters self-identity and worth by acknowledging competencies, skills, and talents. *Tangible support* refers to concrete assistance, where others provide meals, run errands, or take other responsibilities off one's shoulders. *Informational support* includes the advice and guidance from other people about possible solutions to problems. Finally, *nurturance support* is the chance for you to give back to others, the invitation to love and care for others even as they are looking out for you. The combinations among these six categories can be considered the anatomy of social support, the particular muscles in your social relations that lend strength and direction to how you will cope with adversity.

Let's draw the discoveries from research into some practical ideas for how you can get the most out of social support for yourself or for someone else. We present five steps to develop a healthier network: taking stock of social support, naming names, asking for help, persevering, and keeping reciprocity in mind.

### STEP 1. TAKING STOCK OF SOCIAL SUPPORT

Think about the six different dimensions of support: emotional, network, esteem, tangible, informational, and nurturance. Table 3.1 illustrates each with sample statements that help you assess the availability of that aspect of support in your life.

These aids rank differently in importance, depending on a person's history of being helped and the kind of stress being faced. For example, some people grow to maturity relying heavily on praise for accomplishments to reinforce their self-worth; esteem support might be especially gratifying to them. Other people develop habits of depending

---

TABLE 3.1
## *TYPES OF SOCIAL SUPPORT*

EMOTIONAL SUPPORT
_____

I have close relationships that provide me with a sense of emotional
  security and well-being.

I feel a strong emotional bond with at least one other person.

NETWORK SUPPORT
_____

There are people who enjoy the same social activities I do.

I feel part of a group of people who share my attitudes and beliefs.

ESTEEM SUPPORT
_____

I have relationships where my competence and skills are recognized.

There are people who admire my talents and abilities.

TANGIBLE SUPPORT
_____

There are people I can depend on to help me if I really need it.

There are people I can count on in an emergency.

INFORMATIONAL SUPPORT
_____

There is someone I could talk to about important decisions in my life.

There is a trustworthy person I could turn to for advice if I were
  having problems.

OPPORTUNITY FOR NURTURANCE
_____

There are people who depend on me for help.

I feel personally responsible for the well-being of another person.

---

on tangible aid; others on guidance from authority figures like parents
or teachers or clergy; and others on the opportunity to nurture and
care for family and friends. Some people thrive on a few key supports,
others on many. And some acts carry a heavier cargo of meaning than
might appear to an outsider. Running an errand for an ill neighbor
may signal affection or regard that outweighs the tangible aid.

The type of support one needs also depends on the stress at hand.
Moderate illness or injuries belong in one category, separate from life-
threatening diseases and serious disablements. Some physical impairments,
like cancer or AIDS, are culturally stigmatized, arousing fears of con-
tagion, personal vulnerability, or revulsion. Conditions like arthritis

and stroke continue over a long period of time, requiring different sources and types of help than acute, short-term episodes.

Think of your own life, and try responding to the statements in table 3.1 using the answers "agree," "disagree," or "not sure."

The entries can be used to describe the situation you are in, but, importantly, you can also use this exercise in a more diagnostic fashion if you ask yourself: "Do I need to change?" You might discover that you don't have many ties to people in terms of hobbies or social activities. This may be comfortable for you, or you may find this is an area that you wish to develop.

Now you are ready to tackle the step of identifying people who can help.

### STEP 2. NAMING NAMES FOR SOCIAL SUPPORT

Most people have *potential* support systems in families, friends, interest groups, and often coworkers. To figure out the circumstances you face, take a sheet of paper and turn it sideways. Write the six types of support at the top ("emotional," "network," etc.). On the left side of the page, list these three regions of life: (1) home and extended family; (2) friendships, acquaintances, interest groups, and other affiliations; and (3) workplace. Draw vertical and horizontal lines to create eighteen boxes, a grid into which you can enter an inventory of your social support network.

Start by putting the names of people into the boxes. Who can you ask for different kinds of help? Who is likely to provide help spontaneously? Think through daily routines and familiar places of visitation. Recall companions from the gym, bowling league, church or synagogue, or other sites. Some names will belong in more than one box. Some boxes will remain empty.

If you have some blank squares in your grid that represent areas of need, think about people who can help you figure out how to meet that need. For example, we have a friend, an elderly neighbor, who was preparing for a short hospital stay for abdominal surgery. She completed this exercise to find that there were some tangible activities she needed help with. She turned to us and said, "I have everything in order, but I just don't know who I can get to feed and walk my dog. And, I'm reluctant to put him in a kennel. I feel like I have asked everyone I know to do something already. What do you suggest?"

After some discussion, we concluded that she had exhausted her network in terms of asking for favors. We suggested she call the nearby junior high school and ask the principal if he could find someone to care for the dog for the five-day period. Sure enough, a teenager was found, delighted to land her first job. A mentoring relationship grew from this contact, providing a brand-new opportunity for nurturance.

Completing this exercise may call for deep reflection and some detective work. Many writers have observed a loss of community in American society, where a sense of neighborhood has yielded to residential habitats (apartment blocks, condominiums, housing tracts) of mutual strangers who commute to different centers of work, shopping, and recreation. Many locations for informal public life have disappeared. The nest of bars, cafes, beauty parlors, and other hangouts that used to get people through their days has withered.

### STEP 3. ASKING FOR HELP

Asking for support takes courage on anyone's part. Your own experiences may have convinced you that support from some people is more potential than real. Do not become disheartened. There are reasons why many folks are reluctant to ask for support, and why others hold back from giving it.

Asking, of course, risks embarrassment; admitting that you need assistance can jeopardize self-esteem. Feelings of shame are especially inhibiting if you suspect that you may have contributed to your own troubles. Asking will come more easily, though, if you concentrate on just one potential helper at first, and a single thing that you want. Choose someone, if you can, who is unaware of other social supports you may have, who will not retreat behind the "bystander effect"; people are known to be less likely to give help when they see others who might step in.

Ask your one target for a modest favor—simple advice, a single phone call of encouragement at a critical time, or one errand. By limiting your first step, you practice the foot-in-the-door strategy; gaining a small favor at first nurtures larger commitments when you need them later. Even more important, your success at reaching out in this early trial will embolden you to make requests of more people.

People may neglect to offer support unless you clearly invite their attention. The reasons we mentioned earlier—urges to perceive a just world and a heightened sense of personal vulnerability—account for some cases of withdrawal. Equally often, seeing people in distress can leave others feeling helpless: Do we know what to do, or will we only make the situation worse? Would-be helpers are often immobilized by their own lack of confidence or experience with the sufferer's plight. You may have to tell them what you need and how to provide it.

Ronnie Kaye, in her book *Spinning Straw into Gold,* argues that the person whose health is under siege has permission to be honest and open about feelings, to put his or her needs first without feeling guilty. Her story of recovery from breast cancer offers this guidance:

> The second time I faced a breast cancer diagnosis, I was deter-mined not to make the same mistakes (of silence and withdrawal). When I thought of the difficult time that lay ahead, I knew exactly what I would need, and I took action immediately. One by one, I called all my relatives . . . aunts, uncles, cousins, as well as my imme-diate family. "I'm going through a difficult time," I said, "and need your help. I just found out that I have breast cancer again. I am terri-bly frightened, and I feel alone. What I need most of all is a phone call once a week. When you call, I would like you to tell me that my being alive has mattered to you in some way. I need to know that our connection is important to you." Not a day went by without at least one phone call from someone in my family . . . Even though the real-ity of my medical situation hadn't changed, those phone calls made me feel much more secure. I had learned that the best way to get what I needed was to ask for it. Once my family knew exactly what I wanted, they were only too happy to oblige.          (Kaye 1991, 164)

Kaye had arranged for emotional support. Requests might also go out for network support—"I want to continue aerobics with you . . . play golf weekly (or at least ride around the course with the gang) . . . build model ships . . . sew quilts" or whatever. Securing esteem support often means meeting with a boss or coworker and asking him or her to recognize parts of the job one does especially well and to help one continue that level of performance during a period of diminished energy.

In quest of a stronger social network, some general rules apply. Naturally, you will prefer contact with others who are supportive instead of critical—people who can calm you down, celebrate minor achieve-ments in coping, participate in diversions, or encourage your deter-mination to succeed. Anyone shrinks from would-be helpers who point to lapses in attention or fortitude or scold others into trying harder. People seek companions who show respect for the difficulties they face, who resist labeling these circumstances as a catastrophe or, alternatively, minimize them.

Your urge for ties should also acknowledge the special value of social support from people who are not kin. Their words, aid, and feelings are free of any tinges from family history or rivalries. In addition, having two or more clusters of companions, relatively unknown to each other, allows you to withdraw from one set temporarily, if tensions arise, and gain compensatory support from the other. Concentrating too many hopes for social support in a few sources risks an unhealthy dependency, mutual resentments, and a devastating loss if those sources retreat, move, or become ill themselves.

Besieged people who need a sudden boost in social resources can join an interest group—a bridge club, church or synagogue, or support group that focuses on their condition. These providers of network support can quickly help widen other types of social contacts.

### STEP 4. PERSEVERING IN SUPPORT

The necessity for support during a medical crisis may be long-lasting, especially with illnesses like AIDS, some cancers, progressive conditions like arthritis, or permanent injuries. We've already pointed out that even recovery from accidents and short-term conditions takes longer than commonly appreciated. Effective social support is not a topical ointment and a Band-Aid, a quick fix for healing. Even when a patient seems to be recovering nicely, his or her needs may lie camouflaged behind a screen of forced cheerfulness.

Potential givers of support encounter a special challenge when a patient copes in ugly and self-defeating ways. Escapism, wish-fulfillment, anger, hostility, and self-blame may repel onlookers, however realistic or effective these responses to stress might temporarily be. But friends or family in retreat simply inflame poor coping strategies, which further discourages help by others. A downward slide can quickly gain momentum.

The courage to provide social support should be applauded and not just taken for granted. The determination to ask for help should not be misread as a character flaw. Giving and receiving empathic acceptance helps sustain both persons' lives. As we have seen, positive and meaningful relationships lead not only to happiness but to better physical health.

## STEP 5. KEEPING RECIPROCITY IN MIND

Social support often looks different to the giver than to the recipient. Let's take providers first. It's true that they often reap visible payoffs themselves; they may win admiration or affection, for example. Purely altruistic support, though, presents a puzzle. Why would a person reach out to another without the prospect of being rewarded in return?

One explanation has held that selflessly motivated aid may be ingrained in the lore of cultural groups, religions, or families as a way to protect human dignity and the group's cohesiveness. Theorists even speculate that some groups go one step further; they revere altruism on its own merits, and not as a requirement for good standing among fellow members.

A second explanation for altruism takes a decidedly more selfish, even Darwinian tack (Schaller and Cialdini 1988). Psychologists point out that empathy produces sadness or dejection in the observer, seeing another going through tough times. When this happens, the observer reaches out to help the victim out of an urge to lift the observer's heavy heart, to regain a more positive mood. The motive to help, in other words, springs from the helper's emotional needs, more than from a concern for another's welfare. A good deal of research supports this egoistic interpretation of altruism, although the more benevolent theory has its fans, too.

Whatever the case, don't overlook the comforts that extending social support can bring to helpers. These acts make the provider happier, wiping away the negative feelings that witnessing distress brings. Relief from a sorrowful mood is one of the engines that drives altruistic social support. By asking from others (in a discreet, moderate, and courageous way), the sufferer helps others in return.

Thus, providers of help may be motivated in both visible and unconscious ways. The other side, the recipient's point of view, calls for recognition, too. Someone who is ill needs the chance to pay back favors extended, even if in small ways. Altruistic, one-sided help can peter out or grow stale when the parties neglect reciprocity.

This seems paradoxical, but reflect on the following: Interpersonal relationships normally involve a "give and take" between people. Everyone understands this principle when the resources are tangible: money, help with household chores, ride-sharing, and the like. Companionship and emotional support are resources, too, and imbalances in their exchange sometimes spell trouble. Giving more to a relationship than one gets leads to feelings of unfairness and resentment; receiving more than one gives leads to feelings of guilt and shame. Imbalances of either type can dissatisfy and even estrange people.

Casual and close relationships differ in how well people tolerate inequities in the exchange of social support. With casual acquaintances, people hasten to redress the imbalances, uncertain whether the bond would survive without equaling the accounts periodically. On the other hand, close kinship and friendship ties endure temporary inequities because the participants trust that they will have ample time to balance accounts in the future. In fact, tit-for-tat reciprocity actually trivializes the relationship, weakening mutual concern.

Givers of support should understand that the receiver may expect to reciprocate in some way. Givers often need to allow recipients the chance to pay them back with affection, regard, or something else that is prized, if they expect to be granted latitude for giving yet more. Absolute selflessness can make the receiver feel guilty and lead him or her to withdraw, which essentially terminates the possibility of receiving support.

Receivers of support may signal their wish to reciprocate in silent, covert ways. We saw such a case while interviewing Jerry, a volunteer who made visits to homebound seniors, many of whom were enfeebled but still alert. Jerry complained about getting a cool reception from one elderly man. This invalid, Bob, was an eighty-two-year-old retired logger who had spent decades in the Pacific Northwest forests. When the relationship started, Bob was grateful for the time together; but he had turned silent and evasive as these kindnesses continued. We told Jerry about reciprocity and suggested he try it.

Jerry asked Bob to look through some library books of photographs taken in logging camps and lumber towns between 1880 and 1920 and to compare the early industry practices against his own experiences in the woods. Jerry's sixth-grade boy would incorporate these observations into a report due at school. Jerry and Bob's relationship rebounded immediately and continued on a warm footing. Reciprocity gave Bob the chance to pay back his volunteer, and it made a difference.

## SUMMING UP: THE GLOW OF EMPATHIC SUPPORT

Certain helping acts strengthen physical health and boost feelings more powerfully than others. The legendary scholar Carl Rogers provided a cogent explanation. Help has its chance to empower the recipient, he observed, when the giver claims "the intent of promoting the growth, development, maturity, improved functioning, or improved coping with life of the other" (Rogers 1973, 223). The most potent helping, in other words, is other-directed, anchored in the other party's interests and needs. Such aid is not persuasion or influence, although these may be outcomes. This type of aid goes beyond asserting a giver's ego or value system. This help is not ritualistic conformity to the social expectation that people act kindly.

Rogers's ideas seem bold, even unrealistic. How can one assert the power to help someone else, especially in the face of indifference or rejection? How can a helper succeed? Two psychologists, French and Raven, agree with Rogers that the answer is found in *empathy,* the ability to understand someone else's feelings, state of mind, and point of view (Janis 1982). Empathy does not flow simply from similarity: "You have a large family and so do I. So pay attention to what I say." Nor does it rest merely on kindly attentions: "I'm here at your bedside because I like helping people; be grateful and conforming." Empathy is anchored in acceptance of the other and an unflagging commitment to the other's welfare, *as that other person sees it.*

Empathy is counterintuitive and hard to practice. Empathic persons practice what psychologists call "noncontingent regard." This means accepting the other person, weak points as well as strong. This kind of acceptance does not rest on continued demonstration of good works. The other person is treasured—period. "I may see your frailties and shortcomings," the empathic say, "just as you must be able to spot mine. But these count for little alongside the pleasure we can share from knowing and helping each other."

Physical displays of affection nourish empathy. If, for example, one's social customs classify air kissing as a sign of warmth, that will work. A high five is appreciated in some quarters. Others may favor a hearty hug or holding the other in one's arms. A brush of fingers on the cheek, clasping the hand, stroking the hair, or massaging the shoulders can bring a surge of sometimes voiceless appreciation.

The ingredients of empathic support are easy to detect. Empathy is at hand where people share intimate confidences. Can you count on the other to listen to your innermost feelings, even when angry or depressed? Will late-night phone calls be accepted without a resigned tone of voice? Bonds of appreciation grow where there is time for halting, even anguished, accounts of personal troubles. Sometimes you might want to get things off your chest. Other times advice is sought: "How am I handling this situation? What would you do? How do I get out of the pickle I'm in?"

The helping person does not force these intimacies, does not pry when uninvited, or lavish sympathy when understanding is all that is asked. Empathic support also recognizes that all relationships between people contain frictions as well as warmth. Sometimes the closest of friends agree to disagree, valuing their relationship more than personal opinions.

The mortar that binds empathic contacts between people is blended from humble materials. Sometimes these nourishing relationships arise because one of the parties aspires to be like the other. The aspirant, psychologists say, *identifies* with the other individual. The aspirant wants to see himself or herself as like the other—in power, knowledgeability, social skills, appearance, or other features. The target finds this admiration flattering. A friendship blooms.

Other times, contacts arise because one person possesses *assets* that the other values. Access to a circle of friends, opportunities for advancement, and material gifts all work to cement empathic companionship in such situations. Finally, friendships can gain momentum from the harmony that partners see between each other's *values and beliefs*. When people's most-treasured sentiments align, they find cause to spend time together.

Each motive offers legitimate grounds for exchanging empathic social support, because each carries its own obligations for reciprocity. Awareness of these motives unmasks the scaffolding that supports human caring.

## CASES OF SOCIAL SUPPORT AT THE FRONTIERS OF COMMUNICATION TECHNOLOGY

Patients and their family members and friends can create novel and helpful ways to exchange social support, as we have learned in our research applying new information technologies to health care. Some background about our projects underscores the lessons they offer for everyday life. We were inspired by listening to critically ill people recall how they had received their diagnoses and coped with the emotional roller coaster that followed. A common element emerged from these stories. Many patients began to gain control over their situation once they reached out for a crucial bit of information, but it was impossible to predict when they would be ready for this scrap of knowledge, or precisely what kind of information would give them the strength they needed. Patients differed all across the board.

The case of Dr. Ed Rosenbaum is illustrative. He wrote about his fears when he had throat cancer. Picture him twenty-seven days into his thirty-three-day bout with radiation treatment. He is sitting in the waiting room of the X-ray department:

> The waiting room has three boxes. One box has toys for the children. The second has current reading material—not bad for a doctor's office. The third rack has American Cancer Society literature. I have avoided reading the latter, but today I am optimistic. I gingerly take one of the pamphlets, the one on breast cancer. To me that's the safest. I peek through it. It's not too threatening. Nothing there that can hurt me. . . . Finally I have the courage to read the pamphlet on cancer of the larynx.                      (Rosenbaum 1988, 145)

Why, we puzzled, did he shrink from learning about his own condition until the blast of treatments was nearly complete? It appeared that even a physician might shun the medical facts. The information that nudges one patient toward recovery, we discovered across many interviews of our own, is very different from the facts that help another.

Some people struggling with illness want to understand the physiology of their case, like Dr. Rosenbaum, before they can mount an emotional counterattack. Others dread the social isolation that serious illness can bring and wonder how to solidify friendship and family ties. Others want to know what treatments will feel like, how much discomfort a procedure like surgery or a diagnostic test will cause. Yet others need a road map for the coming weeks: When will their treatment sessions take place, how much will these disrupt time at work, when will the doctor check to see how well this is working, and such? Some patients are eager for information early in the game. Some need to wait, as Dr. Rosenbaum did. Some never want to prepare and would rather have events sweep over them.

Under these conditions, ordinary means of communicating information just won't do. With books or pamphlets, frustration often sets in before the patient can find what he or she is looking for. Rarely do sources of advice and the people who need it bump into each other at just the right time. We wondered whether we could repackage and deliver health information not only to be vivid and compelling, but also to be timelier and more responsive to recognized needs. And could we accommodate patients' network of family and friends, too? The communication needs of caregivers and other sources of social support differ dramatically from those of patients. The heaps of "patient education" we have all glanced at seem like feeble gestures to appease everyone—the equivalent of those lumpy socks labeled "one size fits all."

## GIVING PATIENTS THEIR CHOICE IN COMMUNICATION

Fortunately, new technologies are starting to provide solutions to these dilemmas. Interactive multimedia and the Internet offer chances to create many new moments of informational opportunity on demand. We have adapted some of these new tools in order to investigate a common side effect of cancer treatment, hair loss. This is a problem that distressed cancer patients greatly but was routinely dismissed as simply a "temporary" and "cosmetic" issue. With chemotherapy treatment, hair loss is most often temporary, but, it can also be a crushing and graphic reminder of one's frailty and a discouragement to social and sexual contact. Eyebrows, eyelashes, and pubic area may be affected in addition to the head. Cancer survivors and counselors spoke eloquently to us about the shock that hair loss brings. When we turned to booklets intended to ease people through the diagnosis and treatment process, we found skimpy and evasive mentions of this topic, often only a paragraph or two under the formidable heading *alopecia,* the medical term for hair loss. The gulf we found between patients' and most physicians' agendas finds a comical and poignant witness in Gilda Radner:

> The most difficult part of the whole chemotherapy for me was losing my hair. The doctors always tell you that you might not lose your hair because some people don't. But I did. Everything that I always thought I would be strong about made me just the biggest weakling in the world. I couldn't stop crying, couldn't stop feeling ugly. I always said the reason I am so funny is that I am not vain. But I was filled with hatred.
>
> I woke up and the first thing my eyes focused on was hairs all over my pillowcase. I reached into my punk haircut and a bunch of strands came out in my hand. Looking down onto the bathtub floor while I was shampooing, I saw it was covered with hair swirling toward the drain—my hair. I was devastated. It was like the scene from *Psycho* when Janet Leigh is in the shower—I screamed. I became hysterical the way people do in the movies.

The next night we went out to dinner at a friend's house and a clump of my hair fell in my plate at dinner. It looked disgusting. I was trying to get it out of the plate before the hostess noticed, but it wasn't like one hair, it was a little clump of hair in the poached salmon with the special Dijon sauce. It seemed like an event only Roseanne Roseannadanna could make up—me trying to get this hair off the plate and then trying to figure out what to do with the hair.

(Radner 1989, 114–116)

Here, we thought, is a topic that cries out for imaginative communication strategies. With the help of generous grants from the IBM Corporation, we developed and tested a multimedia system for cancer patients. We installed this at hospital treatment centers, at private oncology practices, and in wellness centers that cater to people's social and emotional needs. The system presented a rich variety of full-screen video, graphics, text, and audio covering most of the questions (and answers) that pop into people's minds, with separate sections for patients and for their significant others. Viewers were in total control—choosing sections they wished to see, repeating them, returning to the menu at will, going where they liked. Screens also presented questions about viewers' experiences, opinions, or feelings, and offered them the opportunity to compare their answers to others who had been on the system. Users navigated through the material by making choices on a touch-sensitive screen.

We learned a lot about how to communicate with patients and their loved ones when they are under stress. When people are given the chance to find out *what they want, when they want it,* the effectiveness of their medical treatment improves. Armed with the information that seems vital to them, patients keep more medical appointments, follow the doctor's instructions, and gather emotional courage to face their disease. Importantly, many of our discoveries using this multimedia technology are useful right now, even where people don't have access to an interactive videodisc, or a computer with a CD-ROM player, or feel comfortable browsing the Internet's many sites devoted to health care.

One of the most powerful experiences with our system, we learned, took place when a patient and significant other (close friend, spouse, adult child) viewed together. Today, people can duplicate this experience at home, even without advanced technology such as we used. All it takes is a VCR, remote control, and one of the excellent videocasettes about an illness or its side effects. Videos are available at your local library, doctor's office, pharmacy, or bookstore and cover almost all conditions and diseases. Lessons can even be applied to reading pamphlets or books.

Before getting to this, though, eavesdrop for a moment in the waiting room of a large cancer center in Los Angeles. Hilda, fifty-six and diagnosed with multiple myeloma, and her twenty-four-year-old daughter, Janine, are seated at our video system, shielded from the rest of the room by potted philodendrons. They have accepted an invitation to view the presentation about hair loss and chose to watch together at our attractive display cabinet. They share in pressing the touch-screen to make decisions about chapters to watch and how to answer questions. They have already navigated through some of the material, skipping segments that seemed inapplicable or uninteresting to dwell on portions that meet their curiosities.

Now, Hilda and Janine turn to a video segment of patients talking about their illness, and how widely they discuss their diagnosis, treatment, and feelings with others. A question appears on screen asking: "How do you feel about talking about cancer?"

Hilda immediately presses "I feel comfortable telling most people."

Janine recoils with surprise. "I didn't know you felt that way!" she exclaims. "I was sure you would pick 'Tell no one.'"

Mother and daughter turn to hug each other. A confusion that had clouded their handling of cancer outside the family melts. Our exotic communication technology has achieved its purpose in the most primitive way possible—through reignited human understanding. As this chapter has already made clear, the ill prosper when their significant others are informed and empathic in ways that Janine became that day.

Having witnessed one scene of highly charged co-viewing, it's easy to see how you can duplicate this at home using ordinary television. You want to create occasions where the patient and significant other reveal how each feels about aspects of being ill. The patient and a source of social support should view together, without distractions or time pressures. Sit side-by-side with the remote control handy to both. Discuss ahead of time how you are going to watch the videocassette about the illness or condition. Each of you is going to hit the pause button any time: (1) that you are curious about how the other person feels about what's just been shown or said; or (2) that you have a question or confusion yourself about what's just been shown or said. Watching a videocassette this way will take longer than passive viewing. Both of you should prime yourselves to stop the video periodically—perhaps every four to five minutes—and ask the following questions:

- How does this apply to our situation?
- How do we feel about what has just been presented?
- Is there something else to talk about that has been provoked by the material we've seen?
- What questions should we ask the medical team or other people?

When the cassette is finished, talk about what comes next. What questions, if any, still weigh on your minds? Where could you turn for answers—a physician or nurse, a support group, a book (in the library or in the health section of a well-stocked store)? You want to leave plenty of time for the material to trigger conversation—the sharing of feelings, ideas, reactions, doubts. Keep a notepad handy so that you can record questions or issues that you'll want to revisit.

You can also see how you can "co-consume" written material with a family member or friend. You may want to sit together and read the material aloud, stopping periodically to review and ask the questions listed above. Or, you may want to arrange a time to talk after both you and your support system have read the material. Jot down notes in the margins. Underline sections that you want to discuss.

In making ordinary video or print "interactive," as with any effective communication, the pillars of human motivation come into play. One of these is social comparison: People instinctively like to compare themselves against others' knowledge and feelings when that is possible, and are attentive when situations offer these opportunities. Co-viewing and co-reading make comparison between patient and significant other both immediate and memorable.

The second motivational push comes from involvement in the piece of communication, being engaged by the material, or simply, getting "into the flow." Mihaly Csikszentmihalyi, a psychologist at the University of Chicago, invented this idea to help understand why some individuals pursue their interests passionately—why climbers scale difficult peaks, or chess players hunch over their boards, or amateurs practice artistic skills in music or painting (Csikszentmihalyi 1975, 1991).

People persist in these unrewarded pursuits for the sheer enjoyment of the experience; satisfaction does not depend on recognition by others or money. Importantly, however, such activities will be most

pleasurable when they supply a *manageable degree* of challenge, a balance between one's abilities and the activity's level of difficulty. In the
psychologist's memorable words, the participant is poised between
boredom and anxiety. When the twin conditions of intrinsic gratifica-
tion and manageability are satisfied, people get in the flow.

Co-viewing a video about illness gives the patient a chance to get
into the flow. First, the patient's viewing companion can make the
occasion intrinsically comforting, a time of emotional support and genuine enjoyment. It helps to have snacks and a beverage close at hand.
Second, both parties can use the remote control to steer between boredom and anxiety, pausing to talk over difficult material or to digress
to less threatening topics. The two viewers stay involved by managing
the ebb and flow of information they handle during their visit.

Finally, scores of studies have shown that people's memory for new
information is improved when viewers connect the material to their
own lives (Klein and Kihlstrom 1986). Many of the questions in our
program about hair loss were crafted to spark thinking about episodes
in each viewer's past or to consider present or future feelings or behaviors. Questions that relate to one's own life experiences (how does this
apply to my situation?) promote an organized and coherent memory
for the contents of a message.

It's important to remember that ordinary conversation between
people can become just as involving as an ambitious multimedia presentation. This type of satisfying communication will happen whenever pairs of people (or larger groups) keep participants poised between
boredom and anxiety, experience intrinsic gratifications, and when
questions constantly surface that allow participants to see that the discussion is connecting to real-life experiences. Patient and caregiver can
create this at bedside. So can patient and physician. We need not rely
on video screens and computers for a motivating and rewarding and
informing experience in communication.

## VIDEOCONFERENCING: THE ELECTRONIC HUG

We have experimented with other communication technologies in an
effort to help patients cope with life-threatening conditions. Multimedia
allows patients and their significant others to obtain information at
their own tempo. By contrast, videoconferencing offers untapped possibilities to create a natural setting for the thoughts and feelings that
patients want to share. Videoconferencing, used now almost exclusively

by businesses for meetings, can also unite patients with each other and with medical experts.

For example, the systems can be a way to convene town meetings of people with a common problem, such as the same clinical diagnosis or bereavement. Such gatherings can be larger than the few persons who might assemble for a typical support-group session, including more people, of course, but also more locations and time zones. With larger assemblies, it becomes cost effective to provide the most talented team of support facilitators that one can find.

We have conducted experiments that provide group support to cancer patients via videoconferencing. Our projects took place between two locations, although we envision linkages among more sites in the future. Our experiences reveal important pieces of the scaffolding that sustains social support among the ill.

Just one project illustrates. It involved women with recently diagnosed breast cancer. We wanted to learn whether the potency of support services provided at one location would survive transmission across the miles to another group of strangers. We worked through oncology practices in Los Angeles and in Stamford, Connecticut, to recruit participants for our novel experience of transcontinental support. We invited women to four weekly sessions, where experienced educators in Los Angeles led discussions about coping with cancer and its treatment: what breast cancer is and how it is cured; communication with physicians, family, and friends; dealing with emotions that accompany illness; nutrition and other lifestyle issues; and stress management and relaxation techniques. Each session lasted approximately two hours. The facilitator and educators were all in Los Angeles.

Our groups varied. The Connecticut women were over fifty, postmenopausal, white, parents of adult children, and involved in traditional female careers (teacher, nurse, housewife). Four of the five had been partners in long and apparently happy marriages; one had been divorced twenty years earlier and lived with a female friend. Most were financially secure. The six California women, on the other hand, were under forty-five and premenopausal. Two were Latinas and one Iranian. Three were single, and four were pursuing nontraditional female careers. In economic background, four were midscale, and two were working class. We also recruited six women as controls—who did not take part in any group meetings—for comparison against the Los Angeles and Stamford women. All the women completed questionnaires just before the videoconferencing, immediately after, and five months later. We personally interviewed the participants (not the control-group women), as well.

The three sets of women resembled each other in their medical situations. The groups averaged four to five months postdiagnosis at the project's start. Virtually all were taking adjuvant chemotherapy. One Stamford woman, four Los Angeles women, and four control-group women had undergone mastectomies; the remainder had lumpectomies. But the women's adjustment to their illness, as we measured it, was unrelated to these differences in clinical experience.

Our videoconferences tied two coasts across three time zones, but each Saturday's two-hour session began as a distinctly local experience. The women set aside errands and obligations around the house and drove several miles to a corporate tower sheathed in glass and steel. A multinational company (that prefers to remain anonymous) generously contributed its conference network, including staff. The women wheeled their cars into parking lots vacated for the weekend, checked in with building security for their plastic badges, and rode elevators that opened onto darkened, empty corridors leading to the conference studio. Only when they arrived at this facility did they encounter a familiar face and greeting.

After enjoying coffee and Danish, the women settled into cushioned chairs arranged in a row that fronted a heavy wood table. Eight feet beyond it, two large side-by-side screens displayed the left and the right halves of the other location. From behind smoked glass, video cameras focused on participants, and low silhouette microphones picked up their voices. The four sessions were moderated by a therapist in Los Angeles; for the first three meetings, she was joined by other professionals for part of the program. Thus, women in Los Angeles met the educators face-to-face; participants in Stamford had *only* video and audio contact. The women began as strangers but quickly learned that they could ask and say anything they wished.

Ronnie Kaye, an experienced psychological counselor and cancer support leader, convened all the sessions. She began the first with a cheery greeting and references to her book *Spinning Straw into Gold,* which had been distributed to all participants. Then she asked: "What is the main issue that seems to be difficult for you in this whole experience?" The Connecticut women spoke first.

Unhaltingly, they sketched their concerns about mortality, the dehumanizing aspects of cancer treatment, discomfort at the role-reversal from lifelong caregiver to recipient of others' help, lack of satisfactory communication with physicians, and more. Kaye interspersed the stories with questions that prompted vigorous nods and fuller details. She urged all of the women to phone her with worries right away instead of keeping them bottled up until next week's meeting.

The Los Angeles women joined in, confessing that they were scared and that fears of recurrence were difficult to keep at bay. They shared their apprehensions about forming romantic relationships, and they complained of fatigue, lack of concentration, anxiety attacks, memory loss, and diminished work performance. Kaye asked the women to consider ways that their self-worth depended on fundamental values rather than on possessing breasts or being able to bear children. Women at both ends of the continent dried their eyes and wryly acknowledged the agonies that the others poured forth. The participants grew comfortable addressing each other across the miles. Throughout, Kaye took copious notes and promised that everything would get covered sometime during the four weeks.

After the women's personal observations, Kaye introduced that day's two guest speakers. The first week's session dealt with models of coping and adjustment, based on the physician's research in helping cancer patients improve their immune systems. A spirited argument erupted when the psychiatrist explained that memory loss was due to the psychological stress of the disease; others argued that the chemotherapy drugs were to blame.

This expert relinquished his chair to an oncological nurse, who introduced the benefits of relaxation therapy for fighting fatigue, getting to sleep at night, and countering pain. The two groups of women leaned back in their chairs, closed their eyes, breathed deeply, and brought serene images to mind. They practiced tensing and relaxing different muscle groups.

The guests departed, and the moderator, Kaye, returned to the table, reviewing themes that the discussion had unearthed. She drew women from both cities into vigorous conversation and constructed general principles out of a welter of personal anecdotes. Importantly, she discussed her own background as a cancer survivor who had contended with the same hobgoblins and physical frailties that these women faced. And then time ran out.

Later sessions began with Kaye asking about any "discoveries, achievements, or problems encountered since last week." After a discussion of these issues, she would introduce the guest educator. One was a psychologist whose practice concentrates on how illness affects the family. He asked each woman to describe how her family unit was handling illness and side effects and emphasized that the way in which children adjust to a parent's cancer flows directly from the patient's skill in coping. He observed that men often waited for the woman's invitation toward fondness and sexual pleasure rather than asserting their own.

Another speaker was a clinical oncologist who specialized in treating breast cancer. He stressed the curability of many cancers and demystified some of the statistics describing risk factors. He discussed reasons to examine the lymph nodes, advised in favor of second opinions, and in favor of deliberate choices among options rather than hasty decisions. He talked about the variety of treatments and the broad range of side effects. His presentation prompted many questions about hormone therapy, side effects of tamoxifen, alternative therapies, weight gain, and much more.

Two groups of women a continent apart attended the same four videoconferences. Both groups spoke warmly about their experiences and offered concrete examples of how the sessions had improved their understanding of illness and their personal situation. But the weeks of videoconferencing affected the Stamford and Los Angeles women in profoundly different ways. Contrary to conventional wisdom, the women in distant Connecticut prospered more than those who gathered in Los Angeles, where facilitator and guest experts were just inches away.

Very early in the experiment, the Connecticut women formed a cohesive bond. They agreed to meet at the conference site for lunch before every session and stayed behind after the cameras blinked dark in order to talk about their experiences. Women in Stamford phoned each other during the week. They began carpooling to the sessions. When we interviewed them, women in Stamford peppered their descriptions of program outcomes with the pronouns "we" and "us," instead of "I."

Among the women in Los Angeles, one friendship blossomed for a while, but nothing that approximated an overall group feeling—no lunch gatherings, little phoning between sessions, and no carpooling. Participants in California left the conference facilities immediately after the sessions. Each woman recounted gains she had experienced from an individual perspective, rather than referring to group benefits.

One Stamford woman captured her group's warmth eloquently: "They could put us on a ship and send us out to sea for a week, and we would have a good time." This bonding lasted throughout the four weeks and then slowly withered; the women in Connecticut drifted back to their old friendships. Participants in Los Angeles, by contrast, never fashioned even temporary attachments with their new group. Perhaps their diversity in social background and ethnicity worked against the development of a common spirit.

In short, the two sites participated in the same conferences but embedded the experience in sharply different social fabrics. The differences in peer social support that separated the cities probably explains the gulf we observed in other benefits, measured by more objective indicators.

We inquired into whether the women who attended the conferences improved in emotional well-being more than the women in the control group, across a similar span of time. We looked at three dimensions of psychological adjustment that have become standard in studies of coping with medical problems. The women rated how they were feeling using adjectives that yield these mood scales.

- *Energy* measures vigor and an absence of fatigue. This taps into the women's degree of arousal and activity, as opposed to listlessness and retreat. A minimal energy level is necessary to seek information about coping and to be open to opportunities for positive experiences. Sluggishness, on the other hand, lowers the chances for renewing or novel experiences. The energy scale stands as a crucial indicator of whether or not patients are mobilizing to combat their illness.
- *Tension and depression* can inhibit problem solving and the processing of information. Being fidgety or in a state of hopelessness, even among those whose general energy level might be normal, weakens the opportunities for positive psychological outcomes.
- *Confusion* is the third dimension. Forgetfulness and uncertainty often accompany chemotherapy, although experts argue over how much this results from chemical or from psychological processes.

The three groups of women started on somewhat different psychological footing. All in all, the control group was adapting the best at the start in terms of energy and lack of depression and confusion. Women in Stamford were noticeably less well-off, and Los Angeles was worse yet. Six months later, we found very different results. The women in Stamford stood out, showing gains on all three dimensions. They emerged expressing markedly greater energy and less depression and confusion than the women who had not taken part in the program. In contrast, the women in Los Angeles slipped on two of the three dimensions, compared to the control group. Women in the control group also experienced a decline in their mood states over the six-month period.

These dramatic differences deserve emphasis. The deterioration in moods among women in the control group who did not take part in the conferences suggests that patients who stay away from organized social support and a coping curriculum do not spontaneously improve on their own. The slippage among the Los Angeles women, compared to the powerful gains in Stamford, most likely corresponds to the two cities' differences in socializing outside the sessions. In Stamford, a smaller and more homogeneous city, the group forged bonds; in Los Angeles, a larger and more diverse city, the group did not.

We sum up the experiment this way. It is feasible to deliver a curriculum about coping with life-threatening illness thousands of miles over a video link. Emotions as well as data can survive compression into electronic circuitry. People's well-being, and not just business sales charts, can flourish with videoconferencing.

Benefits from telecommunication surge when the experience helps create social bonding, as our Connecticut women demonstrated. By contrast, inhabiting the same studio with a panel of experts, as our Los Angeles subjects did, is no guarantee of gain. Outreach to help patients— whether technologically based or not—must ignite human contact and understanding while transmitting information, an accomplishment we achieved at a distance at the same time that we stumbled close to home.

Perhaps we could have used humbler tools than interactive television to discover how the healing power of communication can arc across vast distances. One father has told, for example, how his four-year-old with leukemia delighted in using the telephone. The son was called by a young friend, far away in east Texas. Once they were both on the line, however, neither could think of anything to say. The son pointed to the silent receiver: "He's not talking." The father suggested that his son tell his friend something. The boy's face wrinkled in concentration, indicating his friend in Texas had finally spoken. He listened and turned in amazement: "He wants to know what time it is" (Pringle 1992, 117).

## CHAPTER 4

# Appreciating Your Caregiver

THE EATONS always took their vacation planning seriously and made decisions as a family. Lila, Trent, and twelve-year-old Tom would huddle over the kitchen table with maps, color brochures, guide books, and clippings from newspaper articles in hopes of reaching a consensus about where to go each July. This year they decided on a dude ranch in Wyoming.

The week opened with special treats—hiking, fishing, spectacular views, meeting other nature-loving families, campfires, and outdoor grilling. The final day dawned as clear and warm as the others, inspiring the Eatons and several other guests to set out on horseback for a ride into high country. Minutes before reaching their destination, a picnic spot nestled in the Tetons, Lila's horse suddenly reared and threw her to the ground. She landed in a patch of jagged stones and fractured two vertebrae. After an arduous evacuation, Lila spent two weeks bedridden in the Jackson hospital. Doctors there finally allowed her to return to Los Angeles, with instructions to remain flat on her back for three months encircled by a protective brace to ensure that her spine healed in proper alignment.

Lila hadn't reckoned on the extent of her restrictions. She couldn't stand for more than ten minutes at a time, much less cook, clean, drive, resume her work, run errands, or get herself to appointments with the doctor. She couldn't do much of anything except talk, listen to music, read, and watch television. Often, even these simple pastimes were beyond her. In the early weeks of relentless pain, medications left Lila drowsy—bad company for her son and husband. As recovery progressed, she passed back and forth through periods of depression and short-tempered frustration with her situation.

Many readers of this book are the Lila of this story, the physical sufferer of illness or accident. As this chapter will make clear, however, it pays dividends for patients to recognize the trauma that severe health problems bring to people *around the patient,* one of whom usually plays the role of chief caregiver.

Trent had thought he had it tough in Jackson while Lila was hospitalized—unfamiliar town, visits to the hospital, the pressure to entertain his son, the mounting stress of trying to keep up with his own work from a cramped motel room. It didn't take him long to discover that matters could get worse. He was thrilled to get his family back home, but Lila's three-month recuperation had hardly begun before Trent found himself growing frazzled and uncharacteristically brusque. He was trying to juggle all of the household demands, parenting, and his busy professional life. Without recognizing it, Trent had fallen prey to a health-care menace that hovers over many families: the severe shortage of caregiving support for managing an accident or illness. In fact, many caregivers who do spring to the rescue often end up requiring as much attention as the patient. And Trent's trials were relatively easy, compared to many family situations. Lila's health improved steadily, whereas people with chronic conditions require unending, often mounting assistance.

This chapter unpeels the onion of caregiving, revealing its many layered dynamics. You'll learn about the reasons behind the shortage of family caregiving and see how illness encroaches on emotions as well as family living space. Most importantly, you will discover ways that patients and caregivers can join forces in defeating caregiver burnout.

If you're a patient, you can urge family members or other caregivers who make your continued life possible to read these pages as well. Together, you can discuss what you uncover. Share ideas about how you can put the suggestions into practice. You can even consider how to accommodate *your* needs, on occasion, to *their* survival.

When emotional pain and fatigue drive caregivers to the end of their tether, they have nothing left to give the patient at risk. Some even turn vengeful, in masked but cruelly effective ways. Taking the caregiver's point of view before such a crisis erupts helps patient and supporter remain collaborators rather than turning into antagonists.


## WHERE HAVE ALL THE CAREGIVERS GONE?

Studies of caregiving in the United States show that two social trends are at odds with each other, catching individuals and their loved ones in the middle. On the one hand, the need for caregiving is growing; on the other hand, the supply of ready helpers is shrinking.

Hard-earned advances through medicine and improved living conditions (such as nutrition and sanitation) have lengthened life expectancy. Paradoxically, a delay in the onset of serious disease has not materialized to complement this increased span. In fact, improved detection of cardiovascular ailments, cancer, and other maladies now brings news of illnesses earlier in the lifecycle, often during prime years. In a mixed bargain, people live longer but spend more time coping with chronic and disabling conditions.

Just a few numbers illustrate how the demand for caregivers to the elderly has skyrocketed. The prevalence of disorders such as Alzheimer's disease nearly doubles with every five years of life after sixty-five, with half of people over eighty-five exhibiting dementia. Osteoporosis and hip fractures, among other conditions, become increasingly common with age. Forty-five percent of women aged sixty to sixty-nine have multiple chronic disorders; 70 percent of women eighty years or older are so afflicted. And the population is aging overall, with people born in the fertile late 1940s and 1950s now reaching maturity (Eisdorfer 1991).

The control of many chronic illnesses requires caregiving within the family, in addition to medical attention. In decades past, the long-term ill have traditionally depended on women—mothers, wives, and daughters—as caregivers. However, a host of these women now trade hours of home life for careers or just plain jobs to keep the family's financial head above water. In addition, today's smaller family size as well as the trend toward a delayed and bunched period of childbearing leave aging parents with fewer kin to call upon than earlier generations enjoyed. This means, shockingly, that a married couple now may have more living parents than living children.

Geographical separation is another obvious barrier to caregiving. Some children enlist the aid of professional care managers who work with geriatric cases to find services that meet a variety of their needs—living arrangements, physical therapy, and more. A list of providers can be obtained by calling the National Association of Professional Geriatric Care Managers in Tucson, AZ, at 520-881-8008. It's not surprising, perhaps, that national surveys find many children deciding not to lend a hand to infirm parents; they're busy raising their own children, engulfed in their jobs, or simply living too far away. In fact, among parents who are functionally limited, only *one of four* has a daughter or a son who helps with such chores as shopping, meals, getting around, dressing, bathing, taking medications, managing money, or other essentials (Stone and Kemper 1989).

Furthermore, many infants and children who formerly succumbed to illness or disability now survive because of advanced medical technologies, although they live with chronic conditions. A large share of these dependents require continuous caregiving in the home.

Institutions—such as nursing facilities, hospice care, and commercial health agencies that come to the home—have swelled to help meet the needs of patients and caregivers. Volunteer, community-based organizations pick up part of the slack, too, with meal programs, transportation services, and other aid. In spite of this help, there's still a staggering amount of home care needed.

Homegrown assistance to an ill family member has become a dwindling and precious resource that ought to be cherished. Anyone—accident victims like Lila, people ill with a bout of the flu, or the chronically sick or disabled—should not take such help for granted. To recognize and to secure this support, the patient needs to empathize with caregivers, to acknowledge the sacrifices they make and the stresses they endure. The family caregiver is beleaguered and often unsung.

Patients often win sympathy for their pain and limitations—and deservedly so. Only recently has medical and psychological attention been directed to their caregivers, who are collateral targets of illness and disabilities. Begin by imagining someone else's responsibilities. For example, what if *you* were in charge of caring for another person? How would you deal with a parent with Alzheimer's who needed full-time attention in your home, assistance in bathing, and help using the toilet? What if your child had an accident that left her or him debilitated for years? How would you balance your own needs—both physical and emotional—with your obligations to other people?

These are tough questions. To begin to answer them, eavesdrop on a support group that meets each week with an experienced facilitator. Picture the corner dayroom on the third floor of a large, urban hospital. The space is cluttered with unmatched chairs, which we pull into a tight circle because the whoosh of the air-conditioning drowns out soft voices.

Marilyn speaks first, a forlorn-looking woman of forty-eight with tightly curled brown hair. Though employed for years as a medical transcriber, she can no longer work outside the home because caring for her father is so time-consuming. He has five-organ failure, including considerable cognitive loss, and has had numerous short-term hospitalizations for stroke, heart and kidney failure, and respiratory problems. Legally blind, he has been in emotional and physical decline during the two years he has been living with Marilyn and her two children.

As if the stresses from caring weren't enough, a year ago Marilyn's husband of twenty-four years announced that he wanted a divorce. Though Marilyn considers herself completely responsible for her father, she concedes that her nineteen-year-old daughter and eight-year-old son do help with some of the physical caregiving tasks. They are often more forgiving of their grandfather's mental lapses than she is: "One day at dinner he started talking about the 'delicious fish' we were eating— when in fact it was chicken. The kids giggled and encouraged him to eat more. I'm afraid I just lost it—I yelled at him, 'You know that it's not fish, it's chicken. Can't you get anything right?'"

"Maybe I should just put dad in a nursing home," Marilyn continues. "The thought of not having to jump every time he calls is very appealing, but I don't know how long he'd survive in one of those places. The worst of it is, if he did end up staying there a long time we'd be wiped out financially." She noted the irony of her situation: "My father has defied medical expectations many, many times because of the wonderful care he gets from me."

"The truth is," Marilyn adds, "I'm angry all the time and I just hate my father for making me feel this way. One day I decided to play hooky, and I slipped out in the middle of the afternoon and went to a movie. I had just settled into my seat, with my popcorn and drink in hand, when a couple decided to sit directly in front of me in this almost-empty theater. I got up to move, but first I really let them have it—told them they were the rudest, most selfish people I'd ever seen. 'If you do not know what I'm talking about,' I said, 'I suggest you take a look around this theater.'"

The group members nod in sympathy. Danielle, a flamboyant and articulate woman in her early fifties, raises her hand to speak. Her husband, who was diagnosed with colon cancer three years ago, is also manic-depressive, which he controls through medication.

Married for twenty-five years, Danielle runs an art gallery with her husband, who has a son and a daughter from a previous marriage. "But they're no help," she tells the group. "His daughter lives abroad and couldn't care less. His son is like a robot, smart enough, I guess—he's about to graduate from medical school—but a real cold fish. As far as taking care of my husband is concerned, I'm it—for both the cancer and the manic-depressive problem. I do everything—handle all the personal and business finances, run the gallery, and keep an eye on him. I can really relate to what Marilyn said about feeling trapped. There's no such thing as a break. I don't dare leave my husband alone for even a day—he's a real loose cannon."

Danielle's husband has become obsessed with "alternative treatments," pursuing an underground network of healers with potions, pills, injections, and mudlike soups. "That's why I came here tonight," she adds. "I'm at my wit's end about all this stuff he's into. Sure, I want to be supportive, but I don't believe any of these so-called therapies are doing him the slightest good, and my patience is running out. I feel like a prisoner of his madness."

Danielle had listened intently to what Marilyn said about trying to do something for herself, even going to a movie. "I realize how much I need the same thing. And how little hope I have of getting it."

Adults are not the only caregivers, however, as cases outside this support group show. Meet Alonzo, who reminds us that children can get caught up in a complicated web of family obligations. Alonzo lives in a decaying neighborhood in Washington, D.C., with two brothers, two sisters, and his grandmother, who is the primary guardian for all of them. Alonzo was a seventh-grade student when he wrote this essay about his grandmother who has diabetes:

> My grandmother has gangrene in her legs. So now she is sick and I am home watching her. I am trying to be the best I can be. I wash her every day before I leave to go to school. I put her in her wheelchair and read a book or a story to her. After I come home from school, I take her for a little cozy walk around the neighborhood.
>
> Sometimes the homemaker comes and takes care of my grandmother while I am in school. The homemaker cleans the house up

and washes the dishes. Sometimes, when the homemaker does not come, the nurse comes. She bathes my grandmother and wraps her legs.

I'm angry that my grandmother is sick. I miss her being able to walk. When grandmother was well she cooked, cleaned up, mopped the floors, and walked to the stores. She went to the laundromat and did our laundry. She walked around the neighborhood picking up trash, cans, and bottles people had thrown on the streets. She hates a dirty house and a dirty neighborhood.

Now, she's sad. She doesn't like being sick. Her dream is to walk again. It is my dream too.

An indication of a caregiver's need to cry out can be drawn from the effort these people took to express themselves. Marilyn, Danielle, and others in their group traveled across town on rain-slicked and darkened streets to huddle together in a dingy room. Young Alonzo seldom even wrote his name in the weeks before sitting down to compose this essay; his pain pushed him to unprecedented heights of eloquence. These three portraits capture the mixture of resoluteness, resignation, anger, and sadness that is the lot of many caregivers.

## FOR WORSE AS WELL AS BETTER: FAMILIES AND CAREGIVING

Families have been called the bedrock of society, and with good reason. Nonetheless, even in strong and loving homes, relations often balance delicately on points of divided affections and contests over material goods and space. Most siblings are quietly in competition. Imagine a husband and wife, married for many years, who have come to accommodate themselves to each other's needs. Abruptly, a grave accident, a serious diagnosis, or the need to care for an elderly parent crashes rudely into this equation. Nearly always, serious disablement means that everyone has to renegotiate their status, options, and obligations.

### ASSESSING THE CONDITION: WHAT YOU SEE IS WHAT YOU GET

Assistance in the home starts with a drumbeat of physical tasks, each simple but cumulatively an avalanche. Here are notes from the front trenches by one caregiving spouse:

It's difficult having a sick person at home in bed. Every meal, every glass of water, every pill, every cold cloth, every cup of tea, every slipper, every sock, every pajama top, every pencil and paper, every book— every everything has to be fetched.

Then there are the trips. To the drugstore for prescriptions. To the grocery store for soft foods. To the video store, bookstore, and newsstand for things to occupy the patient.

Then there is the laundry. The sheets, towels, washcloths, bed pads, and clothes heap into mediciney mountains at an alarming rate.

Then there is the "help." Help me to the bathroom. Help me to my feet. Help me into the chair. Help me reach the phone. Help me handle my colostomy. Help me clean up the mess I made.

Then there is the cooking. He can have this. He can't have that. Nothing that will make gas. Nothing hard to digest. Nothing with too much sugar or fat. Then there's nothing left that he wants to eat.

Then there is the nursing. Take his temperature. Write it down. Call the doctor. Mete out the pills. Take his blood pressure. Check his incision. Change his dressings.

Then there is the patient. Who isn't. Sick people tend to be self-absorbed. They get bitchy. They want their way. They want attention. They want to complain. They become childish.    (Craig 1991, 69)

The emotional toll from caregiving is often the most serious burden that family members bear and certainly the most easily overlooked. Consider the case of strokes, the third leading cause of death and disability among older persons. Strokes impose special stress because of their unpredictable and uncontrollable nature. One study analyzed the severity of effects on support persons by following them for months after the attack (Schulz, Tompkins, and Rau 1988). One-third of *caregivers* were at risk for serious depression immediately after the patient's stroke, and more than half had reached this state a year later. These alarming symptoms were three times more likely among givers of care than among non-caregivers of the same age.

As might be expected, individuals varied widely. Some caregivers were acutely depressed right after the patient's attack but brightened later. Among others, normal moods deteriorated into severe depression. Caregivers to the most seriously impaired felt pained by the disappearance of the patient's former positive personality, the weakening of social ties, the long-term prognosis for decline, and the loss of a confiding relationship with the patient (Thompson, Bundek, and Sobolew-Shubin 1990). Other illnesses such as Alzheimer's are also marked by widespread depression among caregivers.

In fact, studies of dementia have illuminated a common problem in families, and many of these findings apply to other conditions as well (Boss et al. 1990). When an ill person exhibits increasing physical or mental deterioration, caregivers within the family struggle over ways to define the situation. The most important resolution they must reach involves "boundary ambiguity." The patient is physically present, but what about psychologically? Does the ill person belong, or should the family declare him or her *missing*? Caregivers are immobilized if they cannot clarify whether the ill person is inside or outside the family's psychological net.

Family celebrations and rituals—weddings, holidays, birthdays, and the like—are especially critical times. These occasions traditionally reaffirm family ties and mutual obligations and inevitably draw attention to the patient's status. Sometimes a holiday will go unobserved because there is so much tension over how to handle the situation:

> For the K family Christmas had always been a time when their large family gathered at the home of the parents. This year for the first time the adult children did not spend Christmas together, opting instead to spend it with their own families, and Mr. and Mrs. K went for the day to their eldest daughter's home. The family explained that the change resulted from their experience the Christmas before, which seemed too stressful and confusing for their father who has Alzheimer's disease. Normally he had held the central role in the gathering, deciding when presents were to be handed out and personally selecting each present from under the tree. Last year, however, he had been extremely irritable, had difficulty remembering why the family was gathered together, and spent the time when presents were distributed sitting in another room. The family had difficulty pinpointing how the decision to spend Christmas separately was made for this year, explaining that it simply seemed to be agreed on by everyone.
>
> (Boss, Caron, and Horbal 1988, 135)

Crises of "boundary ambiguity" afflict relationships outside the family, too. A severely impaired friend or workmate challenges everyone with this unspoken question: Should we retain the patient as a member of the in-group? Here's Robert Murphy, who was hospitalized many times during his illness which led to quadriplegia:

> Some people were unable to handle the new ambiguity in their relations with me, and I saw little more of them. Still others visited me in the beginning of my incapacity, but as illness stretched out into permanent disability, many ceased coming. To make matters worse, the dropouts felt guilty, and this made it even more difficult to reestablish ties. One friend rarely drops in on me at home, but he always visits me when I'm in the hospital—and he lives on my block. He is

aware of this and is a bit puzzled by it himself. I suspect that he, and others, do this because the indeterminacy of my status ends when I go to the hospital, where I am no longer betwixt and between. There, I am categorically ill.                                        (Murphy 1990, 169)

How do families deal with "boundary ambiguity"? Clinicians have noted two styles of redefining the ill person's status that originate in more general family norms. Some families have rigid customs about sociability, role obligations, and so on. For example, men are to be commanding and women compliant; children are to defer to elders' opinions; frequent phone calls are expected, as a matter of courtesy. Small deviations are magnified into large transgressions. Other families are more flexible. Gender differences in household chores are minimal, for example. Advice flows freely between generations and in both directions. Members call or write when they have something to share, and they may disagree or argue on occasion.

The first, more structured family recoils from "boundary ambiguity." The patient member is swiftly redefined out of the family whenever she or he crosses the family's threshold of tolerance for aberrant behavior. In the case of Alzheimer's disease, redefinition may come at initial stages of memory loss and confusion or may be delayed until the patient suffers from sleep disturbances and needs constant supervision, or comes even later when the patient can no longer even recognize caregivers. The second, more fluid family bends its ways in the face of boundary problems. Members think of the patient as ill, and not willful, and allow generous latitudes for strange, unpredictable, and unpleasant behaviors. They continue to interact with the patient, inventing unfamiliar but appropriate habits of communication. The patient may not be excluded psychologically until late in the progression of illness, and sometimes not until death.

The important lesson is that stress and depression among caregivers result more from difficulty over resolving the boundary problem than from the severity of the ill person's condition. The patient's mental functioning, ability to perform daily tasks, and behavior problems are not *in themselves* the cause of caregivers' stress. Instead, these symptoms lead families to negotiate their own redefinition of whether the ill person belongs in the family, at varying disease stages. Anxieties reach their high-water mark and remain troublesome as long as considerations of inclusion or exclusion linger unresolved on the agenda.

Carol, a woman in her mid-fifties, is still struggling with the ambiguity and conflicts associated with the care of her son, who was assaulted a year ago and suffered brain damage. She knows very few details of the incident; the police found the young man on the street, and she was notified by emergency-room personnel. He has managed to recoup physically, but he suffers from severe mental and emotional deficits. "My son often becomes extremely violent against me and others in our family. Since he has been home, he has had a number of psychiatric lockups. His thinking is at about the second-grade level."

Should Carol put her son in a mental-health facility? Removing the patient from the home defuses some of the stresses and burdens of immediate care, although placement can spark guilt in family members.

Carol's quandary expands to other situations. Research shows that an objective, clinically exact account of the patient's condition and needs forecasts very little about the amount of stress any caregiver endures. It is the caregiver's *appraisal of circumstances* and that person's resources for coping that count.

One study analyzed married couples in which one of the pair had dementia (Schulz and Williamson 1991). In the two-year study period, a number of the patients were placed in nursing facilities, even though the patients placed under professional care and those who remained at home were very much *alike* in severity of impairment, as measured by tests for memory, behavior problems, and mental functioning. What led some families to place the patient in a nursing home? The caregivers who made the choice to institutionalize their spouses felt the most burdened—that their own health was at risk, that their social life had decayed, or that their ability to work had declined.

Although an outside observer might marvel at the caregiver who seems to manage a patient's acute symptoms with ease, or be shocked by cases where mild demands for care throw family members into panic or deepen resentment, there's actually more to the story. Sometimes a caregiver can snap over just one manifestation of the illness—incontinence, for example—but take other aberrant behaviors in stride. As with most of life, social support helps caregivers adjust their appraisals of the situation and buffers consequences (see chapter 3). And, the importance of financial security hardly needs mention.

Is it irrational for caregivers to feel blue? Are their cranky moods undisguised, selfish demands to gain attention for the sacrifices they make? Maybe, in some situations, but as these cases demonstrate, providing long-term care profoundly affects caregivers' physical and emotional lives. When the patient can understand and acknowledge these issues, he or she starts to create a constructive relationship with caregivers and helps them cope in ways that improve the health of everyone.

## FAMILY SIZE AND HOUSEHOLD SPACE

Less obvious factors also play a role in adjustment to illness or injury. Studies have found vast differences in a caregiver's coping abilities based on the number of people who live in the household (Birkel 1987). Furthermore, the abundance or scarcity of people in the home carries very different implications, depending on whether physical or cognitive limitations afflict the patient.

First consider physical cases in which accident or disease hasn't limited the individual's abilities to communicate lucidly. In these situations, having lots of helping hands around the house can actually inflame tensions and stress. In large families, one person tends to end up carrying the heaviest caregiving load and soon begins to resent it, growing agitated, anxious, sad, and feeling locked in a spiral of declining energy. When the cadre of potential helpers is small, on the other hand, a greater proportion of the family participates; not only do they feel valuable and competent, but the sharing of tasks boosts everyone's morale.

The picture turns around with dementia or other cognitive deficits. In these situations, larger families provide variety in conversational cues and relationships that the patient experiences. Even children can be stimulating to the mentally impaired, and these contacts carry therapeutic value. Compared to small households, therefore, larger families are more likely to help the condition of a patient with cognitive deficits. Larger families provide a greater staff of stand-ins, covering for the primary caregiver when that person must be away shopping or tending to other needs. Thus, caring for the physically challenged may be easier in smaller households, while caring for the mentally challenged is usually easier in larger families.

Adaptation involves more than the sheer number of people at home; the balance between the number of people and the amount of space also makes a difference. Conditions such as spinal cord injury and kidney dialysis speak to this point. Over the long haul, these cases often deprive other family members of their customary space or personal territory. The patient's needs may mean that the household has to reassign rooms and rearrange schedules.

Children may have to sacrifice bedrooms to contain rehabilitation equipment and move in with a resentful sibling, or worse, bunk with a parent. Closets may be given over to storing medical supplies; clothing then transfers to overstuffed drawers or exposed metal racks. The net effect of these displacements is that private space shifts to the patient, and other family members compete for increasingly cluttered wedges of public domain. Everyone becomes irritable as the house seems to get smaller and smaller.

Time, as a psychological commodity, is redivided, too. The patient's transportation to and from treatments may rupture others' work and school schedules. This creates conflicts for family members in valued sectors of their lives. Work and academic performance suffer.

Increased tension in the household can turn normal situations into emergencies. Sullen teenagers, who at other times would be tolerated with a resigned shrug, now become misdiagnosed as maladjusted, or even pathological. Adults who are bored with their jobs, a familiar enough plight, are now seen to be abnormally depressed. Thus, the way in which families share and negotiate their time and space affects their perceptions of one another.

## TAMING THE OVERZEALOUS CAREGIVER

As a patient, you may be coping with a stroke, handicapped by arthritis, or rebounding from cancer, a heart attack, serious accident, or other interruption. Regardless, odds are strong that your caregiver believes you are physically and mentally more limited than you think you are. People around a patient routinely conclude that illness or accident has hit harder than patients themselves do. Understanding these perceptions can help all parties deal with them.

The caregiver becomes overly protective and leaps to your aid in circumstances where it is not needed. The helper may praise you for minor accomplishments or restrict your activities; he or she may constantly do favors or go behind your back to clear paths for you. The patient on the receiving end of over-solicitation can choose among three reactions.

1. You might, for instance, see overprotection as valid evidence that your self-confidence is misplaced; you actually are as feeble or disabled as others think. You might even fume with silent resentment. These interpretations generally grease the slide into depression. Resignation and bitterness at overprotection are quite common, probably explaining a

fair share of the discouragement patients feel, besides the dark emotions that are naturally unleashed by a chronic condition.

2. Another reaction to overprotection takes a more assertive stance. The patient zeroes in on an area where he or she can demonstrate a startling degree of competence. The patient may surprise a caregiver by fixing a tasty meal or cleaning house, taking up a pastime, or reading extensively on a subject. In such ways, a patient announces: "See, I'm a lot healthier than you assume." And the patient argues implicitly: "If I'm good at this, I'm probably more capable than you suspect in other ways, too."

We stumbled upon a novel twist to this strategy when interviewing members of SeniorNet. These older people have immersed themselves in computing and have formed face-to-face clubs as well as virtual groups in cyberspace across the country and the world. Participants are vigorous users of E-mail, exchange and even write software, tutor youngsters, and eagerly await new product releases. Some elderly people with health problems have cultivated this hobby with a calculated purpose in mind: It's their way to leapfrog a generation and inspire awe in a grandchild, who exclaims to an oversolicitous parent: "Wow, Nana's really into computing; she's even surfing the Internet!" This accomplishment halts overprotective caregiving in its tracks. Intellectual activities that become available through computing also provide a way for infirm elders to flex their curiosities and remain engaged with peers and life in general.

3. In a final option against over solicitation, some patients decide to grin and bear it, to quietly tolerate a helper's exaggerated efforts on their behalf.

Individual patients pick their own solution when faced with overzealous caregiving, including clinging to fantasies about their remaining powers. Awareness of this issue, however, gives patients a leg up on potential problems flowing from it. You need not blindly slump into despair when others do more than they should. And you can correctly spot the reason why caregivers sometimes grow hypercritical of their charges and scold them for "trying too much": these helpers are simply misjudging the patient's true capabilities. Other times, caregivers are unable to acknowledge the value of a patient's positive illusions or are intolerant of such thinking.

The shrewd patient doesn't simply react emotionally to overprotection. Rather, preserving the helping relationship reigns as the supreme goal. In these circumstances, the wise patient continues to shower appreciation on caregivers, even while doggedly contesting some of the reasons why their help is extended.

## MEN AND WOMEN: WHO DOES WHAT?

Gender differences in family caregiving piqued the novelist Kaye Gibbons's imagination. She described a man dealing with his spouse's illness this way:

> If you want to see a man afraid just put him in a room with a sick woman who once was strong. . . . And when a man sees a woman like that sick and hurt, especially the kind of man who knows a woman's strength but can't confess it, when he sees her sick or hurt it terrifies him, like he's witnessing a chunk of her universe coming loose and he knows he doesn't have what it takes to stick it back together.
>
> (Gibbons 1989, 13)

Burdens from another's sickness fall unequally on women and men (Kaye and Applegate 1990, 1991). Traditionally, nurturing others in need has been women's work; two-thirds of caregivers of elders are women who spend an average of 16 hours weekly at their tasks. Women become closely involved in hands-on care (bathing, grooming, and toileting) and emotional expression. By comparison, when men pitch in, they lean toward more distant styles of help, such as running errands, doing chores, and assisting with financial and other technical matters. These gender differences are consistent with the fact that women interact more intensively with their extended families than men, throughout many stages in the life cycle (Fitting and Rabins 1985).

This unequal division of support labor shouldn't be surprising for other reasons, too. Women have found themselves conscripted into a lot of unpaid, home-based work. And, of course, sex stereotyping in contemporary societies casts girls in affiliative, nurturing roles from an early age, and expects boys to sacrifice interpersonal closeness to their primary values of competitive achievement. Women typically have more close confidants than men, a sign of their recognition that spending intimate time with others has worth in itself and is not just a tool for attaining other goals.

Social workers who supervise gerontological services expect that coming generations of caregivers will slip into more androgynous styles of helping than their elders. They see the leading edge of this possibility in the greater responsibilities many fathers currently shoulder in the rearing of their children, especially as two-career parenting has become the norm. One can find some evidence for this happening, but many of the surveys that show greater numbers of males accepting the caregiver role and acting in emotionally nurturing ways have been limited to samples of people who participate in social support-group activities. This minority is likely to be nurturant in the first place and not representative overall.

## THE URGE TO COMPARE WITH OTHERS

Caregivers appraise their situation by studying how other caregivers are doing. The more harassed a caregiver feels, the more he or she will draw even further discouragement from any such comparisons. Anticipating such bad feelings, the caregiver may retreat from social contact. A caregiver who just doesn't go out any more, or who avoids trading "war stories" with others in the same situation, may be locked in a downward emotional spiral. The patient can sometimes break this logjam by bringing another patient's caregiver together with his or her own.

People under stress often flail about, looking for solutions to their predicament. Oddly, however, expert advice about an intimidating role pales alongside testimony from more vivid, if sometimes flawed sources: others in similar situations. Hearing about someone else's experience can be more profound than listening to descriptions from a physician, for example. By comparing—taking a look at how others are doing—people construct images through decidedly social means, as we saw with Marilyn and Danielle earlier in this chapter.

What was striking about their meeting, and other support groups we have observed, was the fact that the group leader hardly spoke at all. That night she uttered only four sentences (other than greetings and goodbyes) to propel the conversation forward. The heart of the meeting was the women sharing their experiences. They addressed their urgent quests for coping information to others in the group. The participants appraised each other's stories, which in details were wildly different but had common ground in caregiving challenges. The attendees departed with straighter postures and brighter spirits, exchanging phone numbers for continued contact with each other. They had negotiated a greater understanding of illness and coping out of the fabric of each other's opinions and experiences and not from a clinically "correct" base of knowledge.

It's important to recognize how the urge to compare actually works—whether the comparisons take place in a group, through a conversation in the doctor's waiting room, or while standing at the grocery checkout line. Humans feel driven to form estimates of their capabilities, to judge the correctness of their opinions, and to assess the state of their emotions (Festinger 1954). They do this by asking the question, "How well am I doing?" Other people provide evidence to help banish doubts. The power of these comparative points of view depends, however, on how likeable others are and on how comparable their personal circumstances are to your own. Comparability, you must recognize, is in the eye of the beholder; for example, Marilyn and Danielle were able to imagine similarities that escaped our understanding as mere onlookers. No wonder, then, that strangers begin conversations by signalling cues about their friendliness and exploring similarities, before getting down to matters that invite social comparison.

Your caregiver may seek two different kinds of partners for comparisons: some people who are perceived to be better off, and others thought to be worse off. The key to understanding such comparisons is this: Self-confidence begets positive interpretations of both comparisons, whereas feelings of defeat prompt negative readings across the board. The person who feels at least partly in control of the situation will find reassurance in both upward- and downward-looking views. Upward comparisons to those who are coping better can motivate and bring hope ("Maybe I, too, can reach that point"). Downward comparisons can bring welcome feelings of superiority ("I'm lucky; I could be even worse off!").

On the other hand, people who feel overwhelmed and inadequate tend to discover the less pleasant side to social comparison. The upward gaze reminds them of how poorly they are doing themselves ("She's handling her husband's illness so much more effectively than I am"); the downward look forecasts unpleasant possibilities to come ("I guess that's what I'll look like after another year of taking care of my mother").

The point to underscore is simply this. Caregivers with more than a shred of confidence remaining should be encouraged to seek out other people who shoulder similar burdens. They also should find comparisons outside the family, where upward and downward appraisals won't intermingle with the history of kinship and remembrances of earlier and different times. Patients eager to sustain their caregiver's health don't feel threatened by such contacts; they promote them.

## CAREGIVING: ON SCHEDULE, OFF SCHEDULE, OR BY DESIGN

Students of the human condition are fond of emphasizing two factors that help explain how well people will adapt to altered circumstances. One is whether they chose their new role or had it thrust upon them unwillingly. Second is whether the obligation came as an expected part of growing or maturing, or whether it arrived as a stunning surprise. It's no wonder that these issues arise in caregiving, too.

Some accidents and illnesses, such as when an elderly mother fractures her hip or a parent slips into dementia, are somewhat expected; these can be called "on-schedule" obligations for a caregiver. Few families actually plan ahead for these possibilities, but they quickly acknowledge that their hour as caregiver has arrived. Someone needs to step up to the plate.

An adult child who becomes an on-schedule caregiver for a parent will respond to the situation with a level of willingness that reflects the parent-child relationship. One type of relationship projects a feeling of communal *regard*. Parents merit respect for the experience and judgment they have attained; the caregiver relationship maintains at least the appearance that children are younger and still catching up. Regard means going out of the way to give pleasure to an elder, without necessarily discounting the parent's adult status or assuming a role-reversal in which the caregiver now serves as father or mother to an aged child. In this frame of mind, the caregiver also feels uniquely qualified to provide needed assistance; aid is not just a matter of performing necessary chores, but of infusing these with a respectful and affectionate spirit.

When these feelings are present, the provider acknowledges that the experience of caring returns a sense of warmth to his or her own life and the interrelatedness between generations. Sometimes sons and daughters confess that they spoil or indulge their parent, while making determined efforts to preserve the long-standing generational hierarchy.

A second, contrasting set of attitudes grows out of a relationship based on *exchange* between generations. This usually signifies a less willing caregiver. Feelings emphasize how different the parent has become— in mobility, interests, physical powers, or mental acuity. In these cases, the parent is seen as bringing less to the relationship than before; the parent has become a debtor instead of creditor. This sense of difference, of decay, often combines subtly with the belief that the elder's death would bring sadness, but also relief—that it would be better for everyone. Thoughts of moving the parent to a nursing home occur soon and often. The sons and daughters of this persuasion feel that caregiving has fallen harshly on their backs; they didn't seek this service, and don't play much of a part in shaping its boundaries.

The two sets of attitudes—regard as opposed to exchange—account for the help that some parents receive and some children provide. If imbued with regard, children more patiently pay the deepest costs of care; they will bathe and feed and dress and toilet an elder, and not just lend a hand with shopping, personal finances, and the more antiseptic chores. These caregivers stay the course, putting in long hours over many months and years, if necessary.

On the other hand, children who have an exchange relationship with their parents want to curtail their care when the going gets tough, although lack of affordable options may frustrate these wishes. These helpers make their feelings of unwillingness known through tone of voice and other nonverbal cues, if not in things directly said.

Many social analysts fear that genuine regard may be a waning basis for extending help, an obsolete legacy of agrarian times. Possibly, it is suspected, most adult children now favor a conditional stance toward caregiving; circumstances will govern what is "right" and "wrong," and many situations are "unknowable" until the costs and benefits show their hand. The conviction may have spread that previous generations of caregiving children could radiate more affection and attention because they had time for this. Life is harsher now, more complicated and disconnected. Newer generations can't afford a willingness to care that is anchored in nostalgia.

Whatever the truth in a particular family, on-schedule demands for care are so obvious that anyone can practice ahead of time, imagining how they would be treated if they were the patient, and how they would respond, if called upon to provide help.

## THE SPECIAL DISRUPTIVENESS OF "OFF-SCHEDULE" ILLNESSES

"Off-schedule" occasions for caregiving, on the other hand, strike without warning, or at least seem to. Diagnoses of serious illnesses or accidents interrupt the orderly trajectory of parenting, career building, and other activities. Sometimes such events startle helpers into discovering emotional resources they hadn't suspected they could muster. Other times, helpers themselves are thrown into such chaos that they suffer nearly as much as the patient.

One of the most daunting off-schedule caregiving situations is the young spouse who suddenly faces a partner's need for long-term assistance, an aspect of the marriage contract that didn't seem part of the bargain. We interviewed Michael, forty-four, who has committed years of devoted care to his wife, an unusual case of male-to-female support. Wendy, forty, has diabetes, suffering every possible complication the disease can mete out. While Michael's story is one of courage, it also reveals dark undercurrents of frustrated needs and resentments about the sacrifices he has had to make.

Wendy was diagnosed with Type 1 diabetes (insulin-dependent) at age nine; she met Michael when she was seventeen and married him a year later. Michael told us he was "completely ignorant" about the disease during their courtship, and could recall no medical incidents that caused him any concern. "Just after we announced our engagement, though, my favorite uncle took me aside and warned me not to get married because there would be problems down the road." Michael shrugged him off.

The first five years of marriage were uneventful medically, but Wendy's first pregnancy ended in a miscarriage. That hospitalization was to be the first of more than eighty over the next seventeen years. She has had a kidney transplant, multiple surgeries on her eyes (she has only partial vision in one eye now), neuropathy in both legs, reconstructive surgeries on her feet, and much more. In spite of these formidable challenges, she returned to school to become a licensed therapist, and she and Michael have adopted two children. Michael and Wendy live within minutes of his mother and of her parents and siblings.

Michael's story offers important insights into the dynamics between patient and caregiver.

*Sainthood.* It is well known among their friends and acquaintances that Michael does household chores, chauffeuring, shopping, and other responsibilities associated with parenting two children. He and Wendy are active members of their synagogue. He recalls the "many, many occasions when we've walked into the temple and had people approach us and comment on how great Wendy looks and on what a saint I am. They often add: 'I couldn't do it, how do you do it?' "

This well-intended greeting actually wounds both partners deeply.

For Michael, it raises considerable guilt because, on occasion, he does feel angry toward Wendy, and these are clearly unsaintly feelings. This exalted status also tends to place him out-of-bounds for receiving any help himself. As he puts it, "They notice Wendy and ask if there is anything they can do for her. What am I, chopped liver?"

For Wendy, the conversational opener sparks resentment because it is a reminder of how much she must depend on her husband. For both, references to Wendy's condition reaffirm that the disease drives the conversation, whereas Wendy longs to be defined by her other roles— wife, mother, therapist, fellow congregant.

*Family Ties.*  Two areas of family dynamics bring the most strain to Michael's life. One is rooted in his uncle's early warning. That conversation more than twenty years ago (which Michael shared with Wendy) left a frosty relationship with the uncle that has yet to thaw. It is unlikely to warm now that the uncle's unpleasant forecast has come true.

Another area of tension in this case comes, oddly enough, from the proximity of many close relatives. On the one hand, Michael feels awkward about having to ask for so much help. On the other hand, he is indebted to them for the many times they have pitched in during Wendy's hospitalizations and recoveries. He feels even worse when his in-laws, who have spent long periods taking care of the children, assert their own ideas about child rearing; these major disagreements plunge the entire household into a funk.

*Commitment and Guilt.*  When asked "So, how do you do it?" Michael says, "I'm committed to the person and not to the disease. This disease steals your normal life. The physical part of helping is a pain in the neck, but it's manageable. The emotional part is what's difficult—seeing her suffer, seeing her dealing with doctors and hospitals, and seeing her limitations in terms of the parenting she'd like to do."

Because of Wendy's poor eyesight, Michael must escort and guide her when she walks. One year ago, as they were approaching a restaurant, Michael became distracted for a moment, and Wendy tripped on a small step, breaking her leg. Recovery included major surgery and six months in a cumbersome cast. Michael feels "completely responsible" for the accident and the subsequent trauma. Thus, commitment and guilt go hand in hand.

*Career Mobility.* Michael concedes that he has put his own career aspirations on a back burner. "Promotion in my company requires a willingness to relocate around the country, which isn't possible for me. We
need to be near our families so that they can help out during medical
crises." Michael tries to avoid business trips because his absence leaves
the children with no means of transportation, and Wendy feels more
vulnerable when he is away.

*Sexuality.* Michael looks wistful when this topic is raised. An interview
with another caregiving husband drew this powerful confession about
the least-talked-about liability of spousal disability. Ted, fifty-three, has
assisted his wife through twenty-two years of increasingly debilitating
multiple sclerosis. Issues of sexuality color their relationship. "I feel
guilty," Ted confided, "that I have to remind myself to think of my wife
as a woman."

What does each provider sacrifice in offering care? What motivation sustains these acts: equity, paying someone back for the gifts of
love and resources the other person extended earlier in life, or moral-
ity anchored in society's expectations? What rewards does caregiving offer:
satisfactions from managing another person's time or from strengthening an emotional bond? Somewhere in this brew of motivations,
rewards, and relinquished goals lies the secret of whether anyone, man
or woman, will shoulder the caregiving role.

## THE POWER OF CARING:
## WELFARE MOTHERS AND DISABLED CHILDREN

A third brand of caregiving is by design. It flows from more voluntary
wellsprings, though not always without compensation. We have seen
how a patient-caregiver relationship may galvanize, even inspire people's
lives. The following story explains how—and all the more convincingly because it shows supposedly powerless people mastering challenges that vex more advantaged people in society.

During the past few years, the Judson Center in Royal Oak,
Michigan, has been matching welfare families with developmentally
impaired children, paying the families a small salary to care for the children. Judson has been in operation for more than seventy years, first as
a Baptist orphanage and more recently as an interdenominational center offering a wide range of family services. With help from a state

appropriation, in 1987 the Center began to place severely developmentally disabled children in the foster care of welfare families. This
counterintuitive program now involves twenty-nine youngsters from
infancy through their early twenties, living in nineteen different home
environments, with ten new families qualified but awaiting their placements. Though these numbers don't make much of a dent in Michigan's
backlog of disabled youth, the program's successes demonstrate opportunities for care and human growth across many situations: The foster parents escape from the welfare rolls, the children improve in
dramatic ways, and the government saves considerable amounts of
money.

All the children in this program have mental retardation as a primary diagnosis, but they also suffer from other disabilities, including
cerebral palsy, epilepsy, hearing or vision impairments, or muscular dystrophy. For others, the disabilities are emotional, such as schizophrenia
and depression. Many of the children have been physically or sexually
abused, often for years.

Foster parents are carefully assessed and selected. Each must satisfy
a rigorous screening program that emphasizes three standards: (1) demonstrated parenting skills with their natural children; (2) a strong social support system, from adult children or extended family or from friends in
church or other social groups; and (3) successful completion of an
extensive training program in caring for the severely disabled, leading
to a license by the state of Michigan.

The chemistry that binds this novel mixture of caregiving becomes
clearer from conversations with the families. Sally is a single parent
with two children of her own and three from the Judson Center. She's
reserved, determined, and self-respecting. She welcomed us into her
small but immaculate home. A portrait of Jesus and her framed license
hang on one wall; a stereo and plant anchor the other end of the living room.

Sally beams when talking about the great accomplishments she has
seen with her three Judson children. Her first was Karen, a sixteen-
year-old with cerebral palsy. Karen had been institutionalized for years,
had not been toilet trained, could not feed herself, and would not initiate contact with other people. Four years later, Karen can feed herself and is bowel trained; she has had corrective surgery on her feet and
has taken her first steps. She is able to transfer herself from bed to
wheelchair and even has a "job" delivering lunches at school.

Wally arrived two years later. He was one year old, diagnosed with tuberculosis (TB) of the brain and thought to be terminally ill. He was heavily medicated, tube-fed, and blind in one eye and deaf in one ear. Today he is three years old and functions at an eleven-month level; he crawls and is expected to walk. He speaks in one- and two-word sentences, and he is being toilet trained.

The third child, Quincy, is ten and autistic. He has been in the household for only one year and is learning to dress himself. "I'm teaching him the rules: no plaids with stripes!" Sally says. "But he hasn't quite got the hang of it yet."

Sally's older sister Alice and her husband also participate in the Judson program. They live two houses away. Alice has one child of her own still living at home, two adopted children, a transfer child (with a record of delinquency) from another agency, and one shy ten-year-old from Judson. Both sisters readily acknowledge how much they depend on each other's support and that of their entire family. The children drift from house to house, fully comfortable in either home. Another sister, who has no children of her own, often takes all the youngsters on a Saturday for movies or a visit to an amusement park.

Sally and the other Judson parents are paid an annual salary and an additional payment in benefits to care for each of the children placed in their homes. Judson also funds necessary modifications to the house— a wheelchair ramp, for example, a larger refrigerator, or other needs. Thus, the parents are rewarded for caregiving, a skill in which they and their own children can take pride. The families no longer receive welfare; reproachful glances from neighbors and playground taunts to the kids give way to respect. All of the foster parents told us that getting off welfare was a major incentive to join the program.

The advanced caregiving skills these families practice don't necessarily come naturally. Sally had to learn techniques of behavior modification, emotional coping, and medical supervision, for example. The instruction also includes management. All the parents maintain detailed logs of a child's progress, including incident sheets that report any significant deviations from behavioral or emotional norms, disturbing events, and accidents. These records are required by law, and they reflect the family's attentiveness to their assignment. It's no wonder that Sally and the other families project an air of professionalism; they work purposively toward reaching goals and must document the faltering, as well as confident, steps each child takes.

The self-esteem that Judson parents acquire through caregiving is confirmed by the case of Sharon, forty-six, who with five children of her own, welcomed two Judson placements. Her salary brought material gains within reach, such as purchasing a modest home. But financial advantages are only a small part of this family's rewards. "I'm more of an advocate for myself and my own kids now, much more than before we got Gary and Mandy." Her youngsters from Judson have cerebral palsy and mental retardation, one with an IQ of 40.

"When dealing with my own kids' needs at school," Sharon recalled, "I often felt defensive. The authorities would imply that any problem with my kids was my fault. But it's different with my foster children. I can stand up and ask for certain things because I know I'm not to blame, I'm just here to help them."

Sharon's independence shows in other ways, as well. She is taking community college courses, somehow fitting her studies into an already crowded schedule, with the goal of becoming a social worker. She talked longingly about research assignments, acknowledging that she could spare no time to go to the library. "Any studying or homework I do is done right here at this kitchen table."

She talked at length about her own sons' reactions to their participation in the program. "They were worried at first that I wouldn't have any time left for them, but that passed quickly." What about the cramped quarters? Sharon answered, "I already had two or three boys in each bedroom, so another one or two was not going to make much of a difference."

It took a while for Sharon's family to deal with Gary, who had been abused for much of his first eleven years. His tantrums—aggressive, impulsive, and destructive—often included throwing objects in the house and creating disturbances in public. But progress is being made in this and other ways; Gary attends a special school where he is classified as "trainable."

The Judson program administrator, an experienced social worker, and her staff assist at every turn. She is in touch with the families several times each week; visits are frequent between Judson personnel and the families. Every parent has Judson staff home numbers for off-hours emergencies.

This absorbing case from the front lines of caregiving imparts lessons that apply elsewhere:

1. Taking care of a person whose infirmities seem overwhelming can instill pride of accomplishment. The role of caregiver can bolster self-esteem and self-confidence.

2. Caregiving can be made into a family project where everybody is expected to supply understanding and patience, and to pitch in with meeting household needs. A Judson family's own children become protective of the disabled, insisting that they be treated with respect and shielding them from ridicule in public. Many Judson families report that their own children mature quickly and develop unexpected educational ambitions.

3. The caregiving mothers have become pals, regularly exchanging confidences and emotional support.

The Judson experience, a hothouse of caregiving, supports the earlier points this chapter has made about how patients can help their caregivers. Caregiving can inspire instead of defeat people, if the caregiver sees it as an opportunity. Sharing the burden within family can uncover emotional resources. Social comparison with peers refreshes a caregiver's courage and prompts better ways of meeting common situations.

## WHEN A CHILD IS AT RISK

The Judson foster parents are shining examples of caring for children with a variety of needs. Most caregiving to children, though, helps young patients cope with specific chronic or life-threatening illnesses, where improvements in medical treatment have extended their lives. Conditions such as muscular dystrophy, cerebral palsy, and defective organ functioning now require years of specialized care. Furthermore, care must often be sequenced in fixed steps or exquisitely timed. Surges in physical symptoms may suddenly tax the family's emotional resources.

Parents react with shock to the diagnosis of their offspring's serious illness, and then enter a period of mourning for the loss of a "perfect" child. Nearly half of parents fail to advance beyond this stage of grieving, and this profoundly weakens their ability to provide sensitive and effective care (Marvin and Pianta 1996).

We met such a case in Martha, a twenty-seven-year-old mother whose three-year-old son, Ricky, had cerebral palsy with moderate disability; he could follow his mother around the house. More severely impaired children Ricky's age are unable to scoot, crawl, roll, or walk. We asked Martha to recall when she first realized that Ricky had a medical problem. She told of her feelings at that time and how her feelings had changed. Her words and manner of speech betrayed a lack of resolution.

She seemed stuck in the past, repeating how stunned she and her husband were at the diagnosis. She returned again and again to the existential questions: "What could have caused this to happen to Ricky?" "Why us?" She distorted her son's immediate prospects, believing that he would be able to play normal games with children in the neighborhood. And she voiced unrealistic expectations about the future, confiding at one point that Ricky would probably grow up to become a house painter, like his father and grandfather. Martha's eyes constantly sought for signs of our sympathy; she needed our emotional seal of approval for her grief. Several times during the conversation, she lost her train of thought and became disoriented. She contradicted herself, acknowledging at one point that it would take special efforts to find childhood companions for Ricky.

In contrast to Martha, parents who resolve these sorts of diagnoses recognize their difficulties and can describe how they have stepped forward to cope with them. They suspend the search for ultimate explanations, either biological causes or the reason why lightning struck them. They share a realistic, though not defeated, picture of the child's abilities and future prospects. They relate how they have grown emotionally from the trauma, drawing a contrast between their early teary reactions and feelings now.

Evidence shows that the degree of resolution that parents reach has little to do with the severity of their child's condition. Cases of extreme impairment can be much like milder cases, even within such different conditions as cerebral palsy and epilepsy. Nor does resolution depend on the passage of time since diagnosis. The well educated are no better at achieving closure and understanding than less schooled parents are. Some parents simply remain stuck—often overwhelmed, or angry, or depressed and passive. Others, on the other hand, get on with their lives and their child's future (Pianta et al. 1996).

Resolution makes a clear difference in the child's emotional security. When adults stay mired in grief and confusion, they fail to read the child's needs and other cues accurately. They are uncomfortable interacting with the child in intimate physical settings. They harbor unconscious expectations that the child will function as if he or she were less disabled. They resent sudden caregiving demands, and show it. It is no surprise that their physically challenged child grows anxious and even frantic during brief separations from parents. Caregiving suffers.

Even when parents adjust well to the child's disability, the strain can become unbearable unless they seek respite by hiring day help or by temporarily placing the ill child in a residential facility while they cope with their own needs or simply rest. The former relief may drain a family's finances. As for the latter, many families are unaware of local options for institutionalized services; help is not available in every area, especially rural parts.

Parents may even take courage from a downward transition in the child's condition because some new ground is reached, opening other means of coping. The switch to a wheelchair offers one example. Having to use a powered chair makes it clear that the child lacks stable health and may never be normal. As one father reported: Getting the wheelchair "was pretty low . . . at the same time she became independent, so it was really positive. I thought, 'Oh my God, a wheelchair! This is serious!' But then, finally, when we got the wheelchair, she was suddenly mobile. We were calling her over to us! That's a real God-send; you know, we'd never called her over to us"(Gravelle 1997, 742).

Caregivers of children battle constantly against *chronic sorrow,* ceaseless feelings of grief and even fear. Sorrow and sense of loss intensify whenever the child reaches milestones, such as graduating from primary school or reaching adolescence, when physically normal children are dating. The risks from chronic sorrow mount when parents' crowded schedules restrict their own contacts with acquaintances and other sources of social support, just as they need this balm the most.

Three blessings can come to the aid of a harried parent-caregiver. A first source of caregiver strength can arise when the parent develops *skills as a lay member of the medical team.* As parents learn to operate assistive devices, to inject medicines, to monitor fluid output, and to clear clogged passageways, they overcome feelings of inadequacy. The more that doctors and nurses can provide training and candidly share information about the course of disease, the better for everyone.

At the same time, a caregiver to a child in decline needs more than just medical facts and skills. The child's changing condition requires the caregiver to seek new services, knowledge, and support. Often as not, the parent has to butt heads with yet another bureaucracy, where he or she must retell the child's story to new faces, file a fresh set of forms, and seek another round of reimbursement or technical assistance. As one parent stated: "It's so exhausting and that's what wears me out the most." Many smolder in rage against a cold and complex system of aid that feels like one stone wall after another.

In this second area of assistance, *support groups* of parents are crucial; people who have been through the mill can teach a newcomer their tricks. Nurses often know about these support groups, but may forget to mention the opportunity unless a parent asks. Nurses can also share the names of other families that have faced a similar crisis, once they have sought permission to do so.

Other times, a sympathetic nurse will take a frustrated parent under his or her wing, showing ways to navigate the administrative tangle that can enmesh caregiving. Again, this aid may not appear until prompted by inquiries, such as: "Nurse Jones, I'm having trouble arranging and paying for my child's school tutoring. Do you know anyone who can help me get through this maze?"

When a nurse feels inadequate to this task, he or she may know about publicly funded social agencies or nonprofit groups that offer case-management services. Case management tackles the spectrum of a family's needs comprehensively, not on a piecemeal basis. Managers help caregivers find training in care for their child, locate transportation to the child's school, and negotiate home nursing, legal advice, insurance reimbursement, speech therapy, and the grab bag of other needs. Managers may advise on recreation opportunities and life planning for the child, as well. Much of a manager's time on cases is spent arranging for support services and obtaining financing to cover needs. Direct counseling with parents may be secondary.

When nurses don't know about sources of aid, parents can contact statewide clearinghouses for self-help groups and state and county departments of human services. A telephone call to a major metropolitan pediatric facility can also provide sources of caregiver aid. You can also get in touch with your local chapter of the Case Management Society of America by calling national offices in Little Rock, Arkansas, at 501-225-2229. Members of this organization provide services for a fee to families with a catastrophic medical case (child, adult, or elder).

A third fountain of support comes from efforts to *combat the caregiver's sense of isolation*. Friends and relatives frequently need to come to a parent's rescue. Parents' despair about their ability to continue often flows from a feeling that "I am it." This is the "I am the only person reliable enough to care for the child, capable of giving aid, and available (and affordable) to render continual assistance" syndrome. In fact, a caregiver's sense of loneliness produces just as much stress and surrender as does the seriousness of a child's medical condition. Psychology equals biology in this case. Other people must step up to the plate with encouragement and concrete aid to save a deteriorating situation (see suggestions later in this chapter).

Sometimes, especially in low-income households, grandmothers are roped into helping with chronically ill children. A single parent may have grown overwhelmed, or perhaps both parents are working and can't afford to cut back. Or one or both parents may be dysfunctional—using drugs or acting in frustrated or punishing ways to the child—forcing an older generation to return to responsibilities it never expected to repeat.

Catastrophes are not the norm, of course. More commonly, children fall ill for short periods of time or need hospitalization and rehabilitation that have an end in sight. Nonetheless, the condition may inflate parents' anxiety so much that they become immobilized. Perhaps the sheer strangeness of hospital routines or the bedlam in a brusque and busy clinical setting freezes the parents' instincts for providing positive support. Other times, mothers and fathers put their habits of nurturing and informing the child in cold storage under the mistaken but understandable belief that the medical team has taken charge of parenting.

Parental caregivers who face a frightening predicament, even if short-term, need to start by realizing that their own anxiety is natural. A simple procedure such as injections can distress both parent and child. Aspirations (the removal of body fluids), preoperative procedures, surgeries, and many other interventions agonize parents. Even vague and chronic complaints, such as recurrent abdominal pain in children, leave many parents confused about what to do.

When a caregiver fails to appreciate that his or her own immobilization is normal, friends should come to the rescue with an encouraging talk that moves through four stages.

1. "The hospital or medical team may have talked very little with you—except to explain their services and policies and tell you in general

about diagnosis, what procedures will take place, and when things are likely to happen. You need to know more."

2. "We can talk with doctors and nurses about the typical behaviors of children like yours (age, gender, developmental maturity, medical condition), during and after hospitalization (or the procedure, or experiencing the condition). We can ask how kids usually react. What uncertainties do kids have beforehand, what pain and disorientation during and after? What are the signs that they are coping well or coping poorly?"

3. "We can ask how you, the parent, can take part during hospitalization (or during a procedure or treatment). What chores can you perform that will improve care? Importantly, what can you say and do that will help your child's coping with treatments and side effects—step by step through the entire process toward recovery?"

4. "I've brought along a notebook, so we can write down these ideas. That way, you will have a reminder for review, and a crutch when you are under stress. If you'd rather, we can tape record our discussions with doctors and nurses."

Of course, a parent can make such inquiries on his or her own behalf, and a parent must do so, even where an earlier hospitalization has provided some experience. When the medical team prepares parents for their caregiving role, parents who are active do much better for their children and themselves. They play more with their hospitalized children and bring favored toys and games from home. They bathe their children and touch them more often. They explain tests and procedures, so that their familiar and calming voices supplement those of a newly introduced medical team.

Prepared caregivers can distract the child to help reduce suffering. Common yet effective techniques during a blood drawing include having the child pinch his or her nose or blow on a paper party favor. Caregivers can teach the child skills of *positive self-talk*. This means working with the child before procedures, reciting phrases like "I will feel better in a little while" or "everything is going to be all right" and teaching the child to think these repeatedly when undergoing painful episodes. They teach the child to bring positive fantasies to mind or recall cheerful events when they are alone, in pain, or in darkened rooms.

The prepared caregiver acknowledges for the child that it's "okay to feel scared," but that "I'll be right here, nearby, the whole time."

They reward the child after unpleasant treatments with a hug and kiss, praise for being brave, a special lunch, a small toy, or reading a favorite story together. They understand when the child wants to rehearse a medical experience (injections, surgery) with dolls or enact it in play, and provide time to do this.

Prepared caregivers reinforce their children's progress toward pain-free recovery by awarding happy faces on charts for the good days or investing other tokens (small gifts, privileges) with significance ("I saw this and thought of you, since you have been doing so well"). Realistic goals for a child's improvement must guide these signs of approval; the caregiver should seize upon some small advancement early on, drawing attention to the direction that recovery should take.

In addition, prepared caregivers monitor their children's condition more closely than unprepared parents, alerting nurses and other health professionals to symptoms. On this score, overcommunicating with medical staff is better than hanging back. Terry Pringle's experience with his son's hospitalizations for leukemia makes the point. One day, a nurse "brings a syringe of medication that is clouded, and when I ask if it's supposed to be clear, she says she doesn't know. I suggest she check with the resident. Sighing, she disappears, returning later with a syringe that isn't cloudy" (Pringle 1992, 19).

Of course, no parent facing the emotional roller-coaster of a sick child can keep it together every moment. Sometimes parents lose their cool, even in the most loving and generous families. Again, the Pringles illustrate:

> Eric's whining becomes intolerable and we threaten him with pun-
> ishment we know that we will never deliver if he doesn't shut up, if
> he doesn't act like a big boy. We are as sorry once the words are out
> as we are intent when we say them. Our foul moods feed on them-
> selves. The more we demand of Eric, the less he gives, now refusing
> to walk down the hall while we push the IV pole, insisting instead
> that he be carried. The doctors don't help, telling Eric to get out of
> his mother's lap and to quit acting like a baby.    (Pringle 1992, 21)

Parents need to profit from such flashes of guilt when behaving badly, remembering that prepared and understanding caregivers are more comforting to their children than unprepared ones. They are more useful and skilled participants in their children's recovery, even though lapses are normal. Preparation produces benefits, regardless of the caregiver's style of parenting before the medical emergency or condition arose. Even a parent who is highly anxious by nature, and doubly so because of the episode, does more for the juvenile patient when given the tools. Caregivers can and do become problem solvers.

The child gains, too. The patient becomes less distressed and more cooperative during procedures. Post operative benefits include less need for analgesics, swifter return to fluid intake, and earlier voiding of urine or bowels. The child is better adjusted at home after discharge. Functional health status rebounds more quickly; that is, children whose parental care-giver has taken positive steps get well faster, on average. The patient makes up for lost time at school more rapidly.

Finally, once again, we arrive at the importance of reciprocity. Conventional wisdom argues that children with terminal or serious mental illnesses can never return much to the family member who compromises his or her own life in service. Yet despite reduced oppor-tunities, these patients can (and must) reward their caregivers.

Again, consider the Pringles. The father reads his five-year-old leukemic son a story about another child, diseased with polio and deserted by his parents and taken to live with a faraway foster parent who devotes herself to rehabilitating her new charge. One day, she tells the child that the Lord appeared in her dreams and announced that the child is to walk.

> As I read the words, Eric stands and starts to walk. He has trouble negotiating the turn between the couch and the coffee table and falls back onto the couch. I am amazed by this show of spontaneity. In the past days, he has countered my suggestions that he practice walking with offers to walk "when I get through with my lunch" or "when we get back from a ride" and then he has to sit and consider the act for a few minutes, swinging his legs.
> Now I ask, "What are you doing, E?"
> "Walking."
> "Why?"
> "Because I thought it would make you happy."
> (Pringle 1992, 162–163)

Not all children can pay back in these ways. When children fail to pay back, third persons should step in to prompt them. Even symbolic recognition works wonders. Severely ill children can be coaxed to express affection. "Smile and hug your mother; tell her how grateful you are." "Spend time talking, asking her what she thinks about your favorite TV show (or musical performer, or other interest)." "Show affection to others whom your mother loves—your sister or brother, even though they might have bugged you, or an elder relative."

Children can give simple gifts, such as crayon drawings addressed to their mother or father. They can scrawl thank-you notes. They can agree to take part in family gatherings, making a special effort to dress and come into the living room or join a meal.

Evidence is clear about child-to-parent reciprocity. Family caregivers experience less fatigue and provide greater help to their children (from chores to financial aid and other sacrifices) if the patient acknowledges assistance. Reciprocity counts within bloodlines, even where a young and defenseless patient might be excused from this etiquette.

Those who help a child (or any other patient) pay back the caregiver should understand one more fact of life. Patients tend to think they have been more giving than the recipients of such attention report. A child needs to understand that one thank you doesn't last forever and the memory of one family gathering will fade. Repeated gratitude, spaced across time, makes the difference.

## BEATING THE BLUES

To many people, becoming a caregiver seems like jumping out of an airplane. Nothing before in life has prepared them for the whipping wind and the plunge earthward. Instinctively, they grasp for a parachute. The desperate person, or even just the curious, asks two basic questions: (1) What am I getting into here—what emotions and tasks can I expect to confront? and (2) What do I need to know in order to keep from being overwhelmed?

### REGAINING IMMUNE STRENGTH

This chapter's stories about patients and caregivers add up to a general lesson: Care digs deeply into a family's reserves. Caring also weakens a helper's own physical condition. Ill or disabled patients who wish to appreciate their caregivers must grasp these essentials.

Investigators have found, for example, that spouses and offspring who care for dementia patients have weakened immune systems compared to noncaregivers who otherwise match these supportive people in health status, age, gender, and education. One study followed caregivers of Alzheimer's patients for a period ranging from nine to twenty-four months (Kiecolt-Glaser et al. 1991). These cases averaged five years since onset of the disease; support activities typically consumed eight hours per day. The researchers also studied a comparison group lacking any caregiving responsibilities.

Results were riveting. Caregivers had more days where they were unable to perform normal activities because of their *own* illnesses (primarily upper respiratory tract infections, such as colds) than the matched group. The caregivers reported more doctor visits for their own conditions than did the comparison group. Physiological measures of the caregivers' immune system functioning declined relative to the matched group, over time.

Decay in caregivers' immunity was strongly linked to a lack of social support (Baron et al. 1990). Other studies confirm this finding (see chapter 3). Significant immunological deterioration took place across the study period, even though caregivers had already been lending a hand for many years. Results from this Alzheimer's study are especially disturbing because older caregivers are at greater risk than younger people for potentially irreversible consequences of impaired immune activity.

The way that people express themselves in a caregiving situation also makes a difference for their own health. When people recount highly stressful experiences in a matter-of-fact way, their immune systems weaken, compared to situations in which they vent the emotional side to events. Offering only a cloaked rendition of distressing episodes can be unhealthy; talking about one's feelings openly can boost the immune system. Patients who want to protect their helpers' health can encourage them to blow off steam and turn a deaf ear to the occasional hurtful things that might be said.

Findings from many studies suggest that even healthy and socio-economically advantaged caregivers suffer. Of course, these facts need not discourage extending psychological and material aid. Instead, the evidence should reassure support persons that their anger, resentment, guilt, and depression are perfectly normal. Physical and emotional stresses are to be expected.

One new program of research points the way toward bolstering the immune system so that caregivers can shield themselves against the costs of their service to others. These studies are based on the psychological principle of classical conditioning. The goal is to piggyback a new activity onto one that already acts as a natural stimulus to robust immune functions. In other words, you associate something new with an immune booster that already works, broadening the experiences that will trigger immune strength.

A simple example shows how. Physical exercise usually enhances the performance of people's immune systems. A clever caregiver can capitalize on this by getting in the habit of adding a new activity just *before* exercising. Something entirely different will work, like reading pleasurable things, doing crafts or hobbies, or another activity that is distinctive and recognizable. With repetition, this pairing of a new activity with a natural immune booster teaches the immune system to recognize *both* as appropriate prompts to greater biological efficiency. Soon, the new activity will even arouse immunological defenses on its own. Thus, immune functions become enhanced on more occasions during the day and the week than just when exercise takes place.

Investigators at Trier University in Germany have demonstrated these immunological responses in animals (Buske-Kirschbaum et al. 1992). For example, mice that have been injected with malignant tumors survive longer if their immune systems have been conditioned to respond to an odor that previously had been paired with a chemical immune booster that works naturally on its own. The conditioned stimulus, the odor, begins to work by itself to prompt immune activity, and keep the injected mice alive longer than mice whose immune defenses have not been trained in the additional way (Ghanta et al. 1987).

These hints from research on humans and animals provide the appreciative patient with a vital plan for action. You have a stake in the caregiver's physical and emotional health. Urge your helper to take time off for personal pleasures; encourage activities, such as exercise, that bolster physical health. Make concessions in timing your own needs so that caregivers can link their personal pleasures with naturally healthy pursuits, so that the pairing of activities renews them biologically.

## LAUGHTER: MEDICINE THAT ANYONE CAN PRESCRIBE

In his stage show *Monster in a Box,* the actor and monologist Spaulding Gray quips: "All the world's a hospital, and either you're a patient or a nurse" (Gray 1992, 37). As the U.S. population ages—14 percent will be sixty-five and older by the year 2000—it will be increasingly difficult to escape playing both roles sometime in the normal lifecycle.

Patients as well as their helpers have a vested interest in lightening the burden, and there's an indirect, even sly pathway toward relief that is commonly neglected. Depending on temperament, many people possess a powerful ally for restoring spirits, the funny bone. Shared reminiscences that bring a chuckle belong in this arsenal. Old howlers, too: "Did you hear the story about the rabbi, the priest, and the minister in a lifeboat?" Finding irony in the day's news counts as a strategy. Jests and witticisms and sight gags can help.

The humor we have in mind is diversionary, not focused on making light of the medical condition at stake. In wit and mirth, negative emotions are set aside for a while; or, as Freud suggested, "humor is a means of obtaining pleasure in spite of the distressing affects that interfere with it; it acts as a substitute for the generation of these affects, it puts itself in their place" (Freud 1960, 228). The scholar George Vaillant added that "humor is one of the truly elegant defenses in the human repertoire. Few would deny that the capacity for humor, like hope, is one of mankind's most potent antidotes for the woes of Pandora's box" (Vaillant 1977, 116).

Solid evidence now supports the anecdotal wisdom that positive emotional states strengthen the body's defenses against diseases, defenses that the strains of being a patient or a caregiver often weaken (Cogan et al. 1987; Carroll and Shmidt 1992). First of all, we often find sound general health among people who use humor in dealing with anxiety-provoking events. More significantly, though, laughter at humorous stories raises people's threshold for tolerating discomfort, acting as an antagonist to pain. Laughter buffers stress, relieving depressed moods and making people feel jolly.

One experiment, for example, showed a group of patients two videotapes: a humorous program, *Richard Pryor Live*, followed by an ordinary educational film (Dillon, Minchoff, and Baker 1985). After viewing the humor, salivary immunoglobulin increased, and held up even after the educational presentation. Immunoglobulin is an antibody that protects against respiratory and gastrointestinal tract infections; levels present in saliva are significantly associated with the avoidance of illness. Another study has demonstrated that people with a keen sense of humor maintain high levels of immunoglobulin concentration, even when they are faced with stressful incidents in their lives. By contrast, the immune system among people who are less easily amused suffers from life's hassles.

In short, a desire to improve your physical condition as well as state of mind can send you to the jokebook. A friend of ours, laid up with a blood clot, begged us to escort a mutual acquaintance to his bedside as often as we could. This acquaintance, Arthur, had retired from a career of writing jokes for famous comedians in broadcasting and the movies. He couldn't suppress his instinct for banter, one-liners, and spinning complicated yarns, and the hospital corridor rang with belly laughs. The traffic of caregivers through our friend's room never let up, each hoping that his or her visit would coincide with Arthur's.

Not many caregiving situations duplicate our friend's network and include a professional jokemeister. But reasons to chuckle surround anyone alert enough to find them. If a patient is too distracted to invent punch lines for his or her caregiver, then good friends can step in with their own joke book for inspiration. Listening to stand-up humor performances recorded on CDs or tapes works wonders, as does renting videocassettes of comedic films. Going to a movie may help, or asking a friend to stand in for the caregiver so that he or she can go out for laughs. There are lots of ways to crack a joke, and an entertainment industry stands ready to help.

## GOING TO CAREGIVING SCHOOL

Specialists have developed dozens of programs designed to fortify caregivers and other close friends to meet their responsibilities. Courses develop talents in caring and sometimes also relieve depression and other emotional reactions to the supportive role. Sometimes one-on-one sessions are used, sometimes group meetings. Programs may last for several weeks to several months, usually consisting of a regular series of one- to two-hour encounters.

Formal sessions may achieve their results in different ways. Some are *life satisfaction classes,* focusing on the relationship between pleasant activities and mood. Participants generate their own lists of pleasant events and discuss barriers that prevent them from achieving even greater levels of participation. Class members help other caregivers in the group to think through obstacles and to modify routines of helping in order to plan and carry out positive mood experiences.

Other programs emphasize *problem-solving exercises* for approaching everyday difficulties with patients who are disabled or infirm. Steps include achieving a calm state of mind before addressing a problem, listing potential solutions along with positive and negative points, and testing the chosen solution for satisfaction.

Still other classes explore *anger management,* in which the limitations of extreme reactions are revealed—from agitated venting of emotions to reserved suppression. Sessions start with relaxation training and move on to the identification of hostile, self-defeating talk and how to modify it. Assertiveness training is often included.

Which combination of these sorts of lessons works best for specific caregivers depends on how each person is adapting to the situation. Not everyone needs help in controlling anger, for example. Others are grimly efficient problem solvers but could use a little help in finding some joy in their lives, in lightening up. Others are quick to spot a silver lining but are clumsy problem solvers. Circumstances and needs obviously vary.

Nearly all caregiving courses achieve part of their effect from simply allowing people with a shared concern to talk with each other about their own experiences, fostering social comparisons. A program based at George Washington University takes advantage of this approach (Gonzalez, Steinglass, and Reiss 1987, 1989). This inventive program is called Multiple-Family Discussion Groups (MFDGs) and includes:

- four to six families whose ill members suffer *different* conditions;
- patients as well as caregivers joining together in the group;
- a structured curriculum in addition to opportunities for social comparison, all within only eight weekly sessions.

Multiple-Family Discussion Groups embrace a wide range of conditions—traumas such as spinal cord injury, kidney disease, multiple sclerosis, diabetes, stroke, Parkinson's disease, and chronic back pain, as well as illnesses that involve cognitive and emotional dysfunctions (schizophrenia, dementia, etc.). This ensures that the nuts and bolts of a particular illness get second billing, compared to exploring issues of family adjustment and coping.

Mixing different types of medical conditions and including the patients as well as the caregivers achieve other valued goals. Family members caring for sufferers of chronic medical conditions typically feel guilty about negative feelings they harbor toward the ill person and question the adequacy of their own efforts. Educational components in the MFDGs shift attention away from blaming and adversarial attitudes within families, and toward mutual support and problem solving. Each of the families, wrestling with its own condition, sees its problems reflected in the experiences of others. Feelings of isolation melt away.

By including patients, the format provides a safe forum for the air-ing of long-unspoken feelings within individual families. The presence of other families dilutes harsh and self-critical attitudes and opens discussion. Negative emotions, rarely discussed within families, come into the open, and everyone sees that many of the tensions they have been experiencing are not peculiar to their situation. Nor is stress a mark of family inadequacy.

The educational content of MFDGs has been designed around the following fact: Many long-term, debilitating conditions begin suddenly, and roles and responsibilities may need to change over the course of the illness or recovery from accident. In the first days of a severe heart attack or the first paralytic crisis in multiple sclerosis or the undeniable onset of dementia, the family mobilizes. With the help of professionals, decisions are swiftly made about who will care for the patient, who will fulfill other important family roles, and how lifestyles will change. As crisis fades into chronic care, however, many families should rethink early and hasty decisions. It may be a mistake to get locked into routines established during the height of confusion. Reconsidering the initial coping responses should not be viewed as an attack on family stability or on the earlier judgments made by people who had to respond suddenly.

The MFDG program conceives of the caregivers' stress as flowing from a vicious cycle. The process works this way. Coping with physical or cognitive deficits in the patient produces growing fatigue and loss of morale among caregivers. In time, all but the most serene turn critical and even hostile and find it increasingly difficult to mask these feelings. Caregivers often become overintrusive in managing the ill person, curtailing the patient's daily routines in an attempt to restore family life to normalcy or to maximize their own convenience. As caregivers' resentments become plain and as intrusive management limits the ill person's freedom, the patient reacts by withdrawing psychologically or getting angry. As a result, the ill person's physical and mental capacities may slump even more rapidly, as the section on taming the overzealous caregiver confirmed. Naturally, these reactions depress caregivers, and not just the primary person responsible. Other family members become saddened, matching the caregiver's mood. A wicked spiral sets in.

To combat this, the program asks both patients and caregivers to invoke an especially powerful metaphor. Participants are asked to picture the *illness* (as distinct from the patient) as a two-year-old terrorist who rules over the family with excessive and unpredictable demands and threatens catastrophic revenge if the demands are not met. Group members work together to separate the patient from the illness. They join forces to evaluate current coping strategies and experiment with even fairer and more satisfying ones.

The value of splitting the illness from the patient finds graphic demonstration in conditions like diabetes. Imagine that Jack, who has insulin-dependent diabetes, sinks into a hypoglycemic (low blood sugar) state and begins to act oddly. Sometimes he becomes aggressive, striking loved ones or wrecking household furnishings; other times he acts giddy, out of touch with reality. Rarely does he remember anything about these periods, during which time his wife, Laura, has had to manage alarming, hurtful, and uncontrollable impulses. Later, the couple is left with an ugly stain of emotions to tidy up. Jack resents his wife's nagging attempts at behavior control; his anger mingles with guilt and shame, once he finds out how bizarrely he acted. Laura, on the other hand, feels overwhelmed by helplessness.

These crippling emotions subside, however, if both patient and caregiver can draw a mental perimeter that isolates what happened during hypoglycemic episodes. As Laura explained: "When Jack gets that way, I know it's not him. He's being driven by blood chemistry, and anything he says or does toward me belongs to the out-of-control phase of our lives." Jack, fulfilling his part in this continuing arrangement, rewards Laura for her feats of forgiveness and unflagging willingness to split his Jekyll and Hyde behavior.

In summary, courses about caregiving point to one encouraging conclusion, regardless of the approach they take. Whether by formal instruction or social comparison, people can learn to master new skills. Caregivers can gain confidence in their new and demanding roles—from managing crises such as seizures, to handling mundane tasks such as toileting. Caregivers can reduce the patient's anxieties and their own.

Many community agencies—such as junior colleges, university medical centers, and disease-related associations (cancer, heart, lung, etc.)—offer caregiving classes. Ill people, where they are able, can do themselves and their caregivers a favor by enrolling in such courses, or at the least by making concessions in their own needs so that caregivers can attend.

## DEFEATING FATIGUE

This chapter has already shared many tips for bolstering the caregiver. In addition, we have culled a battle plan for appreciative patients to follow or to plead that others undertake. A wealth of studies confirms that when a patient lacks the insight or energy to launch the fight against caregiver burnout, others must intervene.

Psychologists have interviewed caregivers, asking them to reflect on the problems they face and the actions, feelings, and sentiments that the problems provoke. How have the caregivers tried to manage their difficulties? Results point the way toward controlling anxiety, irascibility, and other disturbances that caregivers experience (Pearlin et al. 1990).

***Sizing Up the Situation.*** If you are a caregiver, getting your thoughts on paper can be indispensable. Find a quiet nook, away from distractions, and try to answer these questions:

- What is your general level of energy? Do you feel exhausted when you go to bed, that you have more things than you can handle, or that you don't have any time just for yourself? Do you feel that you just don't seem to make any progress?
- What is your relationship to the patient: Have you lost the ability to confide in him or her? Are you dealing with someone who no longer knows you well?
- What about goals and activities? Have you lost the chance to do things you planned, or lost contact with people?
- Have family conflicts arisen—over the seriousness of the patient's mental or physical problems, about what things the patient should be able to do for himself or herself, or whether he or she should be placed in a special care facility?
- How do other family members relate to the patient? Do they spend enough time with him or her, assume their fair share of caring, and show appropriate respect and patience? How about your relationships with other family members: Do they phone you enough, show appreciation for what you do, shower you with unwanted advice?
- How has caregiving affected your job performance or your career ambitions? Has caregiving chipped away at your sense of who you are as a person?

- Consider the positive outcomes of caregiving and get these down on paper, too. Perhaps you have gained pride in learning how to deal with a difficult situation, revealed your inner strengths, or grown as a person.

Let the ideas you have written gel for a few days. When you return to your notes, divide the thoughts and feelings into topics you need to discuss with a professional source of advice—physician or other counselor—and those you need to take up directly with family, friends, or colleagues from work. Which should be the topics for intimate talk between caregiver and patient? Each partner may silently crave more candor. Both may be crippled by the tendency to keep mum about conflicts and to bottle emotions until they flare into rage or profound helplessness.

***Getting Social Support to Caregivers.*** Drawing up an inventory of social support can help the caregiver as much as someone beset with a personal health problem. Here, we turn the tables to look at these contacts the other way around, from the standpoint of people who should reach out to comfort the caregiver. Friends and family can ease the caregiving burden by offering to help or extending sympathy. Patients can trigger these overtures, thereby doing themselves a favor. A few concrete suggestions make the point.

1. *For the caregiver who lacks time for "self-indulgent" activities.* A friend or other family member should offer to take over the patient for a half-day, so the caregiver can shop for clothes, visit with friends, go to the library or movies, enjoy a restaurant meal, sit calmly in church, or whatever seems restorative.
2. *For the caregiver who has lost intimate exchange with others.* Suggest substitutions—finding a new partner for confidences, or joining a leisure-time group that can gather, at least occasionally, in the caregiver's home.
3. *For the caregiver with family conflicts.* Nominate a person who is truly detached as a mediator of the most irritating disputes.
4. *For the caregiver whose work has suffered.* Suggest a frank meeting with the boss to negotiate over responsibilities, in light of demands that patient supervision places. Recommend a guidebook about the disease or condition (dementia, spinal cord injuries, etc.) that the caregiver can share with his or her supervisor.
5. *For the caregiver with an impaired sense of self.* Some family member or friend should ask if that person would like to talk about any of these topics

(and respect the response this prompts). Whoever makes this overture should offer tolerant and supportive feedback; reading of caregiving manuals might help show the way.

Sifting through first-person accounts by physicians, caregivers, and patients uncovers nuggets of other helpful ideas, too. Jean Craig's tale of supporting a dying husband includes these insights:

> Any time people have the chance to help with someone bedridden at home, they should. There are few times when help will mean as much. The best thing to do is come as a twosome, with one person staying with the sick person for an hour and the other taking the caretaker out for a drink or a meal.
>
> Remember. It's very hard. When you ask "Is there anything I can do?" you put the onus on the beleaguered caretaker to find a way to let you help. Instead, find a way yourself. (Craig 1991, 70)

Another suggestion comes from a humane physician, with advice that any friend of a caregiver might imitate: "A cancer surgeon I know always holds his patient's hand when he visits—he tells me that, in this way, a *short* visit to the bedside is perceived by the patient as being longer than it really is" (Stone 1990, 27). Friends of caregivers hold hands with them, or touch them in supportive, sincere ways. Visits that include, literally, "reaching out" offer a potent blend of personal warmth and restorative energy.

*Understanding and Hope for Caregivers.* Those who would support caregivers must understand that it is not the patient's actual condition that controls how well the caregiver copes, but rather the caregiver's perspective on the situation. Furthermore, the greatest emotional difficulties often stem from deciding whether the patient still fits into family life and in which ways. All is not bleak: Caregivers can gain in self-esteem from their role, discovering and savoring hidden qualities in themselves. The battle against burnout demands attention to all these features of a difficult and often inescapable role.

## CHAPTER 5

# Protecting Your Choices in Critical Care

IN THIS BOOK you've learned how important it is to take control of your health-care encounters by communicating fully with the medical team—asking questions, using nonverbal tactics, weighing options—and by enlisting the comfort of family and friends. What about the unpleasant, yet commonplace experience of being in a medical situation and *not having the ability* to make decisions and communicate them? For just a moment, imagine that a fateful affliction or accident befalls you. Suppose that an auto crash or a stroke leaves you in a long-term coma. Or Alzheimer's disease overtakes you, muddling your thinking and leaving you unresponsive. In such cases and many others, who would make decisions about medical care that express your preferences?

These types of circumstances motivated all fifty states to develop legal documents called *advance directives;* federal law also encourages their use. Advance directives, accomplished through documents such as a Living Will or a Medical Power of Attorney, became widely available in the 1990s and represent a major advance beyond the basics of informed consent. Advance directives are the forms people use to express the kinds of treatment they would want, and the treatments that they prefer to refuse, if they become unable to make decisions and communicate during a medical crisis. Directives are the patient's surest form of insurance against losing control of health-care choices in case of an incapacitating illness or accident.

Since 1914, the highest courts have recognized the requirement that every competent patient grant permission before medical treatments are administered. Advance directives are a natural extension of those rulings, ensuring patient control even in situations where decision making and communication are impaired.

More recently, ethicists have focused on the benefits and the limits of sophisticated medical technologies and their ability to support life in the face of virulent disease and near-fatal accident. Sometimes in using these technologies, the patient is left with a quality of life that he or she would rather refuse. These situations traumatize families who all too often split into warring camps. One argues that "Mom would never have chosen to live like this," while the other branch protests that "she always wanted to live life to the fullest." Physicians are trapped in the crossfire and often have no recourse except to continue medical treatment indefinitely. Without the patient's expressed wishes to guide them, families often face a residue of bitter feuds and guilt. Confusion and chaos replace dignity in someone's final stage of life.

This chapter shows the way around such a dilemma. You'll learn about advance directives and how they work. Importantly, the following pages will help you explore your feelings and values about critical-care choices and will offer guidance for conversations with family, friends, and professionals. Sharing wishes about life support—whether as a prelude to signing an advance directive or just for its own sake—reduces the chances of family bickering and recriminations later.

## PATIENTS' AND PHYSICIANS' POINTS OF VIEW

When options for critical-care treatment arise and the patient lacks an advance directive, a doctor's care can be unpredictable. Moreover, if the directive is not in the hands of people who can insist that it be honored, the form might as well not exist in the first place. The story of Edward underscores the pivotal importance of a written and available expression of your wishes. He was seventy-eight and a case like many others that hospitals must resolve every day. Edward had a history of severe emphysema from many years of working in heavy industry. He was admitted to the Intensive Care Unit (ICU) with pneumonia, abnormally low blood pressure, and respiratory failure. He was given antibiotics and medications to strengthen circulatory functions; he also required mechanical breathing to survive. Then, he lapsed into a coma. The ICU's lung specialist judged that Edward could never live without a ventilator again. Three weeks later, Edward was still in a coma and showed no signs of improvement, despite the other treatments.

After a recent, prior hospitalization, Edward had told family and doctors that he would never want to prolong his life by artificial means. Recognizing these previously expressed wishes, made *orally but not in writing,* the family asked the attending doctor to withdraw life support. The doctor was faced with the decision: Keep Edward on the ventilator and medications, or suspend such interventions. What will happen?

To feel the significance of this, place yourself in Edward's shoes. Suppose you prayed with your every fiber to be allowed to let go and die peacefully. Now, regrettably, your voice has fallen still; coma has stolen your capacity to make and express decisions. No one can reliably predict how your physician will act. It is far from certain that the doctor would recognize your previously *spoken* wishes, fearing legal repercussions. Chances of this range from nil to probably, depending on factors that would then lie outside your control. And, as you will shortly learn, doctors vary in their own practices for withdrawing life support, even when the decision has been reached to do so.

Your physician might be slow to heed the family's requests, for example, depending on whether he or she has much experience with cases in the ICU. When they judge the situation hopeless, physicians who routinely witness trauma and conflicts over life support tend to conform with patients' stated preferences favoring withdrawal. These doctors are intimately familiar with balancing the restorative promise of high-technology medicine against its power to continue patients in a low quality of life. On the other hand, doctors less familiar with everyday despair in an ICU are reluctant to yield to requests to withdraw treatment, even when they know that a patient has said as much.

One recent survey of doctors showed that they were divided sharply over whether or not to defer to the request from Edward's family. Some would have, while others would not. To retain your voice in these matters, doctors need to see a legally binding advance directive that records the patient's preferences or appoints someone (e.g., family member or friend) as a health-care spokesperson.

## THE COMPLEXITIES OF THINKING ABOUT CRITICAL CARE

Congress passed the Patient Self-Determination Act in 1990, insisting that each of the states refine legal documents called *advance directives.* The Act also required medical providers to distribute these directives to patients during the admissions process—in places like hospitals, nursing homes, hospices, and other care centers—and to offer educational guidance about critical-care choices. Providers could not, however, discriminate in their care of patients according to whether or not they had completed a directive, nor could they compel patients to sign documents.

Three kinds of directives have emerged from approaches that different states have taken. First, all but a handful of states have enacted *Living Will* statutes; these include a document that directs doctors about care preferences when the signer later becomes incapacitated. A second option that most states offer is the *Medical Power of Attorney;* the signer appoints an individual to make health-care decisions, in case the signer becomes incapacitated. Some states allow yet another option, the *Medical Directive,* which is a hybrid of the Living Will and Medical Power of Attorney. Using this form, the signer provides precise instructions for the type of care he or she does or does not want. The individual may also appoint a partner (also called an agent, proxy, surrogate, or attorney-in-fact) to help interpret these instructions.

In spite of the availability and value of advance directives, most people haven't yet completed one. As surveys of U.S. adults show, you have lots of company if you haven't taken action before now (Layson et al. 1994). You may have thought at least fitfully about your future care, especially if you've known other people who received elaborate life support while in a hopeless condition and couldn't stop the heroic medical procedures because they had lost competence. It is also true, by wide margins, that people who want to express their preferences for care seek a less aggressive use of life-sustaining treatments, not a greater use of medical technology. Nonetheless, only about 15 percent of adults have completed an advance directive, compared to approximately 40 percent who have executed a will covering their financial estate.

What is the logjam that stymies advance directives? In order to dig more deeply into people's feeling and clarify misconceptions, we conducted a series of focus groups with seniors (over age fifty-five), as well as one-on-one interviews with individuals of all ages. We have also talked with thousands of people as part of research in collaboration with the American Association of Critical-Care Nurses. Our wide-ranging conversations covered worries about health care, knowledge and feelings about advance directives, experiences watching other people handle critical-care decisions, and more.

From this research program we developed a home-based *Guide to Critical-Care Choices* that helps people decide about medical treatment in case they become incapacitated. The United States Agency for Health Care Policy and Research and several foundations have supported our work. This chapter provides the most important portions of the *Guide* and reflects the exhaustive research that shaped it.

Results of our studies have highlighted the complexities of thinking about critical-care choices (Evans and Clarke 1993). Some of the findings point to a number of important reasons why people are enthusiastic about the protections that directives are designed to provide, but hang back from completing the forms. Other results underscore how frequently people sign the documents but actually misunderstand their intent and legal standing. Out of these hours of talk, a number of themes emerged.

***Seniors Are Comfortable but Still May Be Stymied.***  Contrary to popular belief, older people were more than willing to discuss their preferences about various critical-care situations. Most of them had firmly held beliefs about what they wanted done. Several groups of discussants made their feelings known in a chorus: "When you get to our age, you've had friends who didn't get the type of treatment they wanted from doctors when the time came. We all know about these issues." By contrast, young and middle-aged family members tiptoe around the subject, cloaking it with an unnecessary air of mystery and delicacy. In many cases, elders are reluctant to complete a directive because they sense that younger family members are skittish, unable, or unwilling to face the topic. Thus, seniors refrain from raising the topic, while their younger family members (who could serve as health-care partners) are too timid to open the conversation.

An experience of the novelist Philip Roth demonstrates the problem. His father was in swift decline from a brain tumor when Roth tried to work up the courage to ask him to sign a Living Will while he was still coherent. One evening, Roth recalls, he dined at his father's home, armed with his own Living Will (completed earlier that day) as evidence of the wisdom underlying these documents. However, when the housekeeper ushered the son into his father's bedroom, Roth found an even more wasted and enfeebled man than he had expected from previous visits, profoundly depressed by an embarrassing fall in the bathroom.

"I couldn't do it," Roth confessed, leaving his father's advance directive form sealed in its manila envelope. "Instead of explaining what a Living Will was and why I wanted him to have one, I tried to get his mind as far from death as I could by telling him about a book that I'd just finished reading." The evening passed with reminiscences about Jewish boxers and their championship bouts. Roth left several hours later, thinking that "maybe it was a mistake to force him to face the most bitter of all possibilities" (Roth 1991, 201, 204).

The next day, emboldened by early morning light, the son managed to call his father to read the form's clauses. He almost gagged over phrases like "nasogastric tube feeding," "mechanical respiration," and "heart resuscitation." Finally, he blurted out the bottom-line question: "So? How does it strike you?"

"Send it over and I'll sign," his father said, stunning Roth with his matter-of-fact tone (Roth 1991, 206).

*Exaggerated Expectations.* A second hesitancy to completing directives can be blamed ironically on inflated beliefs that they streamline the emotional anguish over end-of-life decisions. That's unrealistic: A legally-binding document expressing the patient's wishes doesn't banish heartbreak at the moment of truth; a directive does not dilute grief and sorrow. The final event of the Roth family drama, for example, took place at death's bedside, when the son abided by his father's wishes in his recently completed document. In the face of resistance from a stubborn and reluctant doctor, the son asked that his father's breathing machine be turned off. Roth wept and experienced self-doubts. In short, a directive sets down a plan for decision making, but it does not numb human emotions.

*A Gulf Between Patient and Doctor.* To our initial surprise, many people do not want to discuss end-of-life matters with physicians. They either do not have a personal relationship with their doctors, or they don't see the same physician from visit to visit—as in many HMOs. Others suggest that doctors aren't trusted authorities on this topic because they lack training to deal with the issues ("they know about health . . . not death"); because they lack time for unhurried talk; and because the physician may be seen to have a conflict of interest ("the longer I am on a machine, the more money they make," said a number of people). Other people in our discussions resented paying for an office visit in order to discuss their advance directive.

The public's reluctance to turn to physicians for guidance actually runs parallel to doctors' routine behavior. Surveys of physicians commonly show that few initiate contacts, even with elderly patients, about critical care unless they are taking part in a special study that arranges for them to do this. Candidly, doctors are neither trained nor reimbursed for time-consuming talk about the quality of life their patients want to maintain.

It is unfortunate when discussions about end-of-life decisions fail to take place in the clinical setting. Both patients and doctors lose out when doctors resist being drawn into advance planning. After all, it is the doctor who carries out medical decisions and needs to feel confident he or she is complying with a patient's informed and considered wishes.

*Confusion over Terminology and Procedures.*  Many people have very clear feelings concerning life support but remain thoroughly confused by procedures and terminology. To illustrate, many harbor unrealistic ideas about a procedure such as cardiopulmonary resuscitation (CPR)—the nature of this treatment, the benefits, the risks, and the failure rates with frail patients. People who don't understand are hardly to blame. Television has so often dramatized scenes where a patient goes into "cardiac arrest," a medical squad rushes into action with drugs and electric paddles and, within seconds, a normal heart beat is restored on the monitor at bedside. Emergency-room doctors call these depictions the "Hollywood Code," fictional accounts that defy the real danger associated with CPR and the odds of recovery, especially among elderly people.

*Just Signing on the Dotted Line Is Not Enough.*  Many people who had already completed a directive were shocked to discover, once they saw the *Guide,* that their earlier decision had overlooked crucial options. These people had not confronted many issues about quality of life, medical procedures, and preferences about care, usually because the documents they signed and short pamphlets they read failed to disclose important considerations. Sometimes indifferent or uninformed counselors had lulled these individuals into trusting that their signature on a standard form would adequately convey deep values and serious intentions. With the help of the *Guide,* these people explored wishes about care and medical situations they hadn't imagined. Some updated their advance directive; others decided to substitute a Medical Power of Attorney for the original Living Will they had completed. Others were prompted by the materials to initiate discussions with family, medical professionals, clergy, and others. As one woman summed it up: "I used to think of this issue as black and white; now I see the gray areas."

***Don't Hide the Document.*** We have also found another mistake in a disturbing number of cases where people have already executed an advance directive. They have squirreled the forms away, in a desk drawer at home, a safe-deposit box, or elsewhere. These people will be out of luck if a crisis arises where they cannot make decisions for themselves. Doctors will not know what the directive stipulates, or even that it exists. In all likelihood, family members will not think to retrieve it. Instead of archiving a directive—in the way that one preserves financial wills, deeds, and other materials reviewed after death—people need to distribute their health-care document widely. They should send copies to every doctor (general practitioner and specialists, whether in private practice, an HMO, or elsewhere) who might be called upon for care. Copies should go to a spouse or long-term companion, to adult children, other close family, or friends, or clergy. People completing a directive should publicize the news of what they want, so others can learn their wishes firsthand and speak up when the hour of need arrives.

***The Document and the Process of Signing Appear Superficial.*** Ironically, the "apparent" ease of executing an advance directive can seem to trivialize its decisions concerning critical-care choices. Many people have learned that an attorney is not needed to complete the forms. Although this is a reassuring simplification to many, it is an unsettling fact to others who can't believe that an important and binding statement can be issued without a lawyer's consultation and wax seal. Legitimacy of the documents is further weakened in some eyes when forms are provided on tear-off pads, or available over-the-counter in the hospital gift shop. This lends an air of casualness to the directive and the decision making that they don't deserve.

*Men and Women May Differ.*  Gender differences in decision-making strategies complicate the picture. Men are often apprehensive about relin-
quishing control to anyone else. They worry that by nominating their
wife or adult child as their voice, as in a Medical Power of Attorney,
they will be saddling that person with too heavy a burden. Other men
can't abide the thought of handing over any reins of authority. Women,
on the other hand, often think more about the negative consequences
of not completing an advance directive, the messiness this creates in
one's affairs. They want to tidy up the loose ends and get things in order.
But they may have deferred to their husband's values across decades of
marriage. As long as both spouses are alive, conflicting sentiments neu-
tralize the family unit into inaction; nobody takes the first step.

*The Wrong Time to Complete a Directive.*  Federal law requires that hospitals and skilled-nursing facilities ask patients upon admission whether
they have completed an advance directive. If not, the institution is
required to offer educational materials. Nearly all our research participants agreed that the time of admission to a medical facility is the
worst hour to seriously consider critical-care choices for the first time.
In fact, when incoming patients are approached about directives, some
fear that physicians' interest in their welfare depends on whether or
not they sign even though the law mandates otherwise. Our studies
confirm this conclusion: The period of stress over impending medical
procedures is not the occasion to consider advance directives. Such
untimely introduction to advance directives aggravates an already nerve-
wracking situation.

The *Guide* lays these confusions to rest. In the pages that follow,
we urge you to consider issues concerning advance directives at home,
a relaxed and comforting place. You will find easy-to-read sections that
can be shared with other family members or friends. Before you begin,
though, you have a right to understand just how unpredictable end-of-
life care can be, when there are no written instructions to inform the
medical team.

## DOCTORS AND END-OF-LIFE CHOICES
Everyone can take comfort in one irreversible trend. In contrast to
twenty years ago, it is now widely agreed among medical ethicists that
patients may forgo life-sustaining treatments that they do not wish.

Repeated surveys show that the public applauds this principle (Patrick et al. 1997; Singer et al. 1995). In fact, nearly every physician has discontinued at least one form of treatment, with the expectation that the patient would die as a result. They judged the situation medically futile; continued efforts provided "no significant chance for survival *per se* or for a meaningful survival . . . in relation to the patient's values and life goals," as one medical society's official position states it. (Schneiderman, Jecker, and Jonsen 1996; Society of Critical Care Medicine 1997)

There are also grounds to fear that wishes may not be obeyed when the time comes for critical care. Recent surveys of doctors have found a disturbing number who concede that they often overtreat the desperately ill with burdensome and fruitless procedures and provide less pain relief than patients want (Solomon et al. 1993). Some providers simply haven't learned about national recommendations and legal provisions that allow the withholding and withdrawal of such measures as artificial nutrition and hydration if patients want to forgo these. More than a third of clinicians, for example, appear unaware that many dying patients do not experience hunger and that dehydration may actually reduce suffering in the final hours of life (Burge 1996; Fainsinger and Bruera 1997). In other words, numerous practicing physicians have not kept pace with the growing professional consensus behind advance directives, spearheaded by the American Medical Association, the American Association of Critical-Care Nurses, and other major specialty societies.

Professional groups and governmental bodies have written guidelines for the ethical withholding or withdrawing of care for patients who ask that this be done. These measures differ from physician-assisted suicide which occurs when someone initiates procedures (e.g., injections) intended to end life.

We can use Edward's case, recounted earlier, to show how variable a physician's response can be. For example, the physician's ICU experience plays a role. Other characteristics may also affect the doctor's decision to agree to, or resist a plea for, withdrawal of support (Asch, Hansen-Flaschen, and Lauken 1995; Asch and Christakis 1996; Christakis and Asch 1993, 1995). Younger doctors respond to these wishes with greater ease than older ones; their more recent training has highlighted today's respect for patient rights. Teaching and referral hospitals are more likely to honor preferences to end life support than are primary-care facilities.

Doctors' own style of decision making also drives many to pursue extraordinary measures. Some feel personally chagrined when they have been unable to prevent patients from sliding into decline. These physicians tend to keep patients on a ventilator and apply cardiopulmonary resuscitation (CPR), for example, when other providers would hold back from using such treatments to prolong life.

Even doctors' specialty comes into play. Cardiologists tend to view CPR and other intensive care favorably because they work well for patients with acute heart disease. By contrast, cancer patients are less likely to survive CPR. Accordingly, oncologists have learned to be conservative in applying this and other procedures to prolong life (Hanson et al. 1996).

Uncertainty about ending treatments doesn't stop here. The manner by which critically ill patients are allowed to die also varies. A patient may be on several types of support at once, any of which might be withdrawn. Studies have looked closely at how doctors choose among these options, once the decision to allow withdrawal has been made. The results suggest why some doctors, in some situations, may shrink from deciding to withdraw or withhold treatment in the first place. To allow death would require suspending an intervention they are reluctant to deny.

These attitudes are rooted in occupational preferences, much more than in expected discomfort to the dying patient. By wide margins, doctors prefer to withdraw life supports that have been in place for just a few days, over those that have been in place for months, thereby bending to the bias of sunk costs (see chapter 2). They also approve of withdrawing supports required by an underlying disease, more than those necessitated by complications from errors in treatment or diagnostic procedures. They lean toward withdrawing measures that would lead to swift death (a few minutes or hours) over death within a day or two.

Doctors draw other distinctions. They are more willing to suspend the use of blood products and dialysis than mechanical ventilation, tube feeding, and intravenous fluids (see Common Medical Treatments and Glossary of Critical-Care Terminology). Ironically, with effective pain management and palliative care (see below), there is little reason to favor any one measure over others. From a comatose and terminal patient's standpoint, death from chronic organ failure is the same as from acute failure, and death in a few hours no worse than a few minutes.

It's easy to see how conflict aroused by beliefs about the "proper" withdrawal of life support could baffle a medical team. Imagine a severely ill patient who is now in a coma but had earlier expressed the desire to avoid mechanical life supports. A bronchoscopic biopsy of a mass in her lung shows an aggressive and inoperable cancer, which other tests reveal has spread to her brain. Unfortunately, through an error in technique, the bronchoscopy was performed with the wrong biopsy needle, resulting in hemorrhage and the need for mechanical breathing.

Alas, this patient now has two strikes against achieving her medical preferences. First, withdrawal of machine-assisted breathing as a means of ending life support troubles many doctors, whatever the circumstances. On top of that, doctors shy away from withdrawing treatment that has been required because of a clinical mistake. Will this patient's life be allowed to end soon? After all, there's no way to reverse the biopsy error now. Or will she be kept alive for days or weeks, extending her family's emotional pain and draining the patient's financial resources until some other feature of her condition calls for critical care, which can then be withheld?

These are the uncertainties that can shadow people who have neglected to put their wishes about critical care in writing. Confusion and mystery also shroud people's thinking about pain relief during episodes of critical care. You can use your advance directive to instruct others that you want the maximum control of pain, consistent with the level of life support being administered.

Medical breakthroughs in certain conditions have brought new ways to control pain, supplementing or even replacing analgesic drugs that bear a stigma for some patients. For example, care for cancer that has spread to bones has traditionally combined radiation therapy with gradually increased doses of opiates. Now, many cases can be treated with bone-seeking radiopharmaceuticals that suppress pain, leave the patient more alert, and reduce the rate at which new painful sites develop. In the case of pancreatic cancer, surgery may be prescribed for purely palliative purposes, not to control or eliminate the disease.

In many cases, though, strong opiates are required to relieve physical pain and symptoms. Since 1986, the World Health Organization has endorsed a "stepped-care" method of pain control that embraces the use of morphine in medical situations after weaker opiates have been exhausted. Nonetheless, studies show that prescriptions of morphine and other strong opiates fall far short of the amount that one would predict from the numbers and kinds of cancers present in the U.S. population (Rhymes 1996).

Why is this so? Partly, because many patients underreport their pain. Almost half, in some categories of disease, believe that good patients do not complain, or that the discomfort they experience is inevitable (Ward et al. 1993). As one consequence, clinicians routinely underestimate the pain their patients are in. It's not uncommon to find as many as four of ten cancer outpatients, for example, significantly undermedicated, even when pain interferes with daily activities.

Surprisingly as well, some physicians remain unaware of how effective opiates are in suppressing pain, when used in adequate doses; in fact, 75 to 90 percent of cancer pain in terminally ill patients is well controlled using the stepped-care approach (World Health Organization 1986). Furthermore, many patients and their families don't know about hospice care as a medical option (see chapter 2). Physicians at hospices—home-based services as well as residential ones—subscribe to stepped-care and other aspects of effective palliative treatment. In fact, much of today's enthusiasm for doctor-assisted suicide (active euthanasia) might wane if people had greater knowledge about the effectiveness of modern medications and other means of suppressing pain.

Some of health-care professionals' reluctance to prescribe pain medications grows out of a needless concern about addiction among the terminally ill. In addition, doctors are generally overly optimistic when predicting how long their patients will survive; care that relentlessly searches for a cure instead of opting for comfort postpones adequate dosages of pain medications (von Gunten and Twaddle 1996). Doctors may be excessively concerned with respiratory depression, thinking that morphine is only appropriate near death. Some physicians may be unaware that early and liberal use of morphine still leaves the patient with access to stronger agents if pain intensifies. Or more simply, the illegitimate atmosphere surrounding the use of strong opiates, prompted by substance-abuse programs aimed at the healthy, warps clinical judgment.

Patients who grow frustrated with their doctor's schedule of medication need to understand, however, that many factors govern the choice among analgesics—for malignant or nonmalignant pain. The body metabolizes various drugs differently, and people vary in their own metabolic rates. These matters affect a drug's absorption and potency. Convenience of administration may also enter the picture. Medical staffs usually prefer longer intervals of administration over shorter ones. Drugs with similar effects across patients are easier to manage than drugs that vary widely (morphine compared to methadone, for example). Sometimes, doctors need to consider whether the usefulness of a drug declines with sustained or frequent use, compared to short-term administrations.

Some drugs are avoided because they commonly require escalated dosages and may only reveal their toxic side effects long into a period of use, when it's too late to correct the damage. Or, a drug may risk interacting with other medications a patient may be taking. Drugs differ in their cost, and that can influence prescription.

In the final analysis, a patient may need to consult a specialist in palliative care or one in pain management. Each of these fields is a recognized part of the curriculum in most top medical schools. There's nothing embarrassing or out-of-bounds in asking for a referral to such specialists whenever someone suffers persistent pain.

When pain drags on, a patient and family also need frank words with each other. Studies show that caregivers and their ailing loved one differ about as often as they agree concerning pain (Ward, Berry, and Misiewicz 1996). Many caregiver and patient pairs silently disagree about whether pain should be reported to the doctor. They differ in willingness to use strong medications and harbor different fears about side effects like addiction. One denies pain, seeing it as a sure sign that disease is getting worse; the other doesn't share this anxiety. The chances for effective palliative care plunge if such disagreements remain hidden or unresolved.

## ADVANCE DIRECTIVES: MAKING CRITICAL-CARE DECISIONS, STEP-BY-STEP

The following sections bring you highlights from the *Guide,* which separates the process of making critical-care decisions into bite-sized chunks. Completing an advance directive involves examining your feelings about life-support systems, pain, and the effect of your choices on family or friends. People have very different preferences about such matters. For some, decision making may take a few weeks. For others, it may take a shorter or longer period of time. Whatever your situation, the first step is to understand how talking about and completing an advance directive can protect your choices and ease the burden on loved ones.

You can skip around and read the following eight sections in any order that makes sense to you, but we suggest that you at least skim each of the steps.

**1.** Learn about the major types of advance directives.
**2.** Discover your beliefs about critical-care choices.
**3.** Talk with your family, friends, and health-care partner.
**4.** Talk with doctors, nurses, lawyers, or clergy about advance directives.
**5.** Help your partner understand his or her responsibilities.
**6.** Understand some critical-care terminology.
**7.** Express wishes about comfort (palliative) care.
**8.** Complete and distribute your advance directive.

## 1.  *LEARN ABOUT THE MAJOR TYPES OF ADVANCE DIRECTIVES*

Advance directives are written statements, made in advance, that contain your instructions about your health care or appoint someone to make your medical decisions, if you become unable to decide and communicate those wishes for yourself. These documents can describe the kind of care you want; likewise, they can identify treatment and procedures that you prefer to refuse under particular conditions. Physicians and family members can refer to these documents if the need should arise.

A *Living Will* (also called a *Declaration*) is a general term for a document that expresses your wishes about medical treatment at the end of your life. It takes effect only in situations of terminal illness or permanent unconsciousness (check your state's guidelines and forms) and indicates those life-prolonging or life-sustaining treatments that you would like to have withheld or withdrawn. Your written instructions can guide your doctor and act as your voice if you cannot make your own decisions. You do not need a lawyer, loved one, or friend to complete a Living Will document. A copy of the California Living Will is included in Examples of Advance Directives and Wallet Card.

Here are two medical situations—one in which the patient had completed a Living Will and another in which the patient had not.

Charlie, eighty-four years old, had been admitted to the hospital for heart surgery. Following the operation, he was extremely ill. Not only was his heart failing, but his kidneys and lungs were not functioning well. He needed a ventilator to help him breathe and nutrition through a feeding tube inserted down his nose into his stomach. The build-up of toxins made him unable to make coherent decisions.

Charlie had never been married and had few remaining close relatives. A few years ago, he had chosen to write down his preferences concerning future medical care in a Living Will. He stipulated that he didn't want life support or aggressive treatments if he were terminally ill.

The physicians monitored his condition and, after a week, noted that he was deteriorating. Charlie was not conscious. The doctors realized that they must either start kidney dialysis and hope his kidneys improved or allow him to die peacefully. Because Charlie had no family to consult and he was unable to make a decision for himself, his physicians used his Living Will as a guide. They decided further treatment would not provide any benefit but would merely prolong his dying. The physicians decided not to start the dialysis and treated Charlie for any pain and discomfort he might experience.

■

Marilyn, eighty-eight years old, lost her husband years ago but remained in the home in which they spent most of their lives together. Six years ago, when Marilyn was eighty-two, she was diagnosed with breast cancer and treated with surgery, radiation, and chemotherapy. Just recently, her doctors told her that the cancer had spread to her bones and that they would help her deal with the considerable amount of pain that she could expect.

Marilyn consented to chemotherapy, but she did not discuss her feelings about any other treatments—except that she wanted to be as free of pain as possible. She never completed a Living Will stating her preferences.

Marilyn's physical condition began to deteriorate, and she was hospitalized. She became bedridden and unable to eat or drink on her own. Her weight dropped to ninety-six pounds. Importantly, Marilyn also became disoriented and unable to recognize her physicians or a neighbor who often came to see her. Her doctors judged her to be mentally incapacitated.

Marilyn then developed pneumonia. The doctors placed her on tube feeding and treated her with antibiotics, in addition to prescribing pain medication for her advancing cancer. They also continued her chemotherapy; this, along with the life supports—artificial feeding and antibiotics—prolonged Marilyn's survival. She eventually died from her bone cancer two months after a costly hospitalization. Toward the end, she was emaciated and completely noncommunicative.

What do these two cases teach us? First, as in Charlie's case, a Living Will only becomes activated in situations where the patient is terminally ill or permanently unconscious. If Charlie could have made decisions and communicated them, the Living Will would not have been consulted. Marilyn, as well, could have avoided artificial feeding, prolonged chemotherapy, and treatment for pneumonia through a Living Will. Such procedures would have been halted, once two physicians agreed that she had reached a terminal condition. Second, a Living Will allows the signer to list treatments that are not wanted. A third feature of Living Wills is that they do not require naming anyone else in communicating preferences about health care. The signer can complete the form without appointing a family member or friend as the signer's spokesperson. The signer of a Living Will should discuss his or her wishes with others, however, since this will help avoid disagreements and misunderstandings if the Living Will must be consulted.

A *Medical Power of Attorney* is a document in which you choose a person to make medical decisions for you when you are no longer able to decide and communicate for yourself. This document is often called a *Durable Power of Attorney for Health Care Decisions* (see one state's version in Examples of Advance Directives and Wallet Card). It differs from a Living Will in two important ways. First, a Medical Power of Attorney enables you to name a health-care partner who legally expresses your wishes about your medical treatment when you are mentally incapacitated. To complete a Medical Power of Attorney, you must appoint a health-care partner (also called an attorney-in-fact, an agent, a surrogate, or a proxy). Your partner is responsible for carrying out your instructions by talking to your doctor if you are ever so ill that you can't make decisions and communicate for yourself. Second, a Medical Power of Attorney becomes activated *in any situation* in which you are unable to make decisions for yourself (for example, Alzheimer's, a severe stroke, a coma, or many other conditions) whether the circumstances are terminal or not. The Medical Power of Attorney is a broader and a more flexible document than a Living Will, but an individual may not have someone he or she feels comfortable appointing (see Step 3), or perhaps peers are in poor health or unable to handle the responsibility.

Here are two medical situations—one with a Medical Power of Attorney and one without the document.

Linda had Alzheimer's disease. She was unable to make decisions or function on her own and had been in a nursing home for fifteen years. Linda had a Medical Power of Attorney, in which she named her daughter Mary as her partner. In the course of their discussions before completing the Medical Power of Attorney, Linda told her daughter that if she ever needed life-sustaining treatment, she would want the doctors to give her a trial period of treatment to see if her condition improved.

Linda developed pneumonia and became dehydrated and seriously ill. The doctor told Mary that her mother was unable to eat or breathe on her own and recommended antibiotics, a feeding tube, and a ventilator to stabilize her condition. Mary wanted to try everything she could to help her mother, but her father had his doubts. He did not want to see his wife suffer needlessly or become dependent on tubes and machines. However, Mary understood that as her mother's partner in the Medical Power of Attorney she must think of what *her mother* expressed as her wishes, not what she herself or her father might want.

The physician talked with Mary and her father and followed Mary's instructions to pursue treatment for a trial period. He monitored progress over several weeks. When he saw no hope for improvement, he talked to Mary and her father again.

Mary felt that she had allowed a trial period to prolong her mother's life, which is what her mother had wanted. But the treatments were not improving her condition. Mary decided to instruct the doctor to stop treatment and to provide comfort care. Her mother died four days later.

■

Jason, twenty-nine, was in a car accident. When he arrived at the emergency room, physicians discovered heavy bleeding in his head. He was put on a ventilator to help his breathing. After many different tests, Jason's physicians determined that he had severe brain damage. Jason was unresponsive to the touch and voice of his wife and parents. After a month on the ventilator, he remained comatose and unable to communicate with anybody.

Jason's physicians believed he was in an irreversible coma. Jason didn't have a Medical Power of Attorney to help guide his wife, parents, or his doctor about what treatment he would want, and he had never expressed his feelings about life support. The family was confused about what to do. Jason's mother and father could not imagine withdrawing treatment, but they became increasingly distressed and frustrated during visits with their son, who was completely unresponsive. Jason's wife feared even talking with her in-laws about withdrawing life support.

Jason was transferred to a skilled-nursing facility. His breathing was mechanically supported—he was attached to a machine through a tube in his windpipe; his feeding was through a tube placed in his stomach. Five months after the accident, still on life-support systems, Jason died of complications.

What lessons do these two cases convey? First, a Medical Power of Attorney makes it possible for the signer to have his or her wishes honored about medical treatments through a partner who has been legally appointed. Second, a Medical Power of Attorney works well where the signer and partner have talked about preferences and values. Third, when there is no document and there has been no previous discussion about the topic of critical-care treatments and life support, people closest to the patient often feel confused about the best course of action.

Throughout your consideration of an advance directive, be aware that neither a Medical Power of Attorney nor a Living Will takes effect in 911 emergency situations. All 911 paramedics are legally bound to exercise every life-support measure possible from the time they reach the patient until they sign off the case to the medical staff at a hospital. It is not until the patient is *in the hospital* that 911 procedures are no longer in place and instructions in an advance directive can be followed.

There is one exception concerning 911 assistance. In some states, you can obtain an Emergency Medical Services Pre-Hospital Do Not Resuscitate (DNR) Form. Usually, both you and your doctor must sign the form. This DNR order instructs paramedics not to resuscitate you at home or in any other location outside a hospital, including a nursing home or a hospice facility.

You must be aware that state laws and state forms differ. Most states authorize both a Living Will and appointment of a health-care agent. A handful of places authorize only one type of directive. The surest way to obtain current guidelines and documents is to phone your State or County Medical Association (look in the white pages of your telephone directory). Ask about each type of form. Some medical associations lean so heavily toward the Medical Power of Attorney as an advance directive that they do not distribute the Living Will form, but they will usually tell you where you can obtain one. (See table 5.1 for reasons to sign an advance directive.)

2. *DISCOVER YOUR BELIEFS ABOUT CRITICAL-CARE CHOICES*
   It may not be easy to think about future health-care decisions and critical-care choices. However, taking the time now to consider your feelings on these issues will help you make better decisions, which benefit both you and your family. The following exercises can help you discover your feelings about a wide range of medical treatments.

   You can go through the exercises by yourself, keeping your answers

TABLE 5.1
## *TEN GOOD REASONS TO SIGN AN ADVANCE DIRECTIVE*

1. Completing an advance directive is the kindest thing you can do for your family. It gives them the comfort of knowing that they are carrying out your wishes. It also gives them a written tool with which to direct your medical care with physicians, nurses, and other medical staff.

2. Completing an advance directive helps you maintain control of your own health care in any anticipated or unanticipated medical situation in which you are unable to make decisions and speak for yourself. You can maintain a voice in your own care.

3. Through the process of completing an advance directive, you can actually deepen your relationships with loved ones. You will be discussing your values and what quality of life you want to preserve. These conversations are a powerful way to share your love for each other.

4. Simply telling a family member or friend how you feel about health-care treatments may not ensure that your choices will be carried out. Your friends and family can help you protect those choices if you discuss them and then complete an advance directive.

5. The law guarantees your right to make decisions about your medical care, including life support. Without a written statement, you could lose the opportunity to direct your own medical care.

6. Advance directives allow you to avoid lengthy and unpleasant court battles over maintaining or withdrawing life support. Your written wishes, along with discussions about preferences for care with family or friends, will greatly increase the chances you will get the care you want, and prevent treatments you don't want.

7. Even if you don't have someone to name as your health-care partner (as in a Medical Power of Attorney, one type of advance directive), a Living Will can help guide your doctor and loved ones about your wishes if you are ever terminally ill or permanently unconscious.

8. People often take the time to plan for financial matters with a will and estate planning, but health-care matters are equally important. Just as financial planning maintains your control and reassures you about the future, so does planning for health care.

9. The process of completing an advance directive will familiarize you and your loved ones with common medical procedures and treatments. It will make these treatments less overwhelming and unfamiliar if the time ever comes to face them.

10. The process of completing an advance directive will raise your awareness of important beliefs and values that you hold about your quality of life. As you review these beliefs and values, you will be better able to plan your future in satisfying ways.

private. Or, you can share these materials with a close family member or friend. You can even photocopy the following pages, so that another person can read and answer the questions and compare responses with you. You may want to complete all of the exercises or just some of them. In different ways, each activity helps you ask yourself about medical treatments and the quality of life you wish to maintain. There are no right or wrong answers.

*What Would I Want, if This Happened to Me?*  These two case studies can help you explore different issues about quality of life. Read each one and then think about the medical circumstances presented; consider which treatments you would want and the treatments that you would prefer to refuse. Here is a case about a patient with Alzheimer's disease.

> Mrs. H. is a seventy-two-year-old widow with heart problems. She lives alone, and her two adult daughters live out of town. Five years ago, after reading an article in *Reader's Digest,* she told her daughters that "if she ever ended up with dementia [a form of senility or forgetfulness], she would not want to live like that." The topic was not discussed in further detail after that time.
>
> A year later, during one of their visits, her daughters found Mrs. H. forgetful and slightly disheveled. Her memory continued to get worse, and over time she lost the ability to care for herself. After extensive medical and psychological evaluation, she was diagnosed as having Senile Dementia of the Alzheimer's type. Her children decided to place her in a nursing home so that she could receive assistance with her daily activities and hygiene.
>
> Several months ago, Mrs. H. seemed to lose interest in eating. The nursing home asked her children whether their mother would want a feeding tube to provide hydration and nutrition. Without it she could die. The daughters felt conflicted about the decision. On the one hand, they wanted to respect their mother's previously stated wishes. She was a different person now: not caring about her previous interests, nor having any memory of family. On the other hand, their mother seemed to enjoy herself in the nursing home, obtaining pleasure in befriending the home's cat and appreciating the daughters' monthly visits even though she did not recognize either of them. It seemed that the feeding tube might be in her best interests, but the daughters also remembered their earlier discussion with their mother about not wanting to prolong life if she experienced dementia.

This example points out various stages of Alzheimer's disease (see table 5.2). Imagine yourself at each of the following stages. Ask yourself: Would I want life support—such as a machine to help me breathe

TABLE 5.2

## *ILLUSTRATIVE STAGES OF ALZHEIMER'S DISEASE*

| PATIENT'S CONDITION | WOULD YOU WANT LONG-TERM LIFE-SUPPORT? | |
|---|---|---|
| 1. You are able to bathe, groom, and dress yourself. You go outside, but once in a while you get lost and disoriented during grocery shopping.  On occasion, you are unable to recognize your family. | Yes | No |
| 2. You are only able to do daily activities of bathing and grooming with supervision. On numerous occasions you have turned on the gas and forgotten that it's on. Periodically you are able to recognize family or visitors, but mostly you cannot do this. You have accidently destroyed some of your personal property by dropping items. | Yes | No |
| 3. You are bedridden. You cannot bathe or groom yourself and you seldom recognize family members. You cannot communicate your need to use the toilet, so you must use diapers. You have little appetite, but you still smile when you stroke the cat. | Yes | No |
| 4. You are bedridden and rely on a nurse for all your bodily functions and hygiene. You do not respond to touch or to familiar voices. | Yes | No |

and a tube for feeding—on a long-term basis if a medical crisis arose and my physical condition was expected to deteriorate steadily?

Here is a case study about a patient in a coma.

> Mr. F. is in his sixties. He has always been healthy and fit, running two miles in the morning and biking in the afternoons. A few years ago, one of Mr. F.'s friends was in an automobile accident and taken to the hospital. The friend was in a coma and during that time needed a ventilator to help him breathe and a tube for feeding. Mr. F.'s friend came out of the coma after two weeks; he went through some physical and occupational rehabilitation and eventually recovered fully. After this incident, Mr. F. mentioned to his wife that if he was ever in a coma he would want the doctors to be very confident that he

would never come out of it before he was ever taken off "those machines."

A year ago Mr. F. was in a serious accident on his bicycle. Unconscious, he was rushed to the hospital with head injuries. After careful observation and testing for two days, his physicians could not be sure how much brain damage he had sustained. Mr. F. remained in a coma, supported by a ventilator and feeding tube. The physicians continued testing for three weeks and then told Mr. F.'s wife that he most likely was in an irreversible coma and had considerable brain damage, but they couldn't be certain. They also told her that if Mr. F. came out of the coma, they couldn't be sure what state he'd be in or if he'd ever return to his active lifestyle again. The physicians couldn't tell Mrs. F. how long Mr. F. would remain in a coma, saying it could be weeks, months, or years.

Mrs. F. continued to visit her husband every day. When Mrs. F. held her husband's hand, he would seem to respond to her touch. He also opened and closed his eyes. He did not respond to her voice.

Mrs. F. was confused and the doctors could not predict what would happen. She knew a life without exercise and full mental capacities would not be any life for her husband. But, she also remembered when she and her husband discussed their friend's accident, coma, and full recovery. Mrs. F. did not know what to do.

The example of Mr. and Mrs. F. points out the difficulties in predicting outcomes for a person in a coma. Consider the following situations (table 5.3). If an additional medical crisis arose, would you want doctors to intervene in order to prolong your life?

*What Kind of Life Do You Prefer?*   People differ in their feelings about quality and longevity of life. Some people would like to live as long as possible regardless of the quality of life; others want to preserve a certain quality of life even if it means a shorter time alive.

Think about these options and your own feelings. Where do you fall on the scale in table 5.4?

*Health-Care Values Checklist.*   In this exercise (see table 5.5), you will find a number of statements about values (Doukas, Lipson, and McCullough 1989; Doukas and McCullough 1991). Circle "agree," "disagree," or "depends" after each statement. You may want to write comments, questions, or additional thoughts in a notebook. You can skip items if you wish.

Review your answers. These value statements point to some of the

TABLE 5.3
### *ILLUSTRATIVE STAGES OF A COMA*

| PATIENT'S CONDITION | WOULD YOU WANT LONG-TERM LIFE-SUPPORT? | |
|---|---|---|
| 1. You have been in a coma for a week. You randomly respond to touch by squeezing another person's hand. You are not responsive to any verbal instructions. | Yes | No |
| 2. You have been in a coma for a month. You randomly respond to touch by squeezing another person's hand. You are not responsive to anyone's voice. Your arms and legs are abnormally stiff and stretched out. | Yes | No |
| 3. You have been in a coma for a year. Your limbs do not respond to any stimulation— touch, voice, or even pin pricks. Your physical condition has been declining steadily for a year. | Yes | No |

issues you will want to concentrate on as you begin discussions with family, friends, and professionals.

## 3. TALK WITH YOUR FAMILY, FRIENDS, AND HEALTH-CARE PARTNER

Even though a Living Will does not require you to have a legal partner, it is in your best interest to let others know that you have completed such a document. In ideal circumstances, every person who plans ahead for critical care should have someone who can draw the medical team's attention to his or her advance directive, whatever form that takes. This person can press photocopies into doctors' and nurses' hands.

Of course, you are required to designate a health-care partner (surrogate, proxy, agent, or attorney-in-fact) when completing a Medical Power of Attorney. For your own peace of mind, you should talk thoroughly with your partner well ahead of any medical crisis or emergency. Without such consultation, the other person has only a dim idea of what you really want done.

Even spouses often make poor forecasts about each other's care

TABLE 5.4
### QUALITY-OF-LIFE SCALE

| I want to live as long as possible, regardless of how poor the quality of my life gets. | [] [] [] [] [] | I want to preserve a good quality of life, even if I do not live as long. |
|---|---|---|

preferences unless they have sat down and talked about this. It's not unusual for one person to underestimate the other's health status, for example, judging physical or mental impairment to be more serious or unendurable than the patient does. Furthermore, the health-care partner often makes inaccurate guesses about wishes, especially concerning more remote possibilities—such as elective surgery following dementia or willingness to be supported through artificial feeding or breathing over many months.

The fifty states differ somewhat on the qualifications and role of your partner. You will want to ask about these three areas:

1.  *Qualifications.* The partner will have to be an adult. In addition, many states do not allow the partner to be your primary doctor, nurse, or other health-care provider, or employee or operator of a nursing home *unless* this person is related to you by blood, marriage, or adoption. (This is to avoid any possible conflict of interest.) Check state law before appointing a member of the clergy; in some states, an agent is permitted to represent only a specified number of individuals.
2.  *Authority.* Your partner must follow your wishes as they appear on your documents, or as you have specified in discussions. Inquire about whether your partner can make decisions after death about autopsy, disposition of your body, or organ donation. Ask about other areas of authority that your health-care partner can assume.
3.  *Limitations.* Your partner is not allowed to make decisions that are contrary to your instructions as stated in your document. Ask about limitations on your partner's role, such as decisions about commitment to a mental-health facility, psychosurgery, sterilization, abortion, or electroconvulsive therapy.

Most states allow you to choose your health-care partner from a wide range of people: your spouse or domestic partner; an adult child;

## TABLE 5.5
### HEALTH-CARE VALUES CHECKLIST

| | | | |
|---|---|---|---|
| I want to make my own decisions about health care. | Agree | Disagree | Depends |
| I want my doctors to make decisions about my health care. | Agree | Disagree | Depends |
| I want my family to make decisions about my health care. | Agree | Disagree | Depends |
| I want to preserve my dignity, even when I can no longer speak for myself. | Agree | Disagree | Depends |
| If I could not think clearly or recognize people I know, I would not want aggressive medical treatments just to stay alive. | Agree | Disagree | Depends |
| If I could not think clearly or recognize people I know, I would still want life-support treatment in a medical crisis. | Agree | Disagree | Depends |
| I want to try aggressive treatment before giving up. | Agree | Disagree | Depends |
| I want my religious beliefs and traditions followed in all medical situations. | Agree | Disagree | Depends |
| I want to die at home and not in a hospital. | Agree | Disagree | Depends |
| It does not matter to me where I die. | Agree | Disagree | Depends |
| I do not want my family to be financially burdened because of my medical treatments. | Agree | Disagree | Depends |
| I want to tie up all loose ends now in terms of my choices for medical care. | Agree | Disagree | Depends |
| I don't want to be dependent on anyone to carry out my day-to-day functions (such as feeding, going to the bathroom, and personal grooming). | Agree | Disagree | Depends |

*(continued)*

TABLE 5.5
### *HEALTH-CARE VALUES CHECKLIST* (*continued*)

| | | | |
|---|---|---|---|
| I want a comfortable dying process. | Agree | Disagree | Depends |
| I want to be with loved ones at death. | Agree | Disagree | Depends |
| I want to donate my organs for transplantation. | Agree | Disagree | Depends |
| I want to donate my body or organs for medical education and research. | Agree | Disagree | Depends |
| I don't want to be dependent on any technology, such as machines or complex procedures, in order to prolong my life if I am inevitably dying. | Agree | Disagree | Depends |

a parent; a brother or sister; another relative; a close friend; a physician or nurse (other than your own); a clergy member; or an attorney. Several issues guide your selection. As you consider options, think about:

- Who will feel comfortable talking with you about critical-care choices or about death?
- Who has a strong enough personality to insist on what you want in your advance directive?
- Who will not be disturbed by what you want in your Medical Power of Attorney?
- Who understands and respects your values, even though you might feel differently about some things?
- Who will carry out your choices exactly as you have specified them?
- Who can best use his or her judgment for situations that you haven't thought about, and still decide on what you would have wanted?

After reflecting on these questions, you may conclude that no one stands out. If so, you may want to complete a Living Will, which doesn't require a health-care partner.

***Getting the Conversation Going.*** When and how to talk to your partner— or with other loved ones—about your care choices will take some planning. You probably know the best time to bring up an important subject and the best setting. You may want to talk one-on-one with your partner at a prearranged time, or you may prefer a discussion with family members or friends during a holiday gathering or other occasion.

Consider these additional points:

- Set an appointment or date for your discussion ahead of time. Find an occasion that is quiet and not subject to time constraints or other demands. Let your health-care partner know that you would like to talk in a relaxed environment, free of distractions.
- At the beginning of the conversation, reassure the other person(s) that your health has not changed and that this conversation is not prompted by bad medical news from your doctor. The more positive you are, the more likely it is that your partner and/or family will understand that signing these documents is an opportunity for you to maintain control and independence about your future care.
- Consider having more than one meeting with your partner and/or family, and encourage them to have an ongoing dialogue with you. Remember, just as it took you time to reach your decisions, it may take time for your family to be comfortable with your ideas.
- Let your partner and/or family know that you have studied the issues carefully and that signing an advance directive is something you really want to do. Underscore the importance of these documents by explaining the consequences of not signing them.
- Share sections of this chapter with your family and friends.
- Ask your partner and others in your family to support your decisions by simply recognizing them. Even if others do not agree with your specific choices, let them know that you're comforted by the fact that you've made these decisions ahead of time, sparing others needless anguish.

Sometimes starting a conversation itself is the hardest part of the process. You may want to rehearse these lines before you get the ball rolling. You can choose from among these opening sentences:

"Let's talk now about what would happen if I was ever so sick that I couldn't make choices and tell you what I wanted for my health care. With all the decisions that might need to be made, I worry that the family could be left with a terrible burden. The last thing I would ever want would be confusion or disagreements about my preferences."

"I know it's hard for all of us to talk about my death or the possibility of my ever getting so sick that I couldn't make decisions for myself. But we need to talk now so I can know that you and my doctor will understand my wishes and be able to follow them."

"I've been reading about Living Wills and Medical Powers of Attorney, and it's really started me thinking. I had some vague ideas about these documents, but I really didn't understand how they worked. And I certainly didn't know how important they are in helping me maintain control of my care. It's very comforting to know that they are available and recognized by the medical profession and that they're legal documents, just like a regular will for financial matters."

"I recently completed a Medical Power of Attorney and chose (NAME) as my health-care partner in case I can't make decisions for myself because of an illness or accident. I chose (NAME) to relieve all of you of the anguish of making care decisions for me if I'm ever unable to speak for myself. (NAME) and I have spent time together talking and sharing my ideas and choices about the specific types of medical care I want and those that I don't want. I'm confident that if (NAME) ever has to make a decision regarding my treatment, it will really be my decision that is being expressed to my doctors."

In talking with your health-care partner or family, you should discuss personal values and choices about care, using the exercises in Step 2. Or, you may find it more comfortable to guide the conversation in a direction that eventually satisfies these questions:

- Do you understand what kinds of treatments I do and don't want?
- Do you understand how I feel about life and my health, even if I haven't given you directions about specific treatments?
- How do you feel about being my health-care partner? What, if anything, concerns or bothers you about it?
- If a time comes when you need to express my choices, how are you going to tell my family, my doctor, and my clergy member what I want?
- How are we going to talk about my health-care wishes as I get older, in case I change my mind?
- Do you think you can tell the doctors what I want, even if you don't agree with my choices?
- If there's disagreement between what I want and recommendations by family or doctors, do you feel comfortable standing up for my wishes?

At some point during conversations with your health-care partner, both of you should plan to complete the sample medical scenarios that follow. You and your partner will be answering the same questions. The purpose of the exercise is to see how well you and your health-care partner have communicated about your wishes. You want your health-care partner to be able to put himself or herself in your shoes and make the same choices that you would in a difficult medical situation.

You will imagine yourself as the patient and choose one of the preferences listed below each scenario. Your partner will answer each scenario as *he or she thinks you would answer it.* Photocopy the scenarios, so that each of you can work independently. Then, the two of you should compare results, so that you can make sure that your partner understands your preferences and your reasoning behind them.

4. *TALK WITH DOCTORS, NURSES, LAWYERS,*
   *OR CLERGY ABOUT ADVANCE DIRECTIVES*
   You may want to consult with a number of people while completing your Living Will or Medical Power of Attorney. Professionals such as doctors, nurses, lawyers, or clergy members can help you through the process, answering your questions and, most importantly, understanding the choices you've made. You may want to alert your physician that you'd like to spend some extra time at your next appointment going over the critical-care choices you've indicated in your advance directive.

### Questions to Ask Your Doctor.
- What is the procedure for ensuring that my Living Will or Medical Power of Attorney is put in my medical record that you keep? Where else should it be placed?
- What medical issues do you think are relevant to my Living Will or Medical Power of Attorney? Can we discuss any special considerations for my chronic condition (if you have one)?
- Can you explain exactly what happens when a person is on a ventilator?
- What about artificial feeding? How is that accomplished?
- Please explain about CPR and how successful it is under various circumstances. I'd like to learn more about different critical-care treatments and how they work.
- How do you treat patients in pain?
- Does a patient experience pain once life support is withdrawn?
- How will you know if my situation is terminal?
- Do you know what quality of life I want to maintain if I'm ever in need of machines to prolong my life?

## MEDICAL SCENARIOS

*Scenario 1*

Following a car accident, Ms. D., fifty-four, is rushed to the hospital with severe head and spine injuries and multiple internal injuries. In the emergency room, there is a flurry of activity to stabilize her. Medical staff perform life-saving surgery to stop her internal bleeding. The surgeons find that Ms. D.'s liver suffered major damage, and she lost a lot of blood during the operation. She remains in a coma, completely unresponsive to voice or touch. Her physical condition continues to worsen four weeks after the accident. Doctors have determined that she has permanent brain damage, although they do not know the extent. Doctors ask whether they should keep Ms. D. on a ventilator and tube feeding, or withdraw this life support.

- ☐ Stay on life-support machines indefinitely
- ☐ Withdraw life support
- ☐ Continue on life support for a short period, but withdraw if consciousness is not regained
- ☐ Something else

*Scenario 2*

Mr. B., eighty-four years old, has advanced Alzheimer's disease and is unable to make any decisions for himself, including medical decisions. Mr. B. does not recognize his wife, who takes care of his needs for bathing and grooming. Mr. B. has had diabetes for many years and recently developed an infection in his right leg that does not respond to medication. His physicians explain to his wife that the leg has gangrene and must be removed below the knee. If Mr. B.'s leg is not amputated, he will die within a few weeks.

- ☐ Have the surgery to amputate the leg
- ☐ Do not have the surgery to amputate the leg
- ☐ Something else

*Scenario 3*

Mr. G. is seventy-eight and has suffered two heart attacks. The most recent one left him quite frail. He takes a number of different medications to stabilize his condition. He is bedridden and uncommunicative most of the time and has few interests besides occasionally watching TV. His physician has recently diagnosed Mr. G. with colon cancer; aggressive treatment could extend Mr. G.'s life. His physician has tried to get Mr. G. to express an opinion about the medical options, but he is so disoriented and weak that he is unable to make a decision.

*(continued)*

☐ No treatment for cancer, let the disease take its course
☐ Aggressive treatment for cancer, which could include surgery, chemotherapy, and/or radiation
☐ Something else

*Scenario 4*

Mrs. K., sixty-nine, had a severe stroke and fell and broke her hip. She is conscious but has extensive brain damage and is unable to speak or recognize any family members. The doctors are doubtful about her ability to regain speech or recognition, but they feel she could learn to walk again if she had surgery to repair her hip and rehabilitation.

☐ Go ahead with the hip surgery
☐ Tell the doctors not to do the hip surgery
☐ Something else

*Scenario 5*

Mrs. H., seventy-nine years old, has a history of chronic heart disease. Over the past nine years, she has been hospitalized on five separate occasions for a series of small heart attacks. Recently, she was rushed to an Intensive Care Unit (ICU) with a massive heart attack. She is in critical condition but has been stabilized with many medications and the use of a ventilator to help her breathe. Even though she is currently stable, her physicians are worried about her heart stopping because of the extensive damage she has suffered over the years. Physicians need to know whether or not to attempt cardiopulmonary resuscitation (CPR), if her heart fails. Mrs. H. is not strong enough to make decisions or communicate with her medical team.

☐ Ask for cardiopulmonary resuscitation (CPR)
☐ Refuse cardiopulmonary resuscitation (CPR)
☐ Something else

- How do you feel about my choices?
- Would you feel comfortable carrying out my wishes?
- Do doctors really honor advance directives?

If you don't have a primary doctor or you see several doctors as part of an HMO, you may feel uncertain where to start. Try this approach:

- Make an appointment with one of the doctors you see to begin discussing your choices.
- If you are not comfortable with this doctor, ask for two referrals so you can find someone with whom you will feel comfortable.

- If you receive care from several different doctors and/or cannot find a doctor within the HMO with whom you want to discuss your advance directive, discuss your choices with your family, nurses, clergy member, or anyone else with whom you feel comfortable. Then be sure to send copies of your Medical Power of Attorney or Living Will to your doctor(s).
- Staff-based HMOs (see chapter 1) have centralized medical charts for their patients. Each time you see a doctor, even if you see many different doctors at different times, your chart is sent to him or her. Regardless of whether or not you establish a long-term relationship with a doctor, call your HMO to make sure your advance directive is placed in your medical chart.

### Questions to Ask Nurses.
- Is it painful to withdraw life support?
- What kind of comfort can nurses give me if I'm ever on life support? What comfort can they give me if life support is withdrawn?
- Who will talk to my family and my health-care partner about my condition?
- Do doctors really honor advance directives?
- How do you feel about advance directives? Why?

### Questions to Ask Your Lawyer.
Talking to a lawyer is not necessary for these documents to be legally valid, but you may want to consult one if you have specific concerns. Your questions may include the following:

- What is the difference between a will and a Living Will?
- What is the difference between a Living Will and a Medical Power of Attorney, for my situation?
- What could be the impact of prolonged, intensive care on the size or value of my estate?
- If I sign a Medical Power of Attorney, what can my health-care partner legally do?
- Is there anything my health-care partner legally cannot do?

### Views of Clergy on Advance Directives and Questions to Ask.
A wide spectrum of religious authorities within the Judeo-Christian tradition endorse advance directives, as do theological figures in other faiths. You may want to consult your own clergy member or spiritual advisor.

A Protestant minister, who has years of experience counseling people in hospitals and hospice settings, feels strongly that people should retain control of all their health-care decisions, including the last minutes of life. He believes that "Christian people should seriously consider completing an advance directive because we have a responsibility to take care of our bodies. We are created in the image of God (Genesis 1:26–27) and endowed with free will and choice. It is important to exercise these God-given abilities in a responsible way, particularly when it comes to our health. When we complete advance directives, we decide for ourselves, diminishing or eliminating guilt or anxiety for family members at a time of serious illness."

A rabbi of a large congregation spends more and more of his time doing home and hospital visits to members who are seriously ill. His chief concern is that a medical crisis becomes even more traumatic when family members have failed to discuss preferences before the final hours. He is troubled by the family conflicts that erupt, even in cases where everyone is trying to do the right thing. "People come to me in the eleventh hour when there is little time for discussion and when decisions must be made. These kinds of decisions should not come at the last moment but rather when people are clear-headed. I try to tell my congregants that it is when they are healthy that the family must open up to each other and have honest conversations. Tragically, without family discussions and advance directive documents, I see families fighting over which sibling loves papa best, and whether the child who would 'turn off the switch' is the callous one or whether the one who refuses to act is the compassionate one. These situations are surely the furthest from the will of the dying and not in the interest of the family. Now is the time to rehearse for that which is inevitable."

A Catholic priest admitted that many people in his parish are both interested and confused about end-of-life care and that it is becoming an increasingly popular topic for him in one-on-one counseling sessions. He tells his congregants:

> As Catholics we believe that our life is a gift from God over which we have limited power. We have been called to protect and cherish human life and not destroy it. Saint Paul asks us, "Do you not know that you are the temple of God and that the Spirit of God dwells in you?" Our response is our gift to God.
>
> By the same token, we are not morally bound to prolong our lives by means which will inflict serious financial, physical, or emotional hardships on ourselves or our loved ones. Therefore, there is no need to prolong the dying process by every means available to medical science.

A person may appoint a family member or friend as attorney-in-fact in an advance directive to see to it that extraordinary means are not used.

Here are some questions to ask your clergy member:

- What is our religion's stance on the medical treatments I am addressing in my advance directive?
- What is your opinion about the choices and values I'm addressing in my advance directive?
- Does our religion have a position statement on advance directives?
- How would you feel if I indicated in my advance directive that I would like you to pray with me and my family?

5. *HELP YOUR PARTNER UNDERSTAND HIS OR HER RESPONSIBILITIES*

If you decide to complete a Medical Power of Attorney, you will be required to choose a health-care partner. You can help your partner fully appreciate what's being asked by showing him or her this chapter. In particular, Step 5 explains what it means to be a health-care partner, and suggests things that the partner can do to prompt a helpful dialogue with you.

*Information for the Health-Care Partner.*  Your loved one or friend has chosen you as a health-care partner because he or she trusts you to make difficult critical-care decisions. Without your participation, the doctors will not have guidance about the patient's preferences. Completing a Medical Power of Attorney draws you, as partner, and the signer of the document into a special relationship. Of course, the signer will consider his or her feelings about pain, life-support systems, and other medical issues. The signer may also want to weigh the effect of asking you to express his or her wishes, if the need ever arises. It helps both you and the signer to recognize the significance of the assignment you agree to fulfill. Therefore, it is important that the two of you have talked fully about the signer's preferences about medical treatments. It is also important that you talk with the signer about preferences concerning quality of life—the degree of physical and mental health that makes it worthwhile to try to prolong life.

The role as health-care partner has three sets of responsibilities. A health-care partner: (1) learns what medical treatments the signer would want or would not want, and discusses the signer's values about quality of life; (2) helps the signer complete and distribute the Medical

Power of Attorney document; and (3) expresses the signer's choices to physicians in situations where the signer has lost the ability to decide and communicate such choices. In discussing advance directives, critical-care treatments, and quality of life, you and the signer might want to refer to other sections of this chapter.

*Responsibility 1.* Understand the signer's medical preferences and personal values. No one can predict all the different medical circumstances that could arise. What you can do is talk with the signer as he or she goes through the process of thinking about and completing the document. You will learn his or her feelings about the most common types of critical-care procedures, and you will discover the quality of life that the signer feels would justify those means, or make such medical treatments unacceptable. To learn about the signer's preferences, you can also:

- Urge the signer to arrange a scheduled time to discuss the advance directive, when both of you will have ample time to talk.
- Encourage discussion about the signer's values. Earlier sections in this chapter include worksheets to spark your talk, and activities where the signer can write his or her feelings about medical care and quality of life (see exercises in Steps 2 and 3). These prompts can help you to understand the signer's preferences.
- You might also try these sample questions to stimulate conversation: What quality of life is important for you to maintain? Have you read anything or seen anything on television where you've thought, "I don't want to be like that?" When would a situation be hopeless for you? Are there any treatments you would want to try before refusing? Can we go over some of the medical terms and descriptions of treatments in this chapter (see Common Medical Treatments and Glossary of Critical-Care Terminology)? Are there religious or spiritual issues I should know about?
- An earlier section in this chapter contains sample medical scenarios for you and the signer to complete. The exercise presents options for critical care. As the health-care partner, you will try to answer the questions *as you think the signer would answer them.* You can then compare how you answered, on the signer's behalf, against the signer's answers. The exercise will prompt additional discussion.
- Offer emotional support and understanding for these difficult decisions about medical care.

- Remind the signer that by making these decisions he or she is lightening the burden on you and on family and close friends. If a critical-care situation arises, you will know what the signer wants and will be able to carry out his or her wishes.

*Responsibility 2.* Help the signer complete and distribute the document. You do not need a lawyer for this process. The signer needs to obtain the proper forms for his or her state by calling the State or County Medical Association.

- Discuss how to distribute the document to the appropriate people, including doctors, health insurance administrators, yourself as health-care partner, other family members, and friends. It is important to ensure that many people have access to the forms. *Photocopied documents are as legally valid as the original.*
- Put your own copy of the Medical Power of Attorney in an accessible place where you can find it quickly. You will need to have it if a critical-care situation arises for the signer.
- Note the sample wallet card in the Examples of Advance Directives and Wallet Card. Encourage the signer to complete a card like this and place it in his or her wallet.

*Responsibility 3.* If a critical-care situation arises, you will be asked to communicate the signer's preferences. Remember, you are needed as the signer's voice only when he or she has lost the ability to make decisions and communicate them. In such a situation, you can help the signer by taking the following actions:

- Alert the medical team to the Medical Power of Attorney, and hand them copies of the document.
- Be forthright about your job as the health-care partner. Tell the medical team to give you all the information regarding the signer's condition and treatment options. This is your right and responsibility as the signer's legal spokesperson.
- Ask doctors and nurses to describe options and choices for treatment.
- Instruct medical staff about which treatments the signer wants, does not want, or wants for a trial period.
- Communicate with the signer's other loved ones about the situation and treatment options.

There are things you can't do as a partner. Your state's documents will include the limitations on your role and responsibilities.

6. *UNDERSTAND SOME CRITICAL-CARE TERMINOLOGY*
You must understand common treatments for life-support and medical terms that are used in critical-care situations. Two sections help you with these: Common Medical Treatments and the Glossary of Critical-Care Terminology.

7. *EXPRESS WISHES ABOUT COMFORT (PALLIATIVE) CARE*
If you want, add statements to your directive asking for hospice care (see chapter 2) or any other comfort care you desire. Also state your wishes about the use of opiates in the event you suffer intense and prolonged pain.

8. *COMPLETE AND DISTRIBUTE YOUR ADVANCE DIRECTIVE*
The final action for you to take—once you have completed the advance directive that meets your needs—is to make sure that you distribute your document and complete your wallet card.

Make copies of your advance directive document. *These copies have the same legal standing as the original.* It's important to remember that you should not put your document in a safe-deposit box or other remote location, locked away. You want your form available to family and doctors. Don't keep it a secret. The directive can only protect your choices if the appropriate people have access to it.

Develop a list of the people and places that should get copies (doctors, HMOs, health-care partner, family, friends). You should also give copies to family or friends who are likely to go with you, if you are admitted to the hospital Intensive Care Unit (ICU) or emergency room. Then they will be prepared to show your advance directive to the attending physicians.

You might want to write a cover letter to your physician or medical team, when sending the directive, or hand deliver it at your next appointment. Explain that you have just signed the documents, and would like to discuss them. At all times, carry your wallet card that shows that you have a Living Will or Medical Power of Attorney (see Examples of Advance Directives and Wallet Card).

# Lifelong Health

IN THIS BOOK, you have learned many ways to thrive by managing your encounters with the health-care system. We have shared practical results from the frontlines of today's research into well-being. A growing wealth of knowledge about health behavior offers plentiful clues for how people flourish by taking control. You can experiment with new ways of communicating to your doctors. You can weigh choices among treatment options with new insight. You can marshal help within your family and community more purposefully. In short, you can commandeer the fruits of scholarly research.

The medical research we have explored shows how physical health is deeply rooted in people's emotions and habits of thought. A patient's or physician's choice of words, gestures, and feelings really do matter. In subtle and often disguised ways, the human body's biochemical secretions and electrical charges that regulate sickness and health echo activities of the mind.

Three strategies for managing your health care underlie many of the suggestions offered in this book. Regardless of your comfort level or experience with many of the tips we've presented, you can take these final thoughts and apply them to your particular situation. These ideas are deceptively simple—accessible by everyone, but extremely powerful. They might seem obvious, but in a medical situation, it's easy to become stressed and overwhelmed and consequently overlook the obvious. Here are some critical reminders.

## STOP, THINK, AND FEEL

It's normal to react to upheavals such as illness in a conservative, even strangulated way, shutting off thinking and feeling. People want to contain their condition within fixed boundaries. They find reassurance by zeroing in on the present: The health condition is happening now and has no yesterday or tomorrow. They assume that the information already at hand is the only information available. They want to think the condition's impact can be easily contained. They also assume that disability or illness arouses a coherent set of emotions, all of them menacing.

As we've seen in this book, narrow-perspective thinking locks you into a rut. You can benefit from breaking away from habitual meanings and interpretations that you bring to a health problem. Expanded horizons also allow you to learn valuable lessons from illness or disability. You can discover unsuspected strengths and liabilities—how life works for good and ill—and what you can do, even in a reduced state, to uplift others.

Sounds great, but how do you make the transition between restricted, fearful reaction and broader, calm response? The first step is to *stop, think, and feel*. Many of us scamper on our daily treadmill, seldom pausing for reflection. We forsake interludes of quiet alone time, which are necessary to rejuvenate the spirit and make wise decisions. In reading this book, you have reached some choice points, stepping off the treadmill. As you do, try to expand your views about the health problem that vexes you in at least four respects.

- Consider the longest time frame that you can imagine. Might the origin of your current trouble stretch back to a much earlier time of life? Perhaps the disorder is not the abrupt intrusion that it first appears to be. What, do you guess, will be its future consequences, not just tomorrow but down the road?
- Open yourself to a diversity of information about your problem's impact. Reach out to sources that give a variety of types of information about the problem. Recognize that acquaintances, books, magazine columns, professional counselors, religious figures, and other

informants may have useful tidbits and insights to share, even when they disagree.

- Examine your health problem's impact on different spheres and episodes of life. Could it affect performance at work, physical appearance, romantic appeal, your playful interests, or other facets that may not obviously seem connected to physical well-being?

- Allow the full medley of feelings that illness or accident can unleash. Don't resist them. You might alternatively experience sorrow, joy, anxiety, wry pleasure, disillusionment, inspiration, and other perplexing swings in emotion. All are legitimate. Your first instincts, of course, run in the *opposite direction* toward shutting out feelings. This is because illness and accident are anomalous experiences, even traumatic at times. When you stop, think, and feel, you can allow a full range of possibilities that will help you cope.

## CAPTURE THE THERAPEUTIC STRENGTH OF LANGUAGE

It is widely acknowledged that putting experiences into words is healthy. Confiding in friends or a therapist, praying, and writing out thoughts and feelings bring benefits. Divulging, sometimes confessing, is highly meaningful in or outside a religious setting. The advantages of getting stress out in the open have been widely demonstrated.

You can take advantage of this opportunity, even without drawing others immediately into conversation. Many research studies have shown how writing out your thoughts and deepest feelings is therapeutic (Pennebaker 1993b; Hughes, Uhlmann, and Pennebaker 1994). Most of these studies assign people to one of two groups. One set of subjects is required to write for 15 to 20 minutes on several occasions about a personal problem (disability, health challenge, loss of a job, or other distress). They are told to write continuously without regard to grammar, sentence structure, organization, or other niceties. The diary entries are kept strictly confidential. The other set of people is asked to write about some relatively trivial topic. Months later, psychologists compare the two groups.

People assigned to the self-disclosure group turn out to be healthier and have fewer physical complaints and visits to the doctor than the comparison group. The immune functions and other physiological defenses of the self-disclosers have strengthened from the writing experience. Self-disclosers show greater problem-solving skills, too. For example, among people who recently lost jobs, the self-disclosers are twice as likely to have found new positions months later.

You will benefit the most from getting health problems down on paper if you are candid and frank with yourself. Don't shrink from venting dark thoughts, frustrating ideas, or depressing emotions. As you write more about your condition, you will increasingly come to order events in a more coherent pattern. Reasons behind a malady or other condition may appear. A game plan might crystallize.

Many people find that their first attempts to express these experiences on paper are rambling. However, the clarity and coherence of an account will gradually improve. In the short run, you may feel flushed and sweaty in this process. Muscles may tense, you may fidget, and your heart may race. Your writing brings feelings of unease. Don't give up. By persistently writing over several days, you give yourself time to compose a more comprehensive and lucid interpretation of your experience. Temporary anxieties fade. With each new line you write, you will grow more confident and serene.

Writing about a health challenge frees up feelings. This release of energy replaces suppression, which would otherwise build to unhelpful forms of physical arousal. The process works this way. Studies show that a person's efforts to smother thoughts about a distressing situation are doomed to failure; we all know how difficult it is to keep the incident or condition from springing back to mind. What's worse, attempts at inhibiting the feelings actually tax the body biologically. When you suppress thoughts day after day, your blood pressure rises and other systems are kept constantly on alert, even if you don't realize it. It's healthier to release the feelings.

When you translate stress into words, you help yourself assimilate the experience. Threats and anxieties that had been frightening images in the mind take on a linguistic format, and words are friendlier to work with than nervous sensations or ill-defined pictures. Using language to code and express trauma curtails the condition's toxic effects.

Your writing spree can end when you sense that an understandable narrative has emerged, that you have constructed a story about the illness or other condition. With this under your belt, you can go one step further: Share your story with others who have good judgment and who feel warmly toward you. This often elicits helpful ways you might not have imagined for how to cope with what ails you.

## REHEARSE

Many of the tips in this book ask you to step up to the plate and *do something,* not just ruminate about things. For example, we advise that you actually communicate differently with doctors, or ask people for favors, or arrange for someone to substitute for your caregiver. If some of these steps sound intimidating, or if you try them and fail, take heart: You can learn to do them better by practicing.

Rehearsing the conversations that lead to such accomplishments builds the motivation to undertake them by giving you a safe way to test your techniques. Here's the ultimate payoff: Rehearsal in private more than doubles the odds that you will actually attempt the things that would improve health care experiences for you.

Rehearsal begins by imagining yourself taking the desired action and enjoying the positive results that follow. Don't neglect to envision these. After you silently visualize the action and results, try it out loud: Utter the words that express your ideas or wishes. Speak so you hear the sound of your own voice (don't feel embarrassed; successful people talk "to themselves" like this all the time).

You may quaver at first, or speak haltingly or hoarsely; swallow and try again. This time phrases will come more certainly. Practice different sentences. You'll reject awkward expressions, smooth your presentation, and arrive at a comfortable style, a way to clarify ideas that suits your makeup. Pay heed, as well, to how foreign the attempt feels to you. At first, the practice script may appear wildly at variance with your customary behavior—bold where you are usually shy, or persistent where you usually give up easily. If so, divide your new, imagined task into incremental pieces. Ask for small favors, for example, or modest bits of information before requesting more. Be determined and unyielding about one matter before branching into others.

Submit your trial expressions to test. As you experiment with imaginary conversations—talking to a doctor, family member, or substitute caregiver—imagine confronting unexpected or even unwanted responses. What will you say, then, to get back on track? Practice these options. Sometimes, the adverse reaction you imagine can serve an even more constructive purpose; it may suggest that you pursue a fundamentally different aim. Fortunately, you're free as a bird to try out different reactions. You are still in rehearsal, and haven't "opened" your script yet on a real-life stage.

What if you can't even imagine how to begin? Apprehension, or simple lack of experience, may freeze your imagination when you start to rehearse. Don't be alarmed. If you can't think of a way to start the conversation you want, ask a friend for advice. Pose your situation, describe how you wish things were better, and ask the other person what he or she would say to get the ball rolling. Later on, use these ideas to launch your own private rehearsal session. As an example, chapter 5 recognizes that most people are inexperienced at talking about plans for critical care. That's why you'll find a section that suggests "conversational openers" (p. 220) to get the discussion launched.

Talking to yourself in private is best, but don't attempt it while driving to work or during distracting activities. Retreat, instead, to a personal space such as a walk in the park, the bath, or any room when people are away from the house.

Rehearsal will embolden you. With practice, you can aspire to even higher goals than you originally set. Don't be surprised when rehearsing exerts this pull on you. At the start of practicing your questions to the doctor, for instance, you might have aimed for better recall about the treatment program, medications, that sort of thing. After a bit of practice (especially in front of a mirror), you'll start to consider more ambitious accomplishments, such as asking about new options for treatment altogether. Allow your courage to grow.

When you have rehearsed one interchange, you'll get into the swing of things and find it easier to rehearse others. Practicing at better doctor-patient encounters, for instance, will stir your desire to experiment at seeking social support. Your growing flair for simulated conversation will find even wider applications beyond health matters.

## PUTTING IT ALL TOGETHER

One of our research subjects, Hope, shows how you can put it all together. Stopping to think, expressing herself, and rehearsing helped her overcome failed and frustrating medical treatment. She is twenty-seven years old, lives in Minneapolis, and works in computer sales and training. She had been troubled by a tickle in her throat that turned into a persistent and nagging cough, often leading to an inability to talk or project her voice clearly. This was a serious liability in her line of work.

Hope visited her internist who took a throat culture and ruled out a strep infection; she left that appointment with a diagnosis of bronchitis and prescription for a ten-day course of antibiotics. Hope figured that her frantic travel schedule was to blame, and attributed her ailment to a bug that she probably picked up on a recent airline flight. Two weeks later, the condition continued to bother her, and the doctor suggested another course of antibiotics. When this failed to relieve her symptoms, Hope decided to see an ear-nose-throat specialist; perhaps the cough was due to a growth in her throat or on her vocal cords. This physician said the throat looked irritated and took some X rays of her sinuses to check the likelihood of a postnasal drip. He diagnosed laryngitis, urged her to drink lots of fluids, gargle with hot water and salt, and take an over-the-counter cough suppressant.

Weeks of hacking cough spun discouragingly into three months. Hope was annoyed that she had found no relief, and embarrassed that her voice faded at important meetings. She barely had enough strength to get through the required talk of the day, and she found socializing an added burden. She had run out of ideas. She didn't even know what type of doctor to turn to.

Hope decided to write about all these symptoms and her situation in vivid and even hostile words. She thought back to earlier times of her life, when she had been sidelined with a cold or flu. She listed acquaintances with similar experiences, and vowed to call them for advice. She puzzled about the interludes when the coughing seemed to subside, bringing temporary periods of calm. She didn't hold anything back in her writing. She decided to play detective, and methodically wrote about the frequency of her symptoms, the timing and location, and the severity. She analyzed her emotional state: The relationship with her boyfriend was good; her job was satisfying, although she occasionally kicked herself for passing up an opportunity to work at Microsoft; she was planning a friend's baby shower, but that wasn't much of a strain. Was it all in her head?

After this outpouring, a plan began to crystallize in Hope's mind. And you might find similar occasions to use her idea. She dreaded another fruitless trip to her internist's office. Instead, she decided to send a fax. In it, she reminded her physician of symptoms and the consultations they already had; she reviewed how the cough and loss of voice were damaging her life. She presented a list of observations that failed to add up to a pattern to her:

- Antibiotics, cough suppressants, and gargling had not worked; her symptoms continued for more than twelve weeks.

- She actually felt good during her every-other-day swim, but she had trouble during her evening jog.
- She felt worse when she visited her brother and his family.
- Her symptoms grew more acute just prior to her menstrual period.

Hope presented three options for her doctor's consideration:

☐ Arrange another appointment.
☐ Suggest another physician for a consultation.
☐ Something else: _____

The physician chose to call her at home two evenings later to ask a few further questions: Did she have any history of allergies? (Yes, she did have some food allergies as a child and still suffered from seasonal hay fever.) Had she felt any wheezing or shortness of breath? (No, never experienced those symptoms.) Did the symptoms seem to occur at any particular time of day? (The cough was more severe at nighttime and in the early morning hours, often disrupting her sleep.) The physician suggested that Hope might be suffering from asthma and recommended a pulmonary specialist. He explained that Hope should try to arrange an appointment when her symptoms were especially bad, and that the doctor would conduct a breathing test called spirometry to examine her ability to expel air forcefully; a chest X ray would also be required. The specialist might even suggest a scratch test to determine sensitivity to some common allergens.

Hope's story has a happy ending. In fact, she was diagnosed with asthma, which she keeps at bay with a combination of medications, administered through inhalers. She records her symptoms in a diary and has made minor modifications to her lifestyle: Don't jog in cold weather; avoid cigarette smoke and cat dander (the culprits from her brother's home); reduce dust and mold at home; and read food labels carefully for any signs of sulfites. She has learned to adjust her medication to both seasonal pollen fluctuations and monthly menstrual cycles.

All three steps combined to end Hope's needless disability. She thought broadly about her situation. She poured her heart out on paper, which freed her to think about a novel initiative. She rehearsed her communication with the doctor—to the point of composing a thoughtful and interactive message which allowed him unusual latitude in proposing next steps. Concentrate on the broad outlines of this story, not the particulars. As surely as Hope, you can put it all together, too.

# COMMON MEDICAL TREATMENTS

This section introduces you to seven common medical treatments and what they are like. The Glossary in the next section includes medical terms that are used in critical-care situations.

## Antibiotic Medications

*Definition:* Medications to combat serious bacterial infections anywhere in the body. Bacterial pneumonia is an example of a lung infection that can be treated with antibiotics.

*Description:* Antibiotics are usually administered in pill or liquid form or through intravenous (IV) tubes.

*Benefits:* Antibiotics can cure a serious bacterial infection, easing discomfort from fever or pain.

*Limitations:* Antibiotics treat infection but do not correct other underlying health problems. They are not useful for viral or fungal infections.

## Artificial Nutrition and Hydration (Feeding Tubes)

*Definition:* A method of providing nutrition and fluids through a tube, for a patient who cannot eat or drink normally. Also called "feeding tubes" or "tube feeding."

*Description:* There are two methods of tube feeding. Nutrition in liquid form can be given through a small flexible tube passed through the nose to the stomach, or the liquid can be delivered directly to the stomach through a tube that has been surgically inserted by way of the abdomen. The surgical route is usually used when the feeding will be long-term, or when there is trauma to the mouth, throat, or face that makes a nose tube difficult. May be needed on a temporary or permanent basis.

*Benefits:* Ability to prolong life by providing liquids, calories, and minerals needed to maintain bodily functions. Can help a person through a period of recovery, by sustaining life and promoting healing. A stomach tube reduces the risk of the patient's accidentally getting nutritional fluids into the lungs.

*Risks:* The nose tube can make talking and swallowing uncomfortable; it can also cause sores and irritation in the nose. It is possible that an infection can develop at the site of the stomach tube.

### Cardiopulmonary Resuscitation (CPR)

*Definition:* An emergency procedure that restores and maintains breathing and circulation in a person whose heart or breathing has stopped.

*Description:* CPR includes the following methods: forceful compressions of the chest over the heart; assisted breathing through mouth-to-mouth, or a tube in the windpipe attached to a ventilator, or a hand-held breathing bag connected to a mask that is placed over the mouth and nose; intravenous medicines; electric shock to stimulate the heart.

*Benefits:* Survival rate and return to previous condition can be high in previously healthy people if CPR is begun almost immediately.

*Risks:* CPR is less successful with older adults and people with chronic conditions, or if CPR is delayed. When breathing stops, oxygen cannot reach a person's brain, which may cause brain damage and lead to a range of disabilities. Brain damage can occur within a few minutes. Forceful pumping on the chest can cause later pain, broken ribs or breastbone, cuts or bruises of spleen or liver, or rupture of a lung.

### Chemotherapy

*Definition:* Administration of drugs to fight cancer. The goal is to destroy malignant (cancerous or harmful) tumor cells without causing excessive or irreversible damage to the patient's normal cells.

*Description:* Drugs are administered either in pill form, through an injection, or through an intravenous (IV) tube. Chemotherapy can be done in a doctor's office, hospital, or at home.

*Benefits:* Possible that the cancer cells will be destroyed. Disease may go into remission or be cured.

*Risks:* Side effects may include hair loss; nausea; vomiting; sores in the mouth, throat, and intestines; loss of appetite; fatigue; anemia; bleeding; and higher susceptibility to infections. There are drugs that may minimize or prevent some of these risks.

## Comfort (Palliative) Care

*Definition:* A range of treatments intended to relieve pain and suffering, control adverse symptoms, reduce anxiety, and provide comprehensive support.

*Description:* Includes the following: administering pain medicine; hygiene (mouth care and bathing the patient); temperature control; massage; bringing drinks; changing bed linen; turning patient's position; hand holding; stroking; emotional support from family, friends, nurses, and other medical staff; and spiritual support from hospital chaplains and personal religious advisors. Can also include soothing diversions such as music, television, or change of scenery.

*Benefits:* Reduces pain and discomfort. Provides emotional support. Helps create peaceful and nurturing environment.

*Limitation:* Does not correct underlying physical disease processes.


## Dialysis (Hemodialysis or Kidney Dialysis)

*Definition:* Cleaning the blood by machine for patients whose kidneys have failed. Dialysis offers an artificial mechanism for performing some kidney functions.

*Description:* Large tubes are inserted through the arm or groin and into large blood vessels and attached to a portable machine that cleans the blood of excess chemicals, minerals, and impurities and removes excess fluid. Dialysis treatments usually take two to four hours and may be needed as often as daily. They can be done in a hospital or at home. Dialysis may be needed for a temporary period of time or it may be needed permanently.

*Benefits:* Can assume kidney function for the body while the kidneys have time to recover. Dialysis can be used while waiting for a transplant.

*Risks:* Does not cure an underlying kidney condition. If the kidneys don't recover, the patient may need to rely on dialysis forever. Complications of long-term dialysis include anemia that may require blood transfusions, moderate skin itching, and fatigue. Repeated surgery to insert new tubes into the arm or groin is often necessary. Diet must be strictly regulated and people must remain near dialysis facilities at all times.


## Mechanical Breathing (Ventilator)

*Definition:* Breathing with the help of a machine. A ventilator is also called a "respirator."

*Description:* A machine that helps a person breathe when he or she in unable to do so on his or her own. For short-term conditions (for example, after an accident or surgery), a tube is placed either in the mouth or nose and into the patient's windpipe. Medication is often used to ease discomfort during this procedure. For a long-term condition (for example, more than one month), a tube may be placed directly into a hole that has been surgically created in the patient's windpipe. This procedure is called a *tracheotomy*. In a hospital, ventilators are powered by generators so that they continue to function even if there is a loss of the central power supply.

*Benefits:* May only be needed on a short-term basis, for example, following surgery, until the patient can breathe on his or her own. There are people with disabilities who live with ongoing ventilator support.

*Risks:* A nose or mouth tube is uncomfortable and makes it impossible to speak or eat. Pneumonia and other infections are possible, as are sinus infections, mouth wounds, and dry mouth. After a tracheotomy, speaking may be limited to very short periods of time. Patients also have difficulty swallowing.

# GLOSSARY OF
# CRITICAL-CARE TERMINOLOGY

---

This Glossary contains medical terms that are commonly used in critical-care situations.

**Alzheimer's disease.** A disease that causes degeneration of brain tissue. Occurs more often in women than men. Symptoms include: disorientation; progressive, irreversible loss of memory; loss of intellectual functions (such as problem solving and judgment); indifference to surroundings; and speech disturbance. May take anywhere from a few months to many years to progress to a complete loss of intellectual function (see also *Dementia*).

**Brain death.** A permanent loss of all functions of the brain. The body does not move and shows no purposeful response to stimulation (loud noise, painful touch, heat, cold). The body cannot breathe without a ventilator. All protective reflexes such as coughing, blinking, and constriction of the pupils to light have ceased. There is no meaningful electrical activity in the brain or blood flow to the brain. In most of the fifty states, brain death is accepted as the legal definition of death. A standard, systematic medical protocol is used to certify brain death.

**Code.** The term *code* means that the patient's heart stops beating and/or he or she stops breathing and that CPR must be initiated. This event may also be referred to as *Code Blue, Code 99,* or *Code Charlie.* Also referred to as *to code someone,* which means to try to resuscitate that person.

**Coma/comatose.** A coma can be a temporary or a permanent abnormal condition in which the patient is unconscious and cannot be aroused by stimulation such as voice, touch, or pain. The patient is not able to signal what he or she wants. Depending on the depth of coma, there may be bodily movements that occur spontaneously or as a reflex activity, such as withdrawing in response to painful stimulation or squeezing an object placed in the hand. There are many causes of coma including head injury, stroke, brain hemorrhage, tumors, infections, chemical imbalances in the body, and drugs that suppress brain activity. Treatment for coma is specific for the condition causing it, such as antibiotics for infection or surgery for head injury. Recovery from coma depends on the extent of permanent damage to brain tissue caused by the patient's illness or injury. Irreversible damage to those brain tissues responsible for consciousness will result in a permanent coma.

**Decision-making capacity.**  A term used to reflect the ability of a person to make specific decisions; also includes a person's ability to understand relevant information, to reflect on it, and to communicate (verbally or nonverbally) to doctors and nurses. An advance directive *only* takes effect if a patient does *not* have decision-making capacity. A patient who has decision-making capacity will make his or her own decisions regarding treatment by talking or communicating in another way with the physician.

**Dementia.**  A mental state resulting from deterioration of brain tissue. Dementia results from a steady decline in intellectual function—memory, thinking, and judgment—that interferes with a person's normal social and occupational activity. May occur in adults at any age and can be caused by injury or illness severe enough to cause widespread damage to the brain. Often follows hardening of the arteries in the brain, Alzheimer's disease, brain tumors, brain infections, or bleeding into brain tissue.

**Do-not-resuscitate (DNR) order.**  An order in a patient's medical record that instructs physicians and nurses not to attempt to restart a patient's failed heartbeat or breathing using cardiopulmonary resuscitation (CPR). A DNR order is also called *no code*. Such an order can be changed at any time and should be reviewed on a regular basis. However, DNR does not mean no care. The patient will continue to receive treatments, medicines, and nursing care to manage health problems and to provide comfort and emotional support.

**Incapacitated person.**  A person who lacks sufficient mental ability to understand the treatment choices presented, comprehend the alternatives to the treatment, and make and communicate a clear decision. The term can also refer to persons who have been determined by the court to be incompetent.

**Life-sustaining treatment (or life support).**  Any medical procedure or treatment that will support and prolong life. In the case of seriously ill individuals, this can include treatments such as strong medications, cardiopulmonary resuscitation (CPR), a ventilator for mechanical breathing, artificial nutrition and hydration (feeding tubes), or dialysis for kidney failure. Life support can also refer to much simpler treatments like antibiotics and blood transfusions.

***Organ-donation form (or organ-donation card).***  Written instructions indicating a person's wishes to make his or her organs available upon death for transplantation to another person or for donation to medical/educational research. Organs that can be donated include kidneys, heart, liver, lungs, and pancreas. All costs related to donation are paid by the organ procurement program or transplant center and eventually by the recipients of the organs.

***Persistent vegetative state (PVS).***  A state of permanent damage to the parts of the brain that control higher-level functions such as thinking, reasoning, judgment, communication, hunger, and thirst. Patients are persistently unaware of their surroundings and have no verbal or psychological interaction with their environment. A patient in a PVS may appear awake because of spontaneous eye openings or sleep-wake cycles. Patients may be able to breathe on their own because parts of the brain that control more basic bodily functions may not be damaged.

***Terminal condition (or terminal illness).***  There are no universally agreed-upon definitions of these terms. Generally, *terminal* refers to an illness or condition that is incurable and irreversible and in which death is expected to occur within a short time, generally considered less than one year.

***Tissue-donation form (or tissue-donation card).***  Written instructions indicating a person's wishes to make his or her tissues available upon death for transplantation to another person or for donation to medical/educational research. Tissues that can be donated include corneas, skin, bone, middle ear, heart valve plus connective tissue, and blood vessels. All costs related to tissue donation are paid by the tissue procurement program or transplant center and eventually by the recipients of the tissues.

*EXAMPLES OF
ADVANCE DIRECTIVES
AND WALLET CARD*

# CALIFORNIA NATURAL DEATH ACT

*Information, Instructions and Form*

**What is the Natural Death Act?**

In 1976, California adopted the Natural Death Act. This was the first statute in the nation giving legal effect to people's written statements of the medical care they would want if they become terminally ill and unable to speak for themselves. The general name for such a document is an "advance directive." The most familiar type of advance directive is a "Living Will." People have used living wills for many years to express the wish that their dying not be prolonged when recovery is not expected.

In 1991, the California legislature adopted a new Natural Death Act, effective January 1, 1992. This law provides California's version of the living will, called a "Declaration." Whether or not you filled out a "Directive to Physicians" under the old Natural Death Act prior to January 1992, you may wish to fill out a "Declaration" because the old forms were valid only for 5 years and applied only in very limited circumstances. The new law makes it easier for you to exercise your rights.

**What are the major provisions of the Natural Death Act?**

- To execute a valid Declaration you must be at least 18 years old and capable of making decisions about your medical treatment.
- For a Declaration to be implemented:
    - it must have been communicated to your attending physician (you should give your doctor a copy);
    - you must no longer be able to make decisions regarding your medical treatment;
    - your attending physician and one other physician must diagnose that you are permanently unconscious or that you suffer from a terminal illness (one that is incurable and that will result in death within a relatively short time if life-sustaining treatment is not used).
- Any type of medical treatment may be withheld or withdrawn, including food and fluids provided by tubes (unless you indicate otherwise).
- Treatment for comfort and to alleviate pain will still be provided.
- A Declaration will remain valid until you revoke it or write a new one. You may revoke a Declaration at any time, without regard to your mental or physical condition, as long as you can communicate.
- Your physician must put your Declaration in your medical record.
- Your physician must follow your Declaration or transfer your care to another physician.
- A death that results from following a Declaration is not a suicide or homicide.
- You cannot be required to, or prohibited from, writing a Declaration in order to get health care or health insurance, nor can it affect the terms on which you can purchase life insurance.
- Declarations are not effective while a patient is pregnant.

**How does a Declaration compare with a Durable Power of Attorney for Health Care?**

A Declaration just states your wishes but doesn't provide a means of naming someone to make health care decisions on your behalf if you become unable to do so. If you want to specify who among your relatives or close friends will speak for you, you should consider filling out a Durable Power of Attorney for Health Care (DPAHC) instead of a Declaration. If you fill out a valid DPAHC now or later, it will override a Declaration unless the DPAHC specifically states otherwise.

Some people prefer the Declaration because it allows just one thing to be done (withholding and withdrawing life-prolonging treatment) and only under certain circumstances (when you are terminally ill or permanently unconscious). On the other hand, the DPAHC applies to most medical treatments, not just to life-prolonging treatment. And the DPAHC is more flexible in responding to your actual medical condition because it allows the person you name (your agent) to step into your place in making treatment decisions with your doctors if you can't because you are unconscious or very sick. Besides naming an agent you may also specify choices about medical treatment in a DPAHC.

# Instructions for Filling out a Natural Death Act Declaration.

**Before signing a Declaration you may want to talk it over with your family, physician, or other advisors. The form is not complicated, however, and these instructions will help you in filling it out.**

| 1 | *This paragraph declares your wish that treatment be withheld or withdrawn when it merely prolongs an incurable, fatal condition or merely maintains permanent unconsciousness.* It states the basic conditions of a Natural Death Act Declaration. The Declaration will only come into effect when you are no longer able to make health care decisions yourself. **If you WANT feeding and fluids to be provided by a tube to keep you alive, you should cross out the phrase "including artificially administered nutrition and hydration," and place your initials and the date in the margin.**

| 2 | **OPTIONAL:** *Space is provided on the back of the form if you want to spell out your general values as they relate to life-prolongation. Be sure to put your initials and date below the statement.*

There is no way to anticipate exactly what choices may have to be made when you're very sick and can't speak for yourself, so it would be helpful to your doctor and others who have to make medical decisions for you to know the kinds of things you particularly want or don't want. For example, how important are things like maintaining the ability to communicate, avoiding pain, being paralyzed or bed-bound, and so forth? Also, you should realize that a diagnosis of terminal illness or of permanent coma always involves some element of uncertainty. Once the attending physician has reached a diagnosis that is reasonably certain, some people want treatment stopped, while others want to wait or have further testing to eliminate more uncertainty. How do you feel about things like that?

| 3 | The Natural Death Act makes a Declaration ineffective while the declarant is pregnant.

| 4 | Keep the original Declaration and make copies for your doctor and family or whoever might be called in the event of a medical emergency.

| 5 | In this space, write out the date, month, and year when you sign the Declaration.

| 6 | Sign this line in the presence of the people who are serving as your witnesses, and print your name and address legibly on the lines below your signature.

WITNESSES

You will need two witnesses. Neither witness may be a physician or other professional (such as a nurse) who provides health care, or anyone who works for such a person or for a hospital or other health care provider (such as a nursing home or home health agency), or anyone who runs or who works at a community care facility or a residential care facility for the elderly (such as a board-and-care home). **If you are a resident in a long-term care facility (such as a nursing home), one of your witnesses must be a patient advocate or ombudsman designated by the State Department of Aging.**

| 7 | Within these general requirements, the person who signs here can be anyone, including a relative or someone who could inherit something from you.

| 8 | The second witness must be someone who is not named in your will or is not such a close relative that he or she would be entitled under the law to receive part of your estate automatically.

# NATURAL DEATH ACT DECLARATION

1  If I should have an incurable and irreversible condition that has been diagnosed by two physicians and that will result in my death within a relatively short time without the administration of life-sustaining treatment or that has produced an irreversible coma or persistent vegetative state, and I am no longer able to make decisions regarding my medical treatment, I direct my attending physician, pursuant to the Natural Death Act of California, to withhold or withdraw treatment, including artificially administered nutrition and hydration, that only prolongs the process of dying or the irreversible coma or persistent vegetative state and is not necessary for my comfort or to alleviate pain.

2  ☐ By checking this box I indicate that I have written down on the back of this page my general thoughts about the use of life-prolonging treatment and the things I value in life and would hope to obtain from health care, as a guide for those who will give effect to my Declaration.

3  If I have been diagnosed as pregnant, and that diagnosis is known to my physician, this Declaration shall have no force or effect during my pregnancy.

4  I authorize the use of photocopies of this Declaration as though they were originals.

5  Signed this_____day of_____,199___ .

6  Signature _____

   Printed Name_____

   Address _____

   _____

The declarant voluntarily signed this writing in my presence. I am not a health care provider, an employee of a health care provider, the operator of a community care facility, an employee of an operator of a community care facility, the operator of a residential care facility for the elderly, or an employee of an operator of a residential care facility for the elderly.

7  Witness's Signature_____

   Printed Name_____

   Address _____

   _____

The declarant voluntarily signed this writing in my presence. I am not entitled to any portion of the estate of the declarant upon his or her death under any will or codicil thereto of the declarant now existing or by operation of law. I am not a health care provider, an employee of a health care provider, the operator of a community care facility, an employee or an operator of a community care facility, the operator of a residential care facility for the elderly, or an employee or an operator of a residential care facility for the elderly.

8  Witness's Signature_____

   Printed Name_____

   Address _____

   _____

## What should I do with this document once I have filled it out?

Once you and your two witnesses have signed and dated the Declaration, you should give a copy to your physician and ask that it be placed in your medical record. You should also make copies for anyone (such as your next-of-kin) who is likely to know when you are very sick and who might be asked what your wishes about treatment were. You should keep a copy of the Declaration for yourself, with your other important papers - although probably NOT in a safe deposit box, where people may not be able to get it if you were hospitalized. Whenever you go into a hospital, hospice, or nursing facility, or initiate treatment with any home health care agency, take along a copy of your Declaration so that it can be put in your medical record.

## What if I change my mind about my Declaration?

You can revoke your Declaration at any time, even after you become terminally ill. You can do this by tearing it up, by writing "I revoke" on it, or just by saying that you have changed your mind. Make sure that your doctor knows that you have revoked it, and try to tell the other people to whom you gave copies of your Declaration. You can also ask all these people to give you back the copies of your Declaration or to tear them up.

## Declarant's General Statement Of Values To Guide Withdrawal Or Withholding Of Treatment:

_____

_____

_____

_____

_____

_____

_____

_____

**If you write a statement above, put your initials and today's date here:** _____ / _____ / 19 ___

*The information in this form is based on California Health and Safety Code.*
*Sections 7185 to 7194.5, as amended in September 1991, and effective January 1,1992.*

*This document was developed by the California Consortium on Patient Self-Determination, a working coalition*
*of health care provider organizations, health professionals and consumers, bioethics centers, and the State.*

**Permission is granted for health care providers and community organizations to duplicate this form in order**
**to provide single copies at no charge to individuals interested in filling out the form.**

**California Medical Association**
**DURABLE POWER OF ATTORNEY FOR HEALTH CARE DECISIONS**
*(California Probate Code Sections 4600-4753)*

**WARNING TO PERSON EXECUTING THIS DOCUMENT**

This is an important legal document. Before executing this document, you should know these important facts:

This document gives the person you designate as your agent (the attorney-in-fact) the power to make health care decisions for you. Your agent must act consistently with your desires as stated in this document or otherwise made known.

Except as you otherwise specify in this document, this document gives your agent power to consent to your doctor not giving treatment or stopping treatment necessary to keep you alive.

Notwithstanding this document, you have the right to make medical and other health care decisions for yourself so long as you can give informed consent with respect to the particular decision. In addition, no treatment may be given to you over your objection, and health care necessary to keep you alive may not be stopped or withheld if you object at the time.

This document gives your agent authority to consent, to refuse to consent, or to withdraw consent to any care, treatment, service, or procedure to maintain, diagnose, or treat a physical or mental condition. This power is subject to any statement of your desires and any limitations that you include in this document. You may

state in this document any types of treatment that you do not desire. In addition, a court can take away the power of your agent to make health care decisions for you if your agent (1) authorizes anything that is illegal, (2) acts contrary to your known desires or (3) where your desires are not known, does anything that is clearly contrary to your best interests.

This power will exist for an indefinite period of time unless you limit its duration in this document.

You have the right to revoke the authority of your agent by notifying your agent or your treating doctor, hospital, or other health care provider orally or in writing of the revocation.

Your agent has the right to examine your medical records and to consent to their disclosure unless you limit this right in this document.

Unless you otherwise specify in this document, this document gives your agent the power after you die to (1) authorize an autopsy, (2) donate your body or parts thereof for transplant or therapeutic or educational or scientific purposes, and (3) direct the disposition of your remains.

If there is anything in this document that you do not understand, you should ask a lawyer to explain it to you.

## 1. CREATION OF DURABLE POWER OF ATTORNEY FOR HEALTH CARE

By this document I intend to create a durable power of attorney by appointing the person designated below to make health care decisions for me as allowed by Sections 4600 to 4753, inclusive, of the California Probate Code. This power of attorney shall not be affected by my subsequent incapacity. I hereby revoke any prior durable power of attorney for health care. I am a California resident who is at least 18 years old, of sound mind, and acting of my own free will.

## 2. APPOINTMENT OF HEALTH CARE AGENT

*(Fill in below the name, address and telephone number of the person you wish to make health care decisions for you if you become incapacitated. You should make sure that this person agrees to accept this responsibility. The following may not serve as your agent: (1) your treating health care provider; (2) an operator of a community care facility or residential care facility for the elderly; or (3) an employee of your treating health care provider, a community care facility, or a residential care facility for the elderly, unless that employee is related to you by blood, marriage or adoption. If you are a conservatee under the Lanterman-Petris-Short Act (the law governing involuntary commitment to a mental health facility) and you wish to appoint your conservator as your agent, you must consult a lawyer, who must sign and attach a special declaration for this document to be valid.)*

I, _____, hereby appoint:
*(insert your name)*

Name _____

Address _____

Work Telephone (_____) _____  Home Telephone (_____) _____

as my agent (attorney-in-fact) to make health care decisions for me as authorized in this document. I understand that this power of attorney will be effective for an indefinite period of time unless I revoke it or limit its duration below.

(Optional) This power of attorney shall expire on the following date: _____.

© California Medical Association 1995 (revised)

### 3. AUTHORITY OF AGENT

If I become incapable of giving informed consent to health care decisions, I grant my agent full power and authority to make those decisions for me, subject to any statements of desires or limitations set forth below. Unless I have limited my agent's authority in this document, that authority shall include the right to consent, refuse consent, or withdraw consent to any medical care, treatment, service, or procedure; to receive and to consent to the release of medical information; to authorize an autopsy to determine the cause of my death; to make a gift of all or part of my body; and to direct the disposition of my remains, subject to any instructions I have given in a written contract for funeral services, my will or by some other method. I understand that, by law, my agent may not consent to any of the following: commitment to a mental health treatment facility, convulsive treatment, psychosurgery, sterilization or abortion.

### 4. MEDICAL TREATMENT DESIRES AND LIMITATIONS (OPTIONAL)

*(Your agent must make health care decisions that are consistent with your known desires. You may, but are not required to, state your desires about the kinds of medical care you do or do not want to receive, including your desires concerning life support if you are seriously ill. If you do not want your agent to have the authority to make certain decisions, you must write a statement to that effect in the space provided below; otherwise, your agent will have the broad powers to make health care decisions for you that are outlined in paragraph 3 above. In either case, it is important that you discuss your health care desires with the person you appoint as your agent and with your doctor(s).)*

*(Following is a general statement about withholding and removal of life-sustaining treatment. If the statement accurately reflects your desires, you may initial it. If you wish to add to it or to write your own statement instead, you may do so in the space provided.)*

---

I do **not** want efforts made to prolong my life and I do **not** want life-sustaining treatment to be provided or continued: (1) if I am in an irreversible coma or persistent vegetative state; or (2) if I am terminally ill and the use of life-sustaining procedures would serve only to artificially delay the moment of my death; or (3) under any other circumstances where the burdens of the treatment outweigh the expected benefits. In making decisions about life-sustaining treatment under provision (3) above, I want my agent to consider the relief of suffering and the quality of my life, as well as the extent of the possible prolongation of my life.

*If this statement reflects your desires, initial here:* _____

---

Other or additional statements of medical treatment desires and limitations: _____
_____
_____
_____
_____

*(You may attach additional pages if you need more space to complete your statements. Each additional page must be dated and signed at the same time you date and sign this document.)*

### 5. APPOINTMENT OF ALTERNATE AGENTS (OPTIONAL)

*(You may appoint alternate agents to make health care decisions for you in case the person you appointed in Paragraph 2 is unable or unwilling to do so.)*

If the person named as my agent in Paragraph 2 is not available or willing to make health care decisions for me as authorized in this document, I appoint the following persons to do so, listed in the order they should be asked:

*First Alternate Agent:* Name _____

Address _____

Work Telephone ( _____ ) _____     Home Telephone ( _____ ) _____

*Second Alternate Agent:* Name _____

Address _____

Work Telephone ( _____ ) _____     Home Telephone ( _____ ) _____

### 6. USE OF COPIES

I hereby authorize that photocopies of this document can be relied upon by my agent and others as though they were originals.

2

## DATE AND SIGNATURE OF PRINCIPAL
### (You must date and sign this power of attorney)

I sign my name to this Durable Power of Attorney for Health Care  at _____, _____

                                                *(City)*                                 *(State)*

on _____ . _____

          *(Date)*                                      *(Signature of Principal)*

## STATEMENT OF WITNESSES

*(This power of attorney will not be valid for making health care decisions unless it is either (1) signed by two qualified adult witnesses who are present when you sign or acknowledge your signature __or__ (2) acknowledged before a notary public in California. If you elect to use witnesses rather than a notary public, the law provides that none of the following may be used as witnesses: (1) the persons you have appointed as your agent and alternate agents; (2) your health care provider or an employee of your health care provider; or (3) an operator or employee of an operator of a community care facility or residential care facility for the elderly. Additionally, at least one of the witnesses cannot be related to you by blood, marriage or adoption, or be named in your will.  IF YOU ARE A PATIENT IN A SKILLED NURSING FACILITY, YOU __MUST__ HAVE A PATIENT ADVOCATE OR OMBUDSMAN SIGN BOTH THE STATEMENT OF WITNESSES BELOW __AND__ THE DECLARATION ON THE FOLLOWING PAGE.)*

I declare under penalty of perjury under the laws of California that the person who signed or acknowledged this document is personally known to me to be the principal, or that the identity of the principal was proved to me by convincing evidence,* that the principal signed or acknowledged this durable power of attorney in my presence, that the principal appears to be of sound mind and under no duress, fraud, or undue influence; that I am not the person appointed as attorney in fact by this document; and that I am not the principal's health care provider, an employee of the principal's health care provider, the operator of a community care facility or a residential care facility for the elderly, nor an employee of an operator of a community care facility or residential care facility for the elderly.

*First Witness:* Signature _____

Print name _____

Date _____

Residence Address _____

*Second Witness:* Signature _____

Print name _____

Date _____

Residence Address _____

### (AT LEAST ONE OF THE ABOVE WITNESSES MUST ALSO SIGN THE FOLLOWING DECLARATION)

I further declare under penalty of perjury under the laws of California that I am not related to the principal by blood, marriage, or adoption, and, to the best of my knowledge I am not entitled to any part of the estate of the principal upon the death of the principal under a will now existing or by operation of law.

Signature:_____

---

*The law allows one or more of the following forms of identification as convincing evidence of identity: a California driver's license or identification card or U.S. passport that is current or has been issued within five years, or any of the following if the document is current or has been issued within five years, contains a photograph and description of the person named on it, is signed by the person, and bears a serial or other identifying number: a foreign passport that has been stamped by the U.S. Immigration and Naturalization Service; a driver's license issued by another state or by an authorized Canadian or Mexican agency; or an identification card issued by another state or by any branch of the U.S. armed forces.  If the principal is a patient in a skilled nursing facility, a patient advocate or ombudsman may rely on the representations of family members or the administrator or staff of the facility as convincing evidence of identity if the patient advocate or ombudsman believes that the representations provide a reasonable basis for determining the identity of the principal.

## SPECIAL REQUIREMENT: STATEMENT OF PATIENT ADVOCATE OR OMBUDSMAN

*(If you are a patient in a skilled nursing facility, a patient advocate or ombudsman must sign the Statement of Witnesses above and must also sign the following declaration.)*

I further declare under penalty of perjury under the laws of California that I am a patient advocate or ombudsman as designated by the State Department of Aging and am serving as a witness as required by subdivision (e) of Probate Code Section 4701.

Signature: _____       Address: _____

Print Name: _____                 _____

Date: _____                  _____

## CERTIFICATE OF ACKNOWLEDGMENT OF NOTARY PUBLIC

*(Acknowledgment before a notary public is not required if you have elected to have two qualified witnesses sign above. If you are a patient in a skilled nursing facility, you must have a patient advocate or ombudsman sign the Statement of Witnesses on page 3 and the Statement of Patient Advocate or Ombudsman above)*

State of California                                                    )

                                         )ss.

County of _____ )

On this _____ day of _____, in the year _____,

before me, _____,
                        *(here insert name and title of the officer)*

personally appeared _____
                            *(here insert name of principal)*

personally known to me (or proved to me on the basis of satisfactory evidence) to be the person(s) whose name(s) is/are subscribed to this instrument and acknowledged to me that he/she/they executed the same in his/her/their authorized capacity(ies), and that by his/her/their signature(s) on the instrument the person(s), or the entity upon behalf of which the person(s) acted, executed the instrument.

WITNESS my hand and official seal.

_____
    *(Signature of Notary Public)*

**NOTARY SEAL**

## COPIES

YOUR AGENT MAY NEED THIS DOCUMENT IMMEDIATELY IN CASE OF AN EMERGENCY. YOU SHOULD KEEP THE COMPLETED ORIGINAL AND GIVE PHOTOCOPIES OF THE COMPLETED ORIGINAL TO (1) YOUR AGENT AND ALTERNATE AGENTS, (2) YOUR PERSONAL PHYSICIAN, AND (3) MEMBERS OF YOUR FAMILY AND ANY OTHER PERSONS WHO MIGHT BE CALLED IN THE EVENT OF A MEDICAL EMERGENCY. THE LAW PERMITS THAT PHOTOCOPIES OF THE COMPLETED DOCUMENT CAN BE RELIED UPON AS THOUGH THEY WERE ORIGINALS.

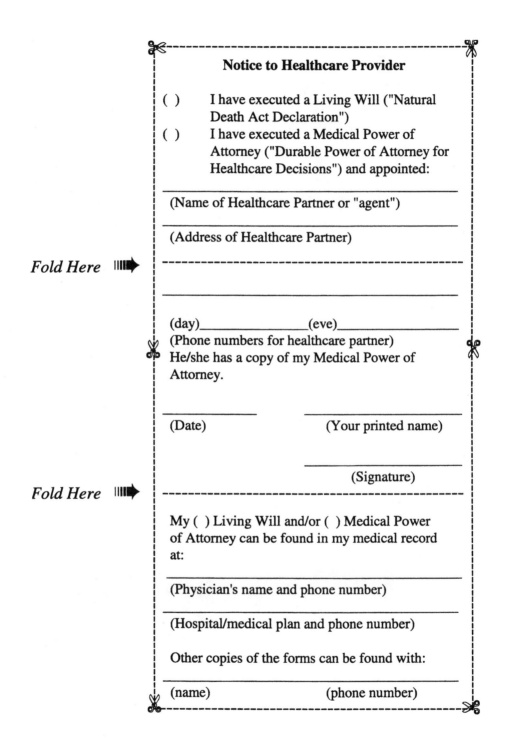

**Notice to Healthcare Provider**

( )     I have executed a Living Will ("Natural Death Act Declaration")

( )     I have executed a Medical Power of Attorney ("Durable Power of Attorney for Healthcare Decisions") and appointed:

_____
(Name of Healthcare Partner or "agent")

_____
(Address of Healthcare Partner)

*Fold Here* ➡

_____

_____

(day)_____(eve)_____
(Phone numbers for healthcare partner)
He/she has a copy of my Medical Power of Attorney.

_____     _____
(Date)           (Your printed name)

             _____
             (Signature)

*Fold Here* ➡

My ( ) Living Will and/or ( ) Medical Power of Attorney can be found in my medical record at:

_____
(Physician's name and phone number)

_____
(Hospital/medical plan and phone number)

Other copies of the forms can be found with:

_____
(name)             (phone number)

# REFERENCES

## Introduction

Benner, P., and J. Wrubel. 1989. *The primacy of caring: Stress and coping in health and illness.* Menlo Park, Calif.: Addison-Wesley.

Callahan, D. 1990. *What kind of life: The limits of medical progress.* New York: Simon and Schuster.

House, J. S., R. C. Kessler, A. R. Herzog, R. P. Mero, A. M. Kinney, and M. J. Breslow. 1990. Age, socioeconomic status, and health. *Milbank Quarterly* 68:383–411.

Moore, G. T. 1992. The case of the disappearing generalist: Does it need to be solved? *Milbank Quarterly* 70:361–379.

Oldenburg, R. 1989. *The great good place.* New York: Paragon.

Sagan, L. A. 1987. *The health of nations: True causes of sickness and well-being.* New York: Basic Books.

Shorter, E. 1985. *Bedside manners: The troubled history of doctors and patients.* New York: Simon and Schuster.

Wofford, J. L., J. A. Pinson, S. J. Folmar, and W. P. Moran. 1995. Health-related messages in consumer magazine advertising. *Journal of General Internal Medicine* 10:488–490.

## CHAPTER 1  *Getting Your Doctor to Pay Attention*

American Hospital Association. 1996. *The Dartmouth atlas of health care in the United States.* Chicago: American Hospital Association.

Anders, G. 1996. *Health against wealth.* Boston: Houghton Mifflin.

Andersen, P. A. 1985. Nonverbal immediacy in interpersonal communication. In *Multichannel integrations of nonverbal behavior,* edited by A. W. Siegman and S. Feldstein. Hillsdale, N.J.: Lawrence Erlbaum.

Anderson, L. A., B. M. DeVellis, and R. F. DeVellis. 1987. Effects of modeling on patient communication, satisfaction, and knowledge. *Medical Care* 25:1044–1056.

Babad, E., F. Bernieri, and R. Rosenthal. 1989. When less information is more informative: Diagnosing teacher expectations from brief samples of behavior. *British Journal of Educational Psychology* 59:281–295.

Baker, R., A. Caplan, L. L. Emanuel, and S. R. Latham. 1997. Crisis, ethics, and the American Medical Association: 1847 and 1997. *Journal of the American Medical Association* 278:163–164.

Bandura, A. 1989. Human agency in social cognitive theory. *American Psychologist* 44:1175–1184.

Barker, P. 1993. *Regeneration.* New York: Plume.

Beckman, H. B., and R. M. Frankel. 1984. The effect of physician behavior on the collection of data. *Annals of Internal Medicine* 101:692–696.

Bensing, J. M., and E. M. Sluijs. 1985. Evaluation of an interview training course for general practitioners. *Social Science and Medicine* 20:737–744.

Bensing, J. 1991. Doctor-patient communications and the quality of care. *Social Science and Medicine* 32:1301–1310.

Blanchard, C. G., M. S. Labrecque, J. C. Ruckdeschel, and E. B. Blanchard. 1988. Information and decision-making preferences of hospitalized adult cancer patients. *Social Science and Medicine* 27:1139–1145.

Blanck, P. D., and R. Rosenthal. 1984. Mediation of interpersonal expectancy effects: Counselor's tone of voice. *Journal of Educational Psychology* 76:418–426.

Blanck, P. D., R. Rosenthal, M. Vannicelli, and T. D. Lee. 1986. Therapists' tone of voice: Descriptive, psychometric, interactional, and competence analyses. *Journal of Social and Clinical Psychology* 4:154–178.

Blau, S. P., and E. F. Shimberg. 1997. *How to get out of the hospital alive: A guide to patient power.* New York: Macmillan.

Bombeck, E. 1989. *I want to grow hair, I want to grow up, I want to go to Boise: Children surviving cancer.* New York: Harper and Row.

Borowsky, S. J., M. K. Davis, C. Goertz, and N. Lurie. 1997. Are all health plans created equal? The physician's view. *Journal of the American Medical Association* 278:917–921.

Bovbjerg, D. H., W. H. Redd, L. A. Maier, J. C. Holland, L. M. Lesko, D. Niedzwiecki, S. C. Rubin, and T. B. Hakes. 1990. Anticipatory immune suppression and nausea in women receiving cyclic chemotherapy for ovarian cancer. *Journal of Consulting and Clinical Psychology* 58:153–157.

Brody, D. S., S. M. Miller, C. E. Lerman, D. G. Smith, C. G. Lazaro, and M. J. Bloom. 1989. The relationship between patients' satisfaction with their physicians and perceptions about interventions they desired and received. *Medical Care* 27: 1027–1035.

Broyard, A. 1990. Doctor talk to me. *New York Times Magazine,* 26 August, 32–33, 36.

Buck, R. 1977. Nonverbal communication of affect in preschool children: Relationships with personality and skin conductance. *Journal of Personality and Social Psychology* 35:225–235.

Buford, B. 1996. The seductions of storytelling. *New Yorker,* 24 June/1 July, 11–12.

Burack, R. C., and R. R. Carpenter. 1983. The predictive value of the presenting complaint. *Journal of Family Practice* 16:749–754.

Burish, T. G., S. L. Snyder, and R. A. Jenkins. 1991. Preparing patients for cancer chemotherapy: Effect of coping preparation and relaxation interventions. *Journal of Consulting and Clinical Psychology* 59:518–525.

Chan, L., T. D. Koepsell, R. A. Deyo, P. C. Esselman, J. K. Haselkorn, J. K. Lowery, and W. C. Stolov. 1997. The effect of Medicare's payment system for rehabilitation hospitals on length of stay, charges, and total payments. *New England Journal of Medicine* 337:978–985.

Cher, D. J., and L. A. Lenert. 1997. Method of Medicare reimbursement and the rate of potentially ineffective care of critically ill patients. *Journal of the American Medical Association* 278:1001–1007.

Classen, D. C., S. L. Pestotnik, R. S. Evans, J. F. Lloyd, and J.P. Burke. 1997. Adverse drug events in hospitalized patients: Excess length of stay, extra costs, and attributable mortality. *Journal of the American Medical Association* 277:301–306.

Cohen, S., and G. M. Williamson. 1991. Stress and infectious disease in humans. *Psychological Bulletin* 109:5–24.

Craig, J. 1991. *Between hello and goodbye.* Los Angeles: Jeremy P. Tarcher.

DiMatteo, M. R. 1979. A social-psychological analysis of physician-patient rapport: Toward a science of the art of medicine. *Journal of Social Issues* 35:12–33.

DiMatteo, M. R. and R. Hays. 1980. The significance of patients' perceptions of physician conduct: A study of patient satisfaction in a family practice center. *Journal of Community Health* 6:18–34.

DiMatteo, M. R., A. Taranta, H. S. Friedman, and L. M. Prince. 1980. Predicting patient satisfaction from physicians' nonverbal communication skills. *Medical Care* 18:376–387.

Eisenberg, D. M., R. C. Kessler, C. Foster, F. E. Norlock, D. R. Calkins, and T. L. Delbanco. 1993. Unconventional medicine in the United States. *New England Journal of Medicine* 328:246–252.

Emanuel, E. J., and L. L. Emanuel. 1992. Four models of the physician-patient relationship. *Journal of the American Medical Association* 267:2221–2226.

Emmons, R. A., and L. A. King. 1988. Conflict among personal strivings: Immediate and long-term implications for psychological and physical well-being. *Journal of Personality and Social Psychology* 54:1040–1048.

Enthoven, A. C. 1993. The history and principles of managed competition. *Health Affairs* 12:24–48.

Evans, S. H., and P. Clarke. 1983. When cancer patients fail to get well: Flaws in health communication. In *Communication yearbook,* edited by R. N. Bostrom. Beverly Hills, Calif.: Sage.

Faden, R. R., C. Becker, C. Lewis, J. Freeman, and A. I. Faden. 1981. Disclosure of information to patients in medical care. *Medical Care* 19:718–733.

Ferber, J. D. 1996. Auto-assignment and enrollment in Medicaid managed care programs. *Journal of Law, Medicine and Ethics* 24:99–107.

Ferguson, T. 1996. *Health online: How to find health information, support groups, and self-help communities in cyberspace.* Reading, Mass.: Addison-Wesley.

Frank, A. 1991. *At the will of the body.* Boston: Houghton Mifflin.

Frankel, R., and H. Beckman. 1989. Evaluating the patient's primary problem(s). In *Communicating with medical patients,* edited by M. Stewart and D. Roter. Newbury Park, Calif.: Sage.

Freud, S. 1964. *The standard edition of the complete psychological works of Sigmund Freud.* Vol. VII. London: Hogarth and the Institute for Psycho-Analysis.

Gergen, K. J. 1996. Beyond life narratives in the therapeutic encounter. In *Aging and biography: Explorations in adult development,* edited by J. E. Birren, G. McNamee, and D. Greenberg. New York: Springer.

Goffman, E. 1971. *Relations in public.* New York: Basic Books.

Grabowski, H., and C. D. Mullins. 1997. Pharmacy benefit management, cost-effectiveness analysis and drug formulary decisions. *Social Science and Medicine* 45: 535–544.

Greenfield, S., S. Kaplan, and J. E. Ware, Jr. 1985. Expanding patient involvement in care: Effects on patient outcomes. *Annals of Internal Medicine* 102:520–528.

Greenfield, S., W. Rogers, M. Mangotich, M. F. Carney, and A. R. Tarlov. 1995. Outcomes of patients with hypertension and non-insulin-dependent diabetes mellitus treated by different systems and specialties: Results from the Medical Outcomes Study. *Journal of the American Medical Association* 274:1436–1474.

Grimaldi, P. L. 1997. New HEDIS means more information about HMOs. *Journal of Health Care Financing* 23:40–50.

Gross, M. 1996. Cancer becomes me: The funny thing about cells run rampant. *New Yorker,* 15 April, 54–55.

Grover, G., C. D. Berkowitz, and R. J. Lewis. 1994. Parental recall after a visit to the emergency department. *Clinical Pediatrics* 33:194–201.

Hall, J. A., D. L. Roter, and C. S. Rand. 1981. Communication of affect between patient and physician. *Journal of Health and Social Behavior* 22:18–30.

Harrigan, J. A. 1985. Self-touching as an indicator of underlying affect and language processes. *Social Science and Medicine* 20:1161–1168.

Harrigan, J. A., J. F. Gramata, K. S. Lucic, and C. Margolis. 1989. It's how you say it: Physicians' vocal behavior. *Social Science and Medicine* 28:87–92.

Harris, M. J., and R. Rosenthal. 1985. Mediation of interpersonal expectancy effects: 31 meta-analyses. *Psychological Bulletin* 97:363–386.

Heath, C. 1986. *Body movement and speech in medical interaction.* Cambridge: Cambridge University Press.

———. 1989. Pain talk: The expression of suffering in the medical consultation. *Social Psychology Quarterly* 52:113–125.

Inui, T. S., and W. B. Carter. 1985. Problems and prospects for health services research on provider-patient communication. *Medical Care* 23:521–538.

Johnson, J. E., D. R. Lauver, and L. M. Nail. 1989. Process of coping with radiation therapy. *Journal of Consulting and Clinical Psychology* 57:358–364.

Kaplan, S. H., S. Greenfield, and J. E. Ware, Jr. 1989a. Assessing the effects of physician-patient interactions on the outcomes of chronic disease. *Medical Care* 27: S110–S127.

———. 1989b. Impact of the doctor-patient relationship on the outcomes of chronic disease. In *Communicating with medical patients,* edited by M. Stewart and D. Roter. Newbury Park, Calif.: Sage.

Kronick, R., D. C. Goodman, J. Wennberg, and E. Wagner. 1993. The marketplace in health care reform: The demographic limitations of managed competition. *New England Journal of Medicine* 328:148–152.

Lear, M. W. 1980. *Heartsounds.* New York: Pocket Books.

Lerner, G. 1985. *A death of one's own.* Madison: University of Wisconsin Press.

Lesar, R. S., L. Briceland, and D. S. Stein. 1997. Factors related to errors in medication prescribing. *Journal of the American Medical Association* 277:312–317.

Levenstein, J. H., E. E. McCracken, I. R. McWhinney, M. A. Stewart, and J. B. Brown.

1986. The patient-centered clinical method 1. A model for the doctor-patient interaction in family medicine. *Family Practice* 3:24–30.

Levine, S., and M. A. Kozloff. 1978. The sick role: Assessment and overview. *Annual Review of Sociology* 4:317–343.

Linden, W., D. L. Paulhus, and K. S. Dobson. 1986. Effects of response styles on the report of psychological and somatic distress. *Journal of Consulting and Clinical Psychology* 54:309–313.

Linden, W., L. Chambers, J. Maurice, and J. W. Lenz. 1993. Sex differences in social support, self-deception, hostility, and ambulatory cardiovascular activity. *Health Psychology* 12:376–380.

Lorber, J. 1975. Good patients and problem patients: Conformity and deviance in a general hospital. *Journal of Health and Social Behavior* 16:213–225.

Lyles, A., B. R. Luce, and A. M. Rentz. 1997. Managed care pharmacy, socioeconomic assessments, and drug adoption decisions. *Social Science and Medicine* 45:511–521.

McConaughy, F. L., S. E. Toevs, and K. M. Lukken. 1995. Adult clients' recall of oral health education services received in private practice. *Journal of Dental Hygiene* 69:202–211.

Matthews, K. T., M. F. Scheier, B. I. Brunson, and B. Carducci. 1980. Attention, unpredictability, and reports of physical symptoms: Eliminating the benefits of predictability. *Journal of Personality and Social Psychology* 38:525–537.

Miller, T. E., C. H. Coleman, and A. M. Cugliari. 1997. Treatment decisions for patients without surrogates: Rethinking policies for a vulnerable population. *Journal of the American Geriatrics Society* 45:369–374.

Milmoe, S., R. Rosenthal, H. T. Blane, and M. E. Chafetz. 1967. The doctor's voice: Postdictor of successful referral of alcoholic patients. *Journal of Abnormal Psychology* 72:78–84.

Mishler, E. G. 1984. *The discourse of medicine: Dialectics of medical interviews.* Norwood, N.J.: Ablex.

National Committee for Quality Assurance. 1997. *The state of managed care quality.* Washington, D.C.: National Committee for Quality Assurance.

Notarius, C. I., and R. W. Levenson. 1979. Expressive tendencies and physiological response to stress. *Journal of Personality and Social Psychology* 37:1204–1210.

O'Sullivan, M., P. Ekman, W. Friesen, and K. Scherer. 1985. What you say and how you say it: The contribution of speech content and voice quality to judgments of others. *Journal of Personality and Social Psychology* 48:54–62.

Parsons, T. 1964. *Social structure and personality.* New York: Free Press.

Paulhus, D. L. 1984. Two-component models of socially desirable responding. *Journal of Personality and Social Psychology* 46:598–609.

Pennebaker, J. W., M. A. Burnam, M. A. Schaeffer, and D. C. Harper. 1977. Lack of control as a determinant of perceived physical symptoms. *Journal of Personality and Social Psychology* 35:167–174.

Pennebaker, J. W., and S. K. Beall. 1986. Confronting a traumatic event: Toward an understanding of inhibition and disease. *Journal of Abnormal Psychology* 95:274–281.

Peterson, C., and A. J. Stunkard. 1989. Personal control and health promotion. *Social Science and Medicine* 28:819–828.

Retchin, S. M., R. S. Brown, S.-C. J. Yeh, D. Chu, and L. Moreno. 1997. Outcomes of stroke patients in Medicare fee for service and managed care. *Journal of the American Medical Association* 278:119–124.

Rodwin, M. A. 1995. Conflicts in managed care. *New England Journal of Medicine* 332:604–607.

———. 1997. The neglected remedy: Strengthening consumer voice in managed care. *American Prospect* September–October:45–50.

Rosenbaum, E. 1988. *A taste of my own medicine: When the doctor is the patient.* New York: Random House.

Rosenthal, G. E., D. L. Harper, L. M. Quinn, and G. S. Cooper. 1997. Severity-adjusted mortality and length of stay in teaching and nonteaching hospitals. *Journal of the American Medical Association* 278:485–490.

Rosenthal, R., P. D. Blanck, and M. Vannicelli. 1984. Speaking to and about patients: Predicting therapists' tone of voice. *Journal of Consulting and Clinical Psychology* 52:679–686.

Rosenthal, R., and L. I. Benowitz. 1986. Sensitivity to nonverbal communication in normal, psychiatric, and brain-damaged samples. In *Nonverbal communication in the clinical context,* edited by P. D. Blanck, R. Buck, and R. Rosenthal. University Park: Pennsylvania State University Press.

Rubin, H., B. Gandek, W. H. Rogers, M. Kosinski, C. McHorney, and J. E. Ware. 1993. Patients' ratings of outpatient visits in different practice settings: Results from the Medical Outcomes Study. *Journal of the American Medical Association* 270:835–840.

Ryer, J. C. 1997. *Health net: Your essential resource for the most up-to-date medical information online.* New York: John Wiley.

Safran, D., A. R. Tarlov, and W. Rogers. 1994. Primary care performances in fee-for-service and prepaid health care systems: Results from the Medical Outcomes Study. *Journal of the American Medical Association* 271:1579–1586.

Sheldon, K. M., and T. Kasser. 1995. Coherence and congruence: Two aspects of personality integration. *Journal of Personality and Social Psychology* 68:531–533.

Shorter, E. 1985. *Bedside manners: The troubled history of doctors and patients.* New York: Simon and Schuster.

Shreve, E. G., J. A. Harrigan, J. R. Kues, and D. K. Kagas. 1988. Nonverbal expressions of anxiety in physician-patient interactions. *Psychiatry* 51:378–384.

Steinberg, A. J. 1997. *The insider's guide to HMOs: How to navigate the managed-care system and get the health care you deserve.* New York: Plume.

Taylor, S. E. 1979. Hospital patient behavior: Reactance, helplessness, or control? *Journal of Social Issues* 35:156–184.

Tepper, D. T., Jr., and R. F. Haase. 1978. Verbal and nonverbal communication of facilitative conditions. *Journal of Counseling Psychology* 25:35–40.

Verhaak, P. F. 1986. Variations in the diagnosis of psychosocial disorders: A general practice observation study. *Social Science and Medicine* 23:595–604.

———. 1988. Detection of psychologic complaints by general practitioners. *Medical Care* 26:1009–1020.

Waitzkin, H. 1984. Doctor-patient communication: Clinical implications of social scientific research. *Journal of the American Medical Association* 252:2441–2446.

———. 1985. Information giving in medical care. *Journal of Health and Social Behavior* 26:81–101.

Ware, J. E., M. S. Bayliss, W. H. Rogers, M. Kosinski, and A. R. Tarlov. 1996. Differences in 4-year health outcomes for elderly and poor, chronically ill patients treated in HMO and fee-for-service systems. *Journal of the American Medical Association* 276:1039–1047.

Weil, T. P. 1996. The blending of competitive and regulatory strategies: A second opinion. *Journal of Health Care Finance* 23:46–56.

West, C. 1983. "Ask me no questions. . . . " An analysis of queries and replies in physician-patient dialogues. In *The social organization of doctor-patient communication,* edited by S. Fisher and A. D. Todd. Washington, D.C.: Center for Applied Linguistics.

Wurman, R. 1985. *Medical access.* Los Angeles: Access Press.

Zuckerman, M., B. M. DePaulo, and R. Rosenthal. 1986. Humans as deceivers and lie detectors. In *Nonverbal communication in the clinical context,* edited by P. D. Blanck, R. Buck, and R. Rosenthal. University Park: Pennsylvania State University Press.

## CHAPTER 2 *Making the Best Medical Decisions*

Ader, R., D. Felten, and N. Cohen. 1990. Interactions between the brain and the immune system. In *Annual review of pharmacology and toxicology,* edited by R. George, A. K. Cho, and T. F. Blaschke. Palo Alto, Calif.: Annual Reviews.

Allen, A. 1990. Nurses' evaluations of patient attributions for the cause and future of their illness. *Journal of Applied Social Psychology* 20:1225–1255.

Alloy, L. B., C. Peterson, L. Y. Abramson, and M.E.P. Seligman. 1984. Attributional style and the generality of learned helplessness. *Journal of Personality and Social Psychology* 46:681–687.

American Hospital Association. 1996. *The Dartmouth atlas of health care in the United States.* Chicago: American Hospital Association.

Andersen, B. L., J. T. Cacioppo, and D. C. Roberts. 1995. Delay in seeking a cancer diagnosis: Delay stages and psychophysiological comparison processes. *British Journal of Social Psychology* 34:33–52.

Andersen, R. M. 1995. Revisiting the behavioral model and access to medical care: Does it matter? *Journal of Health and Social Behavior* 36:1–10.

Angell, M. 1996. *Science on trial: The clash of medical evidence and the law in the breast implant case.* New York: W. W. Norton.

Appelbaum, P. S., C. W. Lidz, and A. Meisel. 1987. *Informed consent: Legal theory and clinical practice.* New York: Oxford University Press.

Arendt, J., D. S. Minors, and J. M. Waterhouse, eds. 1989. *Biological rhythms in clinical practice.* London: Butterworth.

Arkes, H. R. 1991. Costs and benefits of judgment errors: Implications for debiasing. *Psychological Bulletin* 110:486–498.

Arkes, H. R., and C. Blumer. 1985. The psychology of sunk cost. *Organizational Behavior and Human Decision Processes* 35:124–140.

Arkes, H. R., D. Faust, T. J. Guilmette, and K. Hart. 1988. Eliminating the hindsight bias. *Journal of Applied Psychology* 73:305–307.

Arkes, H. R., L. T. Herren, and A. M. Isen. 1988. The role of potential loss in the influence of affect on risk-taking behavior. *Organizational Behavior and Human Decision Processes* 42:181–193.

Atlas, G. D., and C. Peterson. 1990. Explanatory style and gambling: How pessimists respond to losing wagers. *Behavior Research and Therapy* 28:523–529.

Babkoff, H., T. Caspy, M. Mikulincer, and H. C. Sing. 1991. Monotonic and rhythmic influences: A challenge for sleep deprivation research. *Psychological Bulletin* 109:411–428.

Badwe, R. A., W. M. Gregory, M. A. Chaudary, M. A. Richards, A. E. Bentley, R. D.

Rubens, and I. S. Fentiman. 1991. Timing of surgery during menstrual cycle and survival of premenopausal women with operable breast cancer. *Lancet* 337: 1261–1264.

Banks, S. M., P. Salovey, S. Greener, and A. J. Rothman. 1995. The effects of message framing on mammography utilization. *Health Psychology* 14:178–184.

Baron, J. 1988. *Thinking and deciding.* Cambridge: Cambridge University Press.

Baron, R.A. 1990. Environmentally induced positive affect: Its impact on self-efficacy, task performance, negotiation, and conflict. *Journal of Applied Social Psychology* 20:368–384.

Ben-Eliyahu, S., R. Yirmiya, J. C. Liebeskind, A. N. Taylor, and R. P. Gale. 1991. Stress increases metastatic spread of a mammary tumor in rats: Evidence for mediation by the immune system. *Brain, Behavior, and Immunity* 5:193–205.

Beninger, R. J. 1983. The role of dopamine in locomotor activity and learning. *Brain Research Reviews* 6:173–196.

Benzion, U., A. Rapport, and J. Yagil. 1989. Discount rates inferred from decisions: An experimental study. *Management Science* 35:270–284.

Block, R. A., and D. R. Harper. 1991. Overconfidence in estimation: Testing the anchoring-and-adjustment hypothesis. *Organizational Behavior and Human Decision Processes* 49:188–207.

Bodenhausen, G.V. 1990. Stereotypes as judgmental heuristics: Evidence of circadian variations in discrimination. *Psychological Science* 1:319–322.

Brown, J. D., and K. L. McGill. 1989. The cost of good fortune: When positive life events produce negative health consequences. *Journal of Personality and Social Psychology* 57:1103–1110.

Brun, W., and K. H. Teigen. 1988. Verbal probabilities: Ambiguous, context-dependent, or both? *Organizational Behavior and Human Decision Processes* 41:390–404.

Burns, M. O., and M.E.P. Seligman. 1989. Explanatory style across the life span: Evidence for stability over 52 years. *Journal of Personality and Social Psychology* 56:471–477.

Calabrese, J. R., M. A. Kling, and P. W. Gold. 1987. Alterations in immunocompetence during stress, bereavement, and depression: Focus on neuroendocrine regulation. *American Journal of Psychiatry* 144:1123–1134.

Christakis, N. A. 1994. Timing of referral of terminally ill patients to an outpatient hospice. *Journal of General Internal Medicine* 9:314–320.

Christakis, N. A., and J. J. Escarce. 1996. Survival of Medicare patients after enrollment in hospice programs. *New England Journal of Medicine* 335:172–178.

Christensen, C. 1989. The psychophysics of spending. *Journal of Behavioral Decision Making* 2:69–80.

Christensen-Szalanski, J.J., and G.B. Northcraft. 1985. Patient compliance behavior: The effects of time on patients' values of treatment regimens. *Social Science and Medicine* 21:263–273.

Clark, D. M., and J. D. Teasdale. 1985. Constraints on the effects of mood on memory. *Journal of Personality and Social Psychology* 48:1595–1608.

Cohen, B. J., and S. G. Pauker. 1994. How do physicians weigh iatrogenic complications? *Journal of General Internal Medicine* 9:20–23.

Cohen, S., D.A.J. Tyrrell, and A.P. Smith. 1991. Psychological stress and susceptibility to the common cold. *New England Journal of Medicine* 325:606–612.

Connors, A. F., N.V. Dawson, H. R. Arkes, and M. J. Roach. 1990. Decision making in SUPPORT: Physician perceptions and preferences. *Journal of Clinical Epidemiology* 43:59S–62S.

Creyer, E., and W.T. Ross. 1993. Hindsight bias and inferences in choice: The mediating effect of cognitive effort. *Organizational Behavior and Human Decision Processes* 55:61–77.

Cutrona, C. E., D. Russell, and R. D. Jones. 1984. Cross-situational consistency in causal attributions: Does attributional style exist? *Journal of Personality and Social Psychology* 47:1043–1058.

Dafter, R. E. 1996. Why "negative" emotions can sometimes be positive. *Advances* 12:6–19.

Davis, C. G., D. R. Lehman, R. C. Silver, C. B. Wortman, and J. H. Ellard. 1996. Self-blame following a traumatic event: The role of perceived avoidability. *Personality and Social Psychology Bulletin* 22:557–567.

Davison, K. P., and J.W. Pennebaker. 1996. Emotions, thoughts, and healing: After Dafter. *Advances* 12:19–23.

Day, R. P., M. G. Hewson, P. J. Kindy, and J. Van Kirk. 1993. Evaluation of resident performance in an outpatient internal medicine clinic using standardized patients. *Journal of General Internal Medicine* 8:193–198.

Denig, P., F. M. Haaijer-Ruskamp, H. Wesseling, and A. Versluis. 1993. Towards understanding treatment preferences of hospital physicians. *Social Science and Medicine* 36:915–924.

DiCaccavo, A., and F. Reid. 1995. Decisional conflict in general practice: Strategies of patient management. *Social Science and Medicine* 41:347–353.

Dreifuss-Kattan, E. 1990. *Cancer stories: Creativity and self-repair.* Hillsdale, N.J.: Analytic Press.

Eisenberg, D. M., R. C. Kessler, C. Foster, F. E. Norlock, D. R. Calkins, and T. L. Delbanco. 1993. Unconventional medicine in the United States. *New England Journal of Medicine* 328:246–252.

Eraker, S. A., and H. C. Sox. 1981. Assessment of patients' preferences for therapeutic outcomes. *Medical Decision Making* 1:29–39.

Evans, D. A., M. R. Block, E. R. Steinberg, and A. M. Penrose. 1986. Frames and heuristics in doctor-patient discourse. *Social Science and Medicine* 22:1027–1034.

Fagley, N. S., and P. M. Miller. 1990. The effect of framing on choice: Interactions with risk-taking propensity, cognitive style, and sex. *Personality and Social Psychology Bulletin* 16:496–510.

Feinstein, A. R. 1995. The chagrin factor and qualitative decision analysis. *Archives of Internal Medicine* 145:1257–1259.

Fischoff, B. 1982. Debiasing. In *Judgement under uncertainty: Heuristics and biases,* edited by D. Kahneman, P. Slovic, and A. Tversky. Cambridge: Cambridge University Press.

Folkard, S., R. A. Wever, and C. M. Wildgruber. 1983. Multi-oscillatory control of circadian rhythms in human performance. *Nature* 305:223–226.

Garland, H. 1990. Throwing good money after bad: The effect of sunk costs on the decision to escalate commitment to an ongoing project. *Journal of Applied Psychology* 75:728–731.

Geisler, M. W., and J. Polich. 1992. P300, food consumption, and memory performance. *Psychophysiology* 29:76–85.

Gillooly, P. B., M. H. Smolensky, D. L. Albright, B. Hsi, and D. R. Thorne. 1990.

Circadian variation in human performance evaluated by the Walter Reed Performance Assessment Battery. *Chronobiology International* 7:143–153.

Gotay, C. C., and B. D. Bultz. 1986. Patient decision making inside and outside the cancer care system. *Journal of Psychosocial Oncology* 4:105–114.

Grayboys, T. B., B. Biegelsen, S. Lampert, C. M. Blatt, and B. Lown. 1992. Results of a second-opinion trial among patients recommended for coronary angiography. *Journal of the American Medical Association* 268:2537–2540.

Gregory, W. L., R. B. Cialdini, and K. M. Carpenter. 1982. Self-relevant scenarios as mediators of likelihood estimates and compliance: Does imagining make it so? *Journal of Personality and Social Psychology* 43:89–99.

Haaga, D.A.F., and B. L. Stewart. 1992. Self-efficacy for recovery from a lapse after smoking cessation. *Journal of Consulting and Clinical Psychology* 60:24–28.

Heine, S. J., and D. R. Lehman. 1995. Cultural variation in unrealistic optimism: Does the West feel more invulnerable than the East? *Journal of Personality and Social Psychology* 68:595–607.

Heller, R. F., H. D. Saltzstein, and W. B. Caspe. 1992. Heuristics in medical and non-medical decision-making. *Quarterly Journal of Experimental Psychology* 44A: 211–235.

Hewson, M. G., P. J. Kindy, J. Van Kirk, V. A. Gennis, and R. P. Day. 1996. Strategies for managing uncertainty and complexity. *Journal of General Internal Medicine* 11: 481–485.

Hirt, E. R., N. Murray, H. Sujan, and M. Sujan. 1990. The influence of mood on categorization: A cognitive flexibility interpretation. *Journal of Personality and Social Psychology* 59:411–425.

Holahan, J., C. Winterbottom, and S. Rajan. 1995. A shifting picture of health insurance coverage. *Health Affairs* 14:253–264.

Horne, J. A., and O. Ostberg. 1977. Individual differences in human circadian rhythms. *Biological Psychology* 5:179–190.

Hrushesky, W.J.M. 1996. Menstrual cycle timing of breast cancer surgery. *Recent Results in Cancer Research* 140:27–40.

Hrushesky, W.J.M., S. A. Gruber, R. B. Sothern, R. Hoffman, D. Lakatua, A. Carlson, F. Cerra, and R. Simmons. 1988. Natural killer cell activity is age, estrous- and circadian-stage dependent and correlates inversely with metastatic potential. *Journal of the National Cancer Institute* 80:1232–1237.

Hrushesky, W.J.M., A. Z. Bluming, S. A. Gruber, and R. B. Sothern. 1989. Menstrual influence on surgical cure of breast cancer. *Lancet* 2:949–952.

Hrushesky, W.J.M., R. Langer, and F. Theeuwes, eds. 1991. *Temporal control of drug delivery.* New York: New York Academy of Sciences.

Hutt, J., and G. Weidner. 1993. The effects of task demand and decision latitude in cardiovascular reactivity to stress. *Behavioral Medicine* 18:181–188.

Idler, E. L., S.V. Kasl, J. H. Lemke. 1990. Self-evaluated health and mortality among the elderly in New Haven, Connecticut, and Iowa and Washington Counties, Iowa 1982–1986. *American Journal of Epidemiology* 131:91–103.

Isen, A. M., and B. Means. 1983. The influence of positive affect on decision-making strategy. *Social Cognition* 2:18–31.

Isen, A. M., and K. A. Daubman. 1987. Positive affect facilitates creative problem solving. *Journal of Personality and Social Psychology* 52:1122–1131.

Isen, A. M., and N. Geva. 1987. The influence of positive affect on acceptable level of risk:The person with a large canoe has a large worry. *Organizational Behavior and Human Decision Processes* 39:145–154.

Isen, A. M., T. E. Nygren, and F. G. Ashby. 1988. The influence of positive affect on the subjective utility of gains and losses: It's just not worth the risk. *Journal of Personality and Social Psychology* 55:710–717.

Isen, A.M., and R. A. Baron. 1991. Positive affect as a factor in organizational behavior. In *Research in organizational behavior,* edited by L. L. Cummings and B.M. Staw. Greenwich, Conn.: JAI Press.

Isen, A. M., A. S. Rosenzweig, and M. J. Young. 1991. The influence of positive affect on clinical problem solving. *Medical Decision Making* 11:221–227.

Isen, A. M., P. M. Niedenthal, and N. Cantor. 1992. An influence of positive affect on social categorization. *Motivation and Emotion* 16:65–78.

Janis, I. L. 1989. *Crucial decisions.* New York: Free Press.

Johnson, C. H., and J. W. Hastings. 1986. The elusive mechanism of the circadian clock. *American Scientist* January–February:29–36.

Kahneman, D. 1991. Judgment and decision making: A personal view. *Psychological Science* 2:142–145.

Kahneman, D., and A. Tversky. 1982. The psychology of preferences. *Scientific American* 246:160–173.

———. 1984. Choices, values, and frames. *American Psychologist* 39:341–350.

Kahneman, D., and D. T. Miller. 1986. Norm theory: Comparing reality to its alternatives. *Psychological Review* 93:136–153.

Kamen, L. P., and M.E.P. Seligman. 1987. Explanatory style and health. *Current Psychological Research and Reviews* 6:207–218.

Kaplan, S. H., S. Greenfield, B. Gandek, W. H. Rogers, and J. E. Ware, Jr. 1996. Characteristics of physicians with participatory decision-making styles. *Annals of Internal Medicine* 124:497–504.

Keenan, G. 1987. Decision making under stress: Scanning of alternatives under controllable and uncontrollable threats. *Journal of Personality and Social Psychology* 52:639–644.

Keren, G., and P. Roelofsma. 1995. Immediacy and certainty in intertemporal choice. *Organizational Behavior and Human Decision Processes* 63:287–297.

Kobak, K. A., L. H. Taylor, S. L. Dottl, J. H. Greist, J. W. Jefferson, D. Burroughs, J. M. Mantle, D. J. Katzelnick, R. Norton, H. J. Henk, and R. C. Serlin. 1997. A computer-administered telephone interview to identify mental disorders. *Journal of the American Medical Association* 278:905–910.

Korda, M. 1996. *Man to man: Surviving prostate cancer.* New York: Random House.

Kraft, M., and R.J. Martin. 1995. Chronobiology and chronotherapy in medicine. *Disease-a-Month* 41:501–575.

Kreuter, M. W., and V. J. Stretcher. 1995. Changing inaccurate perceptions of health risk: Results from a randomized trial. *Health Psychology* 14:56–63.

Kronick, R., D. C. Goodman, J. Wennberg, and E. Wagner. 1993. The marketplace in health care reform: The demographic limitations of managed competition. *New England Journal of Medicine* 328:148–152.

Lamm, S. H. 1995. Silicone breast implants and long-term health effects: When are data adequate? *Journal of Clinical Epidemiology* 48:507–511.

Landerman, L. R., B. J. Burns, M. S. Swartz, H. R. Wagner, and L. K. George. 1994. The relationship between insurance coverage and psychiatric disorder in predicting use of mental health services. *American Journal of Psychiatry* 151:1785–1790.

Landman, J. 1993. *Regret: The persistence of the possible.* New York: Oxford University Press.

Langer, E. J. 1983. *The psychology of control.* Beverly Hills, Calif.: Sage.

———. 1989. *Mindfulness.* Reading, Mass.: Addison-Wesley.

———. 1992. Matters of mind: Mindfulness/mindlessness in perspective. *Consciousness and Cognition* 1:289–305.

———. 1994. The illusion of calculated decisions. In *Beliefs, reasoning, and decision making: Psycho-logic in honor of Bob Abelson,* edited by R. C. Schank and E. J. Langer. Hillsdale, N.J.: Lawrence Erlbaum.

Leventhal, E. A., H. Leventhal, P. Schaefer, and D. Easterling. 1993. Conservation of energy, uncertainty reduction, and swift utilization of medical care among the elderly. *Journal of Gerontology* 48:P78–P86.

Levi, F., C. Canon, Y. Touitou, A. Reinberg, and G. Mathe. 1988. Seasonal modulation of the circadian time structures of circulating T and natural killer lymphocyte subsets from healthy subjects. *Journal of Clinical Investigation* 81:407–413.

Levi, F., A. Reinberg, and C. Canon. 1989. Clinical immunology and allergy. In *Biological rhythms in clinical practice,* edited by J. Arendt, D. S. Minors, and J. M. Waterhouse. London: Butterworth.

Levin, I. P., R. D. Johnson, P. J. Deldin, L. M. Carstens, L. J. Cressey, and C. R. Davis. 1986. Framing effects in decisions with completely and incompletely described alternatives. *Organizational Behavior and Human Decision Processes* 38:48–64.

Lin, E. H., and C. Peterson. 1990. Pessimistic explanatory style and response to illness. *Behavior Research and Therapy* 28:243–248.

Lindsey, P. A., and J. P. Newhouse. 1990. The cost and value of second surgical opinion programs: A critical review of the literature. *Journal of Health Politics, Policy, and Law* 15:543–570.

Lipkus, I. M., C. Dalbert, and I. C. Siegler. 1996. The importance of distinguishing the belief in a just world for self versus for others: Implications for psychological well-being. *Personality and Social Psychology Bulletin* 22:666–677.

Loewenstein, G. 1988. Frames of mind in intertemporal choice. *Management Science* 34:200–214.

Loewenstein, G., and J. Elster, eds. 1992. *Choice over time.* New York: Russell Sage.

Logue, A. W. 1988. Research on self-control: An integrating framework. *Behavioral and Brain Sciences* 11:665–679.

Lynn, J. 1996. Caring at the end of our lives. *New England Journal of Medicine* 335:201–202.

McCall, T. B. 1995. *Examining your doctor: A patient's guide to avoiding harmful medical care.* New York: Birch Lane.

McFarlane, J., C. L. Martin, and T. M. Williams. 1988. Mood fluctuations: Women versus men and menstrual versus other cycles. *Psychology of Women Quarterly* 12:201–223.

McKinlay, J. B. 1996. Some contributions from the social system to gender inequalities in heart disease. *Journal of Health and Social Behavior* 37:1–26.

McKinlay, J. B., D. A. Potter, and H. A. Feldman. 1996. Non-medical influences on medical decision-making. *Social Science and Medicine* 42:769–776.

McNeil, B. J., S. J. Pauker, H. C. Sox, and A. Tversky. 1982. On the elicitation of preferences for alternative therapies. *New England Journal of Medicine* 306:1259–1262.

Mangione, S., and L. Z. Nieman. 1997. Cardiac auscultatory skills of internal medicine and family practice trainees: A comparison of diagnostic proficiency. *Journal of the American Medical Association* 278:717–722.

Mann, L. 1992. Stress, affect, and risk taking. In *Risk-taking behavior,* edited by F. Yates. Chichester: Wiley.

Marteau, T. M. 1989. Framing of information: Its influence upon decisions of doctors and patients. *British Journal of Social Psychology* 28:89–94.

Mazur, D. J. 1988. Why the goals of consent are not realized: Treatise on informed consent for the primary care physician. *Journal of General Internal Medicine* 3:370–380.

Mazur, D. J., and D.H. Hickam. 1990a. Interpretation of graphic data by patients in a general medicine clinic. *Journal of General Internal Medicine* 5:402–405.

———. 1990b. Treatment preferences of patients and physicians: Influences of summary data when framing effects are controlled. *Medical Decision Making* 10:2–5.

———. 1993. Patients' and physicians' interpretations of graphic data displays. *Medical Decision Making* 13:59–63.

Mazur, D. J., and J. F. Merz. 1993. How the manner of presentation of data influences older patients in determining their treatment preferences. *Journal of the American Geriatrics Society* 41:223–228.

———. 1994. How age, outcome severity, and scale influence general medicine clinic patients' interpretations of verbal probability terms. *Journal of General Internal Medicine* 9:268–271.

Medvec, V. H., S. F. Madey, and T. Gilovich. 1995. When less is more: Counterfactual thinking and satisfaction among Olympic medalists. *Journal of Personality and Social Psychology* 69:603–610.

Meyerowitz, B. E., and S. Chaiken. 1987. The effect of message framing on breast self-examination attitudes, intentions, and behavior. *Journal of Personality and Social Psychology* 52:500–510.

Moore, D. S. 1990. Uncertainty. In *On the shoulders of giants: New approaches to numeracy,* edited by L. A. Steen. Washington, D.C.: National Academy Press.

Morahan, P. S., and D. M. Murasko. 1989. Viral infections. In *Natural immunity in disease processes,* edited by D. S. Nelson. New York: Academic Press.

Mumford, M. D., and S. B. Gustafsan. 1988. Creativity syndrome: Integration, application, and innovation. *Psychological Bulletin* 103:27–43.

Murray, N., H. Sujan, E. R. Hirt, and M. Sujan. 1990. The influence of mood on categorization: A cognitive flexibility interpretation. *Journal of Personality and Social Psychology* 59:411–425.

Nardone, D. A., G. K. Johnson, A. Faryna, J. L. Coulehan, and T. A. Parrino. 1992. A model for the diagnostic medical interview. *Journal of General Internal Medicine* 7:437–442.

Neck, C. P., and G. Moorhead. 1995. Groupthink remodeled: The importance of leadership, time pressure, and methodical decision making procedures. *Human Relations* 48:537–557.

Neufeld, K. R., L. F. Degner, and J. A. Dick. 1993. A nursing intervention strategy to foster patient involvement in treatment decisions. *Oncology Nursing Forum* 20:631–635.

Nisbett, R. E., H. Zukier, and R. E. Lemley. 1981. The dilution effect: Non-diagnostic information weakens the implications of diagnostic information. *Cognitive Psychology* 13:248–277.

Nolen-Hoeksema, S., J. S. Girgus, and M.E.P. Seligman. 1991. Sex differences in depression and explanatory style in children. *Journal of Youth and Adolescence* 20:233–245.

Paauw, D. S., M. D. Wenrich, J. R. Curtis, J. D. Carline, and P. G. Ramsey. 1995. Ability of primary care physicians to recognize physical findings associated with HIV infection. *Journal of the American Medical Association* 274:1380–1382.

Pear, R. 1996. Word for word/HMO contracts: The tricky business of keeping doctors quiet. *New York Times*, 22 September, E7.

Peterson, C., A. Semmel, C. von Baeyer, L. Y. Abramson, G. I. Metalsky, and M.E.P. Seligman. 1982. The attributional style questionnaire. *Cognitive Therapy and Research* 6:287–300.

Peterson, C., and M.E.P. Seligman. 1987. Explanatory style and illness. *Journal of Personality* 55:237–265.

Peterson, C., M.E.P. Seligman, and G. E. Vaillant. 1988. Pessimistic explanatory style is a risk factor for physical illness: A thirty-five-year longitudinal study. *Journal of Personality and Social Psychology* 55:23–27.

Peterson, C., and L. M. Bossio. 1991. *Health and optimism.* New York: Free Press.

Petros, T. V., B. E. Beckwith, and M. Anderson. 1990. Individual differences in the effects of time of day and passage difficulty on prose memory in adults. *British Journal of Psychology* 81:63–72.

Petty, R. E., D. W. Schumann, S. A. Richman, and A. J. Strathman. 1993. Positive mood and persuasion: Different roles for affect under high- and low-elaboration conditions. *Journal of Personality and Social Psychology* 64:5–20.

Plous, S., and P. G. Zimbardo. 1986. Attributional biases among clinicians: A comparison of psychoanalysts and behavior therapists. *Journal of Consulting and Clinical Psychology* 54:568–570.

Polich, J., and M. W. Geisler. 1991. P300 seasonal variation. *Biological Psychology* 32: 173–179.

Polister, P. E. 1989. Cognitive guidelines for simplifying medical information: Data framing and perception. *Journal of Behavioral Decision Making* 2:149–165.

Powe, N. R., C. A. Steiner, G. F. Anderson, and A. Das. 1996. Awareness of providers' use of new medical technology among private health care plans in the United States. *International Journal of Technology Assessment in Health Care* 12:367–376.

Price, R. 1995. *A whole new life: An illness and a healing.* New York: Plume.

Reader's Digest. 1995. *Know your rights, and how to make them work for you.* Pleasantville, N.Y.: Reader's Digest Association.

Redelmeier, D. A., and A. Tversky. 1990. Discrepancy between medical decisions for individual patients and for groups. *New England Journal of Medicine* 322:1162–1164.

———. 1992. On the framing of multiple prospects. *Psychological Science* 3:191–193.

Reinberg, A., and M. Smolensky. 1983. *Biological rhythms and medicine: Cellular, metabolic, physiopathologic, and pharmacologic aspects.* New York: Springer.

Robinson, E. J., and M. J. Whitfield. 1985. Improving the efficiency of patients' comprehension monitoring. *Social Science and Medicine* 21:915–919.

Roelofsma, P., and G. Keren. 1995. Framing and time-inconsistent preferences. In *Contributions to decision making-1,* edited by J. P. Caverni, M. Bar-Hillel, F. H. Barron, and H. Jungermann. Amsterdam: Elsevier.

Roenneberg, T., and J. Aschoff. 1990. Annual rhythm of human reproduction: I. Biology, sociology, or both? and II. Environmental correlations. *Journal of Biological Rhythms* 5:195–239.

Roese, N. J., and J. M. Olson. 1993. Self-esteem and counterfactual thinking. *Journal of Personality and Social Psychology* 65:199–206.

———. 1993. The structure of counterfactual thought. *Personality and Social Psychology Bulletin* 19:312–319.

———, eds. 1995. *What might have been: The social psychology of counterfactual thinking.* Mahwah, N.J.: Lawrence Erlbaum.

Rosenberg, S. N., S. A. Gorman, S. Snitzer, E. V. Herbst, and D. Lynne. 1989. Patients' reactions and physician-patient communication in a mandatory surgical second-opinion program. *Medical Care* 27:466–477.

Rosenberg, S. N., D. R. Allen, J. S. Handte, T. C. Jackson, L. Leto, B. M. Rodstein, S. D. Stratton, G. Westfall, and R. Yasser. 1995. Effect of utilization review in a fee-for-service health insurance plan. *New England Journal of Medicine* 333: 1326–1330.

Rosenthal, N. E., and M. C. Blehar, eds. 1989. *Seasonal affective disorders and phototherapy.* New York: Guilford.

Rybash, J. M., and P. A. Roodin. 1989. The framing heuristic influences judgements about younger and older adults' decision to refuse medical treatment. *Applied Cognitive Psychology* 3:171–180.

Schaubroeck, J., and E. Davis. 1994. Prospect theory predictions when escalation is not the only chance to recover sunk costs. *Organizational Behavior and Human Decision Processes* 57:59–82.

Sedek, G., and M. Kofta. 1990. When cognitive exertion does not yield cognitive gain: Toward an informational explanation of learned helplessness. *Journal of Personality and Social Psychology* 58:729–743.

Seligman, M.E.P. 1995. The effectiveness of psychotherapy: The Consumer Reports study. *American Psychologist* 50:965–974.

Seligman, M.E.P., and P. Schulman. 1986. Explanatory style as a predictor of productivity and quitting among life insurance sales agents. *Journal of Personality and Social Psychology* 50:832–838.

Sherman, S. J., R. B. Cialdini, D. F. Schwartzman, and K. D. Reynolds. 1985. Imagining can heighten or lower the perceived likelihood of contracting a disease: The mediating effect of ease of imagery. *Personality and Social Psychology Bulletin* 11: 118–127.

Showers, C., and N. Cantor. 1985. Social cognition: A look at motivated strategies. *Annual Review of Psychology* 36:275–305.

Siminoff, L. A., and J. H. Fetting. 1991. Factors affecting treatment decisions for a life-threatening illness: The case of medical treatment of breast cancer. *Social Science and Medicine* 32:813–818.

Sinclair, R. C. 1988. Mood, categorization breadth, and performance appraisal: The effects of order of information acquisition and affective state of halo, accuracy, information retrieval and evaluations. *Organizational Behavior and Human Decision Processes* 42:22–46.

Smith, C. S., C. Reilly, and K. Midkiff. 1989. Evaluation of three circadian rhythm questionnaires with suggestions for an improved measure of morningness. *Journal of Applied Psychology* 74:728–738.

Sox, H. C., Jr., M. A. Blatt, M. C. Higgins, and K. I. Marton. 1988. *Medical decision making.* Boston: Butterworth.

Steiner, C. A., N. R. Powe, G. F. Anderson, and A. Das. 1997. Technology coverage decisions by health care plans and considerations by medical directors. *Medical Care* 35:472–489.

Stone, A. A., S. M. Hedges, J. M. Neale, and M. S. Satin. 1985. Prospective and cross-sectional mood reports offer no evidence of a "Blue Monday" phenomenon. *Journal of Personality and Social Psychology* 49:129–143.

Sutherland, H. J., V. Dunn, and N. F. Boyd. 1983. The measurement of values for states of health with linear analog scales. *Medical Decision Making* 3:477–487.

Sutherland, H. J., G. A. Lockwood, D. L. Tritchler, F. Sem, L. Brooks, and J. E. Till. 1991. Communicating probabilistic information to cancer patients: Is there "noise" on the line? *Social Science and Medicine* 32:725–731.

Svenson, O., and A. J. Maule, eds. 1993. *Time pressure and stress in human judgment and decision making.* New York: Plenum Press.

Swartz, K., J. Marcotte, and T. D. McBride. 1993. Personal characteristics and spells without health insurance. *Inquiry* 30:64–76.

Sweeney, P. D., K. Anderson, and S. Bailey. 1986. Attributional style in depression: A meta-analytic review. *Journal of Personality and Social Psychology* 50:974–991.

Taylor, S. E., and J. D. Brown. 1988. Illusion and well-being: A social psychological perspective on mental health. *Psychological Bulletin* 103:193–210.

Taylor, S. E., and S. K. Schneider. 1989. Coping and the simulation of events. *Social Cognition* 7:174–194.

Thaler, R. H. 1992. *The winner's curse: Paradoxes and anomalies of economic life.* New York: Free Press.

Travis, C. B., R. H. Phillippi, and B. E. Tonn. 1989. Judgment heuristics and medical decisions. *Patient Education and Counseling* 13:211–220.

Tversky, A., and D. Kahneman. 1981. The framing of decisions and the psychology of choice. *Science* 211:453–458.

———. 1983. Extensional versus intuitive reasoning: The conjunction fallacy in probability judgment. *Psychological Review* 90:293–315.

———. 1986. Rational choice and the framing of decisions. *Journal of Business* 59:S251–S278.

———. 1992. Advances in prospect theory: Cumulative representation of uncertainty. *Journal of Risk and Uncertainty* 5:297–323.

U.S. Bureau of the Census. March 1990–1994. *Current population survey.* Washington, D.C.: U.S. Department of Commerce.

Vanderford, M. L., D. H. Smith, and T. Olive. 1995. The image of plastic surgeons in news media coverage of the silicone breast implant controversy. *Plastic and Reconstructive Surgery* 96:521–538.

Verplanken, B. 1993. Need for cognition and external information search: Responses to time pressure during decision making. *Journal of Research in Personality* 27:238–252.

Visintainer, M. A., J. R. Volpicelli, and M.E.P. Seligman. 1982. Tumor rejection in rats after inescapable or escapable shock. *Science* 216:437–439.

Wagner, J. 1986. *The search for signs of intelligent life in the universe.* New York: Harper and Row.

Weil, T. P. 1996. The blending of competitive and regulatory strategies: A second opinion. *Journal of Health Care Finance* 23:46–56.

Weiner, B. 1985. "Spontaneous" causal thinking. *Psychological Bulletin* 97:74–84.

Weinstein, N. D. 1980. Unrealistic optimism about future life events. *Journal of Personality and Social Psychology* 39:806–821.

———. 1984. Why it won't happen to me: Perceptions of risk factors and susceptibility. *Health Psychology* 3:431–457.

———. 1987. Unrealistic optimism about susceptibility to health problems: Conclusions from a community-wide sample. *Journal of Behavioral Medicine* 10:481–500.

Whyte, G. 1993. Escalating commitment in individual and group decision making: A prospect theory approach. *Organizational Behavior and Human Decision Processes* 54:430–455.

Willich, S. N., T. Linderer, K. Wegscheider, A. Leizorovicz, I. Alamercery, and R. Schroder. 1989. Increased morning incidence of myocardial infarction in the ISAM study: Absence with prior beta-adrenergic blockade. *Circulation* 80:853–858.

Wong, P.T.P., and B. Weiner. 1981. When people ask "why" questions, and the heuristics of attributional search. *Journal of Personality and Social Psychology* 40:650–663.

Yates, J. F., and L. G. Zukowski. 1976. Characterization of ambiguity in decision making. *Behavioral Science* 21:19–25.

Zullow, H. M., G. Oettingen, C. Peterson, and M.E.P. Seligman. 1988. Pessimistic explanatory style in the historical record: CAVing LBJ, presidential candidates, and east versus west Berlin. *American Psychologist* 43:673–682.

Zullow, H. M. 1991. Pessimistic rumination in popular songs and newsmagazines predict economic recession via decreased consumer optimism and spending. *Journal of Economic Psychology* 12:501–526.

## CHAPTER 3 *Seeking the Right Kind of Social Support*

Baekeland, F., and L. Lundwall. 1975. Dropping out of treatment: A critical review. *Psychological Bulletin* 82:738–783.

Bandura, A. 1989. Human agency in social cognitive theory. *American Psychologist* 44:1175–1184.

———. 1991. Social cognitive theory of self-regulation. *Organizational Behavior and Human Decision Processes* 50:248–287.

Baron, R. S., C. E. Cutrona, D. Hicklin, D. W. Russell, and D. M. Lubaroff. 1990. Social support and immune function among spouses of cancer patients. *Journal of Personality and Social Psychology* 59:344–352.

Batson, C. D., M. H. Bolen, J. A. Cross, and H. E. Neuringer-Benefiel. 1986. Where is the altruism in the altruistic personality? *Journal of Personality and Social Psychology* 50:212–220.

Batson, C. D., S. C. Sympson, J. L. Hindman, P. Decruz, R. M. Todd, J. L. Weeks, G. Jennings, and C. T. Burris. 1996. "I've been there, too": Effect on empathy of prior experience with a need. *Personality and Social Psychology Bulletin* 22:474–482.

Beery, T. A. 1995. Gender bias in the diagnosis and treatment of coronary artery disease. *Heart and Lung* 24:427–435.

Bellah, R. N., R. Madsen, W. M. Sullivan, A. Swidler, and S. M. Tipton. 1985. *Habits of the heart.* New York: Harper and Row.

Bergelson, B. A., and C. L. Tommaso. 1995. Gender differences in clinical evaluation and triage in coronary artery disease. *Chest* 108:1510–1513.

Bloom, J. R. 1982. Social support, accommodation to stress, and adjustment to breast cancer. *Social Science and Medicine* 16:1329–1338.

Boyce, W. T. 1985. Social support, family relations, and children. In *Social support and health,* edited by S. Cohen and S. L. Syme. New York: Academic Press.

Broadhead, W. E., B. H. Kaplan, S. A. James, E. H. Wagner, V. J. Schoenbach, R. Grimson, S. Heyden, G. Tibblin, and S. H. Gehlbach. 1983. The epidemiologic evidence for a relationship between social support and health. *American Journal of Epidemiology* 117:521–537.

Cafferata, G. L., J. Kasper, and A. Bernstein. 1983. Family roles, structure, and stressors in relation to sex differences in obtaining psychotropic drugs. *Journal of Health and Social Behavior* 24:132–143.

Carkhuff, R. R. 1969. *Helping and human relations: A primer for lay and professional helpers.* New York: Holt, Rinehart and Winston.

Chapman, N. J., and D. L. Pancoast. 1985. Working with the informal helping networks of the elderly: The experiences of three programs. *Journal of Social Issues* 41:47–63.

Clarke, P., S. H. Evans, and K. Hoyes. 1991. Memory for communication: An application of encoding strategies. Paper presented at the Annual Meeting of the International Communication Association, May 1991, Chicago.

Cohen, S. 1988. Psychosocial models of the role of social support in the etiology of physical disease. *Health Psychology* 7:269–297.

Cohen, S., and T. A. Will. 1985. Stress, social support, and the buffering hypothesis. *Psychological Bulletin* 98:310–357.

Cohen, S., and E. Lichtenstein. 1990. Partner behaviors that support quitting smoking. *Journal of Consulting and Clinical Psychology* 58:304–309.

Colon, E. A., A. L. Callies, M. K. Popkin, and P. B. McGlave. 1991. Depressed mood and other variables related to bone marrow transplantation survival in acute leukemia. *Psychosomatics* 32:420–425.

Counte, M. A., and G. L. Glandon. 1991. A panel study of life stress, social support, and the health services utilization of older persons. *Medical Care* 29:348–361.

Coyne, J. C., and A. DeLongis. 1986. Going beyond social support: The role of social relationships in adaptation. *Journal of Consulting and Clinical Psychology* 54:454–460.

Crandall, C. S., and D. Moriarty. 1995. Physical illness stigma and social rejection. *British Journal of Social Psychology* 34:67–83.

Csikszentmihalyi, M. 1975. *Beyond boredom and anxiety.* San Francisco: Jossey-Bass.

———. 1991. *Flow: The psychology of optimal experience.* New York: HarperCollins.

Cutrona, C. E. 1986. Behavioral manifestations of social support: A microanalytic investigation. *Journal of Personality and Social Psychology* 51:201–208.

———. 1989. Ratings of social support by adolescents and adult informants: Degree of correspondence and prediction of depressive symptoms. *Journal of Personality and Social Psychology* 57:723–730.

Cutrona, C. E., and D. W. Russell. 1990. Type of social support and specific stress: Toward a theory of optimal matching. In *Social support: An interactional view,* edited by I. G. Sarason, B. R. Sarason, and G. R. Pierce. New York: Wiley.

Dakof, G. A., and S. E. Taylor. 1990. Victims' perceptions of social support: What is helpful from whom? *Journal of Personality and Social Psychology* 58:80–89.

Evans, S. H., and P. Clarke. 1986. Social support and adherence to a diet and exercise program. Report to the Pritikin Foundation. Santa Monica, Calif.

———. 1990. Pictures with a thousand words: Using interactive videodiscs to help cancer patients get well. Report to the IBM Corporation. Yorktown Heights, N.Y.

Feingold, A. 1994. Gender differences in personality: A meta-analysis. *Psychological Bulletin* 116:429–456.

Fiore, J., J. Becker, and D. B. Coppel. 1984. Social network interactions: A buffer or a stress. *American Journal of Community Psychology* 11:423–439.

Franks, P., and C. M. Clancy. 1993. Physician gender bias in clinical decision making: Screening for cancer in primary care. *Medical Care* 31:213–218.

Gerin, W., C. Pieper, R. Levy, and T. G. Pickering. 1992. Social support in social interaction: A moderator of cardiovascular reactivity. *Psychosomatic Medicine* 54:324–336.

Goethals, G. R., and P. R. Solomon. 1989. Interdisciplinary perspectives on the study of memory. In *Memory: Interdisciplinary approaches,* edited by P. R. Solomon, G. R. Goethals, C. M. Kelley, and B. R. Stephens. New York: Springer.

Gottlieb, B. H., and A. E. Coppard. 1987. Using social network therapy to create support systems for the chronically mentally disabled. *Canadian Journal of Community Mental Health* 6:117–131.

Greenwald, A. G., and M. R. Banaji. 1989. The self as a memory system: Powerful, but ordinary. *Journal of Personality and Social Psychology* 57:41–54.

Heller, K., M. G. Thompson, P. E. Trueba, and J. R. Hogg. 1991. Peer support telephone dyads for elderly women: Was this the wrong intervention? *American Journal of Community Psychology* 19:53–74.

Hibbard, J. H., and C. R. Pope. 1991. Effect of domestic and occupational roles on morbidity and mortality. *Social Science and Medicine* 32:805–811.

———. 1993. The quality of social roles as predictors of morbidity and mortality. *Social Science and Medicine* 36:217–225.

Hislop, T. G., N. E. Waxler, A. J. Coldman, M. Elwood, and L. Kan. 1987. The prognostic significance of psychosocial factors in women with breast cancer. *Chronic Disease* 40:729–735.

House, J. S., C. Robbins, and H. L. Metzner. 1982. The association of social relationships and activities and mortality: Prospective evidence from the Tecumseh community health study. *American Journal of Epidemiology* 116:123–140.

House, J. S., K. R. Landis, and D. Umberson. 1988. Social relationships and health. *Science* 241:540–545.

Janis, I. L., ed. 1982. *Counseling on personal decisions: Theory and research on short-term helping relationships.* New Haven, Conn.: Yale University Press.

Jemmott, J. B., C. Hellman, D. C. McClelland, S. E. Locke, L. Kraus, R. M. Williams, and C. R. Valeri. 1990. Motivational syndromes associated with natural killer cell activity. *Journal of Behavioral Medicine* 13:53–73.

Kaye, R. 1991. *Spinning straw into gold.* New York: Simon and Schuster.

Kiecolt-Glaser, J. K., and R. Glaser. 1989. Interpersonal relationships and immune function. In *Mechanisms of psychological influence on physical health,* edited by L. L. Carstensen and J. M. Neale. New York: Plenum.

Klaus, M. H., J. H. Kennell, S. S. Robertson, and R. Sosa. 1986. Effects of social support during parturition on maternal and infant morbidity. *British Medical Journal* 293:585–587.

Klein, S. B., and J. F. Kihlstrom. 1986. Elaboration, organization, and the self-reference effect in memory. *Journal of Experimental Psychology: General* 115:26–38.

Korda, M. 1996. *Man to man: Surviving prostate cancer.* New York: Random House.

Krzysztof, K., and F. H. Norris. 1993. A test of the social support deterioration model in the context of natural disaster. *Journal of Personality and Social Psychology* 64:395–408.

Kulik, J. A., and H. I. M. Mahler. 1987. Effects of preoperative roommate assignment on preoperative anxiety and recovery from coronary-bypass surgery. *Health Psychology* 6:525–543.

————. 1989a. Social support and recovery from surgery. *Health Psychology* 8:221–238.

————. 1989b. Stress and affiliation in hospital setting: Preoperative roommate preferences. *Personality and Social Psychology Bulletin* 15:183–193.

Lepore, S. J., G. W. Evans, and M. L. Schneider. 1991. Dynamic role of social support in the link between chronic stress and psychological distress. *Journal of Personality and Social Psychology* 61:899–909.

Lester, D. 1977. The use of the telephone in counseling and crisis prevention. In *The social impact of the telephone,* edited by I. d. S. Pool. Cambridge, Mass.: MIT Press.

Levy, R. L. 1983. Social support and compliance: A selective review and critique of treatment integrity and outcome measurement. *Social Science and Medicine* 17:1329–1338.

Levy, S. M., R. B. Herberman, T. Whiteside, K. Sauzo, J. Lee, and J. Kirkwood. 1990. Perceived social support and tumor estrogen/progesterone receptor status as predictors of natural killer cell activity in breast cancer patients. *Psychosomatic Medicine* 52:73–85.

Lipkus, I. M., C. Dalbert, and I. C. Siegler. 1996. The importance of distinguishing the belief in a just world for self versus for others: Implications for psychological well-being. *Personality and Social Psychology Bulletin* 22:666–677.

Lynch, J. J. 1979. *The broken heart: The medical consequences of loneliness.* New York: Basic Books.

McNair, D. M., M. Lorr, and L. F. Droppleman. 1981. *EDITS manual for the profile of mood states.* San Diego, Calif.: Educational and Industrial Testing Service.

Manne, S. L., and A. J. Zautra. 1989. Spouse criticism and support: Their association with coping and psychological adjustment among women with rheumatoid arthritis. *Journal of Personality and Social Psychology* 56:608–617.

Meagher, D. M., F. Gregor, and M. Stewart. 1987. Dyadic social-support for cardiac surgery patients: A Canadian approach. *Social Science and Medicine* 25:833–837.

Meichenbaum, D., and D. C. Turk. 1987. *Facilitating treatment adherence.* New York: Plenum.

Morisky, D. E., D. M. Levine, L. W. Green, S. Shapiro, R. P. Russell, and C. R. Smith. 1983. Five-year blood pressure control and mortality following health education for hypertensive patients. *American Journal of Public Health* 73:153–162.

Neuling, S. J., and H. R. Winefield. 1988. Social support and recovery after surgery for breast cancer: Frequency and correlates of supportive behaviors by family, friends, and surgeon. *Social Science and Medicine* 27:385–392.

Oldenburg, R. 1989. *The great good place.* New York: Paragon.

Orth-Gomer, K., and J. V. Johnson. 1987. Social network interaction and mortality: A six year follow-up study of a random sample of the Swedish population. *Journal of Chronic Diseases* 40:949–957.

Ostergren, P. O., B. S. Hanson, S. O. Isacsson, and L. Tejler. 1991. Social network, social support and acute chest complaints among young and middle-aged patients in an emergency department—a case-control study. *Social Science and Medicine* 33:257–267.

O'Sullivan, P., S. H. Evans, and P. Clarke. 1991. Emotion-laden health communication in videoconferencing: A case study. Paper presented at the Annual Meeting of the International Communication Association, May 1991, Chicago.

Patterson, J. T. 1987. *The dread disease: Cancer and modern American culture.* Cambridge, Mass.: Harvard University Press.

Payer, L. 1988. *Medicine and culture.* New York: Penguin.

Penninx, B. W., T. van Tilburg, D. M. Kriegsman, D. J. Deeg, A. J. Boeke, and J. T. van Eijk. 1997. Effects of social support and personal coping resources on mortality in older age: The longitudinal aging study Amsterdam. *American Journal of Epidemiology* 146:510–519.

Porritt, D. 1979. Social support in crisis: Quantity or quality? *Social Science and Medicine* 13A:715–721.

Pringle, T. 1992. *This is the child.* Dallas: Southern Methodist University Press.

Pritikin, N., and P. M. McGrady, Jr. 1979. *The Pritikin program for diet and exercise.* New York: Grosset and Dunlap.

Radner, G. 1989. *It's always something.* New York: Simon and Schuster.

Roberts, H. 1997. Socioeconomic determinants of health. Children, inequalities, and health. *British Medical Journal* 314:1122–1125.

Rogers, C. R. 1973. The characteristics of a helping relationship. In *Interpersonal dynamics,* edited by W. G. Bennis, D. E. Berlew, E. H. Schein, and F. I. Steele. Homewood, N.J.: Dorsey.

Rook, K. S. 1984. The negative side of social interaction: Impact on psychological well-being. *Journal of Personality and Social Psychology* 46:1097–1108.

———. 1987. Reciprocity of social exchange and social satisfaction among older women. *Journal of Personality and Social Psychology* 52:145–154.

———. 1991. Facilitating friendship formation in late life: Puzzles and challenges. *American Journal of Community Psychology* 19:103–110.

Rosenbaum, E. 1988. *A taste of my own medicine: When the doctor is the patient.* New York: Random House.

Russell, D., C. E. Cutrona, J. Rose, and K. Yurko. 1984. Social and emotional loneliness: An examination of Weiss's typology of loneliness. *Journal of Personality and Social Psychology* 46:1313–1321.

Salomon, G. 1981. *Communication and education: Social and psychological interactions.* Beverly Hills, Calif.: Sage.

Schaller, M., and R. B. Cialdini. 1988. The economics of empathic helping: Support for a mood management motive. *Journal of Experimental Social Psychology* 24:163–181.

Schank, R. C. 1990. *Tell me a story: A new look at real and artificial memory.* New York: Charles Scribner's Sons.

Schultz, R., and S. Decker. 1985. Long term adjustment to physical disability: The role of social support, perceived control, and self-blame. *Journal of Personality and Social Psychology* 48:1162–1172.

Seeman, T. E., G. A. Kaplan, L. Knudsen, R. Cohen, and J. Guralnik. 1987. Social network ties and mortality among the elderly in the Alameda County study. *American Journal of Epidemiology* 126:714–723.

Shye, D., J. P. Mullooly, D. K. Freeborn, and C. R. Pope. 1995. Gender differences in the relationship between social network support and mortality: A longitudinal study of an elderly cohort. *Social Science and Medicine* 41:935–947.

Sontag, S. 1978. *Illness as metaphor.* New York: Farrar, Straus, and Giroux.

Sosa, R., J. Kennell, M. Klaus, S. Robertson, and J. Urrutia. 1980. The effect of a supportive companion on perinatal problems, length of labor, and mother-infant interaction. *New England Journal of Medicine* 303:597–600.

Stewart, M. J. 1989. Social support: Diverse theoretical perspectives. *Social Science and Medicine* 28:1275–1282.

———. 1990. Expanding theoretical conceptualizations of self-help groups. *Social Science and Medicine* 31:1057–1066.

Telch, C. F., and M. J. Telch. 1986. Group coping skills instruction and supportive group therapy for cancer patients: A comparison of strategies. *Journal of Consulting and Clinical Psychology* 54:802–808.

Thoits, P. A. 1991. Stress, coping, and social support processes: Where are we? What next? *Journal of Health and Social Behavior* 36 (extra issue):53–79.

Thomas, P. D., J. M. Goodwin, and J. S. Goodwin. 1985. Effect of social support on stress-related changes in cholesterol level, uric acid level, and immune function in an elderly sample. *American Journal of Psychiatry* 142:735–737.

Uchino, B. N., J. K. Kiecolt-Glaser, and J. T. Cacioppo. 1992. Age-related changes in cardiovascular response as a function of a chronic stressor and social support. *Journal of Personality and Social Psychology* 63:839–846.

Umberson, D. 1992. Gender, marital status and social control of health behavior. *Social Science and Medicine* 34:907–917.

Verbrugge, L. M. 1985. Gender and health: An update on hypotheses and evidence. *Journal of Health and Social Behavior* 26:156–182.

Veroff, J., E. Douvan, and R. A. Kulka. 1981. *The inner American: A self-portrait from 1957 to 1976*. New York: Basic Books.

Waxler-Morrison, N., T. G. Hislop, B. Mears, and L. Kan. Effects of social relationships on survival for women with breast cancer: A prospective study. *Social Science and Medicine* 33:177–183.

Weiss, R. S. 1974. The provisions of social relationships. In *Doing unto others,* edited by Z. Rubin. Englewood Cliffs, N.J.: Prentice-Hall.

Weitzman, L. J. 1985. *The divorce revolution.* New York: Free Press.

Williams, K. B., and K. D. Williams. 1983. Social inhibition and asking for help: The effects of number, strength, and immediacy of potential help givers. *Journal of Personality and Social Psychology* 44:67–77.

Wortman, C. B. 1984. Social support and the cancer patient: Conceptual and methodologic issues. *Cancer* 53:2339–2360.

Wortman, C. B., and D. R. Lehman. 1985. Reactions to victims of life crises: Support attempts that fail. In *Social support: Theory, research, and applications,* edited by I. G. Sarason and B. R. Sarason. Dordrecht: Martinus Nijhoff.

Young, R. F., and E. Kahana. 1993. Gender, recovery from late life heart attack, and medical care. *Women and Health* 20:11–31.

CHAPTER 4    *Appreciating Your Caregiver*

Ahmann, E. 1994. Family-centered care: Shifting orientation. *Pediatric Nursing* 20:113–117.

Albert, S. M. 1992. Psychometric investigation of a belief system: Caregiving to the chronically ill parent. *Social Science and Medicine* 35:699–709.

Allen, A. 1990. Nurses' evaluations of patient attributions for the cause and future of their illness. *Journal of Applied Social Psychology* 20:1225–1255.

Baron, R. S., C. E. Cutrona, D. Hicklin, D. W. Russell, and D. M. Lubaroff. 1990. Social support and immune function among spouses of cancer patients. *Journal of Personality and Social Psychology* 59:344–352.

Betz, C. L., O. A. Unger, B. Frager, L. Test, and C. Smith. 1990. A survey of self-help groups in California for parents of children with chronic conditions. *Pediatric Nursing* 16:293–296.

Birkel, R. C. 1987. Toward a social ecology of the home-care household. *Psychology and Aging* 2:294–301.

Boaz, R. F. 1996. Full-time employment and informal caregiving in the 1980s. *Medical Care* 34:524–536.

Boss, P., W. Caron, and J. Horbal. 1988. Alzheimer's disease and ambiguous loss. In *Chronic illness and disability,* edited by C. S. Chilman, E. W. Nunnally, and F. M. Cox. Newbury Park, Calif.: Sage.

Boss, P., W. Caron, J. Horbal, and J. Mortimer. 1990. Predictors of depression in caregivers of dementia patients: Boundary ambiguity and mastery. *Family Process* 29:245–254.

Bowers, J. A. 1988. Family perceptions of care in a nursing home. *Gerontologist* 28:361–368.

Brody, E. M. 1985. Parent care as a normative family stress. *Gerontologist* 25:19–29.

Buske-Kirschbaum, A., C. Kirschbaum, H. Stierle, H. Lehnert, and D. Hellhammer. 1992. Conditioned increase of natural killer cell activity (NKA) in humans. *Psychosomatic Medicine* 54:123–132.

Buunk, B. P., R. L. Collins, S. E. Taylor, N. W. Van Yperen, and G. A. Dakof. 1990. The affective consequences of social comparison: Either direction has its ups and downs. *Journal of Personality and Social Psychology* 59:1238–1249.

Cacioppo, J. T. 1994. Social neuroscience: Autonomic, neuroendocrine, and immune responses to stress. *Psychophysiology* 31:113–128.

Campbell, L. A., S. E. Kirkpatrick, C. C. Berry, and J. J. Lamberti. 1995. Preparing children with congenital heart disease for cardiac surgery. *Journal of Pediatric Psychology* 20:313–328.

Carroll, J. L., and J. L. Shmidt. 1992. Correlation between humorous coping style and health. *Psychological Reports* 70:402.

Chapman, N. J., and D. L. Pancoast. 1985. Working with the informal helping networks of the elderly: The experiences of three programs. *Journal of Social Issues* 41:47–63.

Clements, D. G., L. G. Copeland, and M. Loftus. 1990. Critical times for families with a chronically ill child. *Pediatric Nursing* 16:157–161.

Cogan, R., D. Cogan, W. Waltz, and M. McCue. 1987. Effects of laughter and relaxation on discomfort thresholds. *Journal of Behavioral Medicine* 10:139–144.

Cohen, S., and E. Lichtenstein. 1990. Partner behaviors that support quitting smoking. *Journal of Consulting and Clinical Psychology* 58:304–309.

Counte, M. A., and G. L. Glandon. 1991. A panel study of life stress, social support, and the health services utilization of older persons. *Medical Care* 29:348–361.

Cousins, N. 1979. *Anatomy of an illness.* New York: Norton.

Craig, J. 1991. *Between hello and goodbye.* Los Angeles: Jeremy P. Tarcher.

Crimmins, E. M., Y. Saito, and D. Ingegneri. 1989. Changes in life expectancy and disability-free life expectancy in the United States. *Population and Development Review* 15:235–267.

Dillon, K. M., B. Minchoff, and K. H. Baker. 1985. Positive emotional states and enhancement of the immune system. *International Journal of Psychiatry in Medicine* 15:13–18.

Dura, J. R., K. W. Stukenberg, and J. K. Kiecolt-Glaser. 1991. Anxiety and depressive disorders in adult children caring for demented parents. *Psychology and Aging* 6:467–473.

Eisdorfer, C. 1991. Caregiving: An emerging risk factor for emotional and physical pathology. *Bulletin of the Menninger Clinic* 55:238–247.

Emery, C. F., E. J. Burker, and J. A. Blumenthal. 1991. Psychological and physiological effects of exercise among older adults. In *Annual Review of Gerontology and Geriatrics,* edited by K. W. Schaie and M. P. Lawton. New York: Springer.

Esterling, B. A., M. H. Antoni, M. Kumar, and N. Schneiderman. 1990. Emotional repression, stress disclosure responses, and Epstein-Barr viral capsid antigen titers. *Psychosomatic Medicine* 52:397–410.

Festinger, L. 1954. A theory of social comparison processes. *Human Relations* 57:271–282.

Fitting, M. D., and P. V. Rabins. 1985. Men and women—Do they give care differently? *Generations* 10:23–26.

Fraley, A. M. 1990. Chronic sorrow: A parental response. *Journal of Pediatric Nursing* 5:268–273.

Freud, S. 1960. *Jokes and their relation to the unconscious.* New York: W. W. Norton.

Fries, J. F. 1989. The compression of morbidity: Near or far? *Milbank Quarterly* 67:208–232.

Gallagher, D., A. Wrabetz, S. Lovett, S. DelMaestro, and J. Rose. 1989. Depression and other negative affects in family caregivers. In *Alzheimer's disease treatment and family stress: Directions for research,* edited by E. Light and B. Lebowitz. Washington, D.C.: National Institute of Mental Health.

Gallagher-Thompson, D., S. Lovett, and J. Rose. 1991. Psychotherapeutic interventions for stressed family caregivers. In *New techniques in the psychotherapy of older patients,* edited by W. A. Myers. Washington, D.C.: American Psychiatric Press.

Gatz, M., V. L. Bengston, and M. J. Blum. 1990. Caregiving families. In *Handbook of the psychology of aging,* edited by J. E. Birren and K. W. Schaie. San Diego, Calif.: Academic Press.

Ghanta, V., R. N. Hiramoto, B. Solvason, and N. H. Spector. 1987. Influence of conditioned natural immunity on tumor growth. *Annals of the New York Academy of Sciences* 496:637–646.

Gibbons, K. 1989. *A virtuous woman.* New York: Vintage Books.

Gonzalez, S., P. Steinglass, and D. Reiss. 1987. *Family-centered interventions for people with chronic disabilities.* Washington, D.C.: George Washington University Medical Center.

———. 1989. Putting the illness in its place: Discussion groups for families with chronic medical illnesses. *Family Process* 28:69–87.

Gottlieb, B. H., and A. E. Coppard. 1987. Using social network therapy to create support systems for the chronically mentally disabled. *Canadian Journal of Community Mental Health* 6:117–131.

Gravelle, A. M. 1997. Caring for a child with a progressive illness during the complex chronic phase: Parents' experience of facing adversity. *Journal of Advanced Nursing* 25:738–745.

Gray, S. 1992. *Monster in a box.* New York: Vintage.

Haley, W. E., E. G. Levine, S. L. Brown, J. W. Berry, and G. H. Hughes. 1987. Psychological, social and health consequences of caring for a relative with senile dementia. *Journal of the American Geriatrics Society* 35:405–411.

Helgeson, V. S. 1993. Implications of agency and communion for patient and spouse adjustment to a first coronary event. *Journal of Personality and Social Psychology* 64:807–816.

———. 1994. Relation of agency and communion to well-being: Evidence and potential explanations. *Psychological Bulletin* 116:412–428.

Horne, J. 1991. *A survival guide for family caregivers.* Minneapolis, Minn.: CompCare.

Horwitz, A. V., S. C. Reinhard, and S. Howell-White. 1996. Caregiving as reciprocal exchange in families with seriously mentally ill members. *Journal of Health and Social Behavior* 37:149–162.

Jacono, J., G. Hicks, C. Antonioni, K. O'Brien, and M. Rasi. 1990. Comparison of perceived needs of family members between registered nurses and family members of critically ill patients in intensive care and neonatal intensive care units. *Heart and Lung* 19:72–78.

Joslin, D., and A. Brovard. 1995. The prevalence of grandmothers as primary caregivers in a poor pediatric population. *Journal of Community Health* 20:383–401.

Kaye, L. W., and J. S. Applegate. 1990. Men as elder caregivers: A response to changing families. *American Journal of Orthopsychiatry* 60:86–95.

———. 1991. Components of a gender-sensitive curriculum model for elder caregiving: Lessons from research. *Gerontology and Geriatrics Education* 11:39–56.

Kiecolt-Glaser, J. K., R. Glaser, E. C. Shuttleworth, C. S. Dyer, P. Ogrocki, and C. E. Speicher. 1987. Chronic stress and immunity in family caregivers for Alzheimer's disease victims. *Psychosomatic Medicine* 49:523–535.

Kiecolt-Glaser, J. K., J. R. Dura, C. E. Speicher, O. J. Trask, and R. Glaser. 1991. Spousal caregivers of dementia victims: Longitudinal changes in immunity and health. *Psychosomatic Medicine* 53:345–362.

King, S., C. Collins, B. Given, and J. Vredevoogd. 1991. Institutionalization of an elderly family member: Reactions of spouse and nonspouse caregivers. *Archives of Psychiatric Nursing* 5:323–330.

Kruglanski, A. W., and O. Mayseless. 1990. Classic and current social comparison research: Expanding the perspective. *Psychological Bulletin* 108:195–208.

Kurtz, M. E., J. C. Kurtz, C. W. Given, and B. Given. 1995. Relationship of caregiver reactions and depression to cancer patients' symptoms, functional states and depression—A longitudinal view. *Social Science and Medicine* 40:837–846.

Lawton, M. P. 1975. The Philadelphia Geriatric Center morale scale: A revision. *Journal of Gerontology* 30:85–89.

Lawton, M. P., E. M. Brody, and A. R. Saperstein. 1991. *Respite for caregivers of Alzheimer patients: Research and practice.* New York: Springer.

McClelland, D. C. 1989. Motivational factors in health and disease. *American Psychologist* 44:675–683.

Manne, S. L., W. H. Redd, P. B. Jacobsen, K. Gorfinkle, and O. Schorr. 1990. Behavioral intervention to reduce child and parent distress during venipuncture. *Journal of Consulting and Clinical Psychology* 58:565–572.

Manton, K. G. 1991. The dynamics of population aging: Demography and policy analysis. *Milbank Quarterly* 69:309–338.

Manton, K. G., and E. Stallard. 1991. Cross-sectional estimates of active life expectancy for the U.S. elderly and oldest-old populations. *Journal of Gerontology* 46:S170–S182.

Manton, K. G., L. S. Corder, and E. Stallard. 1993. Estimates of change in chronic disability and institutional incidence and prevalence rates in the U.S. elderly population from 1982, 1984, and 1989 national long-term care survey. *Journal of Gerontology* 48:S153–S166.

Marcenko, M. O., and L. K. Smith. 1992. The impact of a family-centered case management approach. *Social Work in Health Care* 17:87–100.

Martin, R. A., and H. M. Lefcourt. 1983. Sense of humor as a moderator of the relation between stressors and moods. *Journal of Personality and Social Psychology* 45:1313–1324.

Martin, R. A., and J. P. Dobbin. 1988. Sense of humor, hassles, and immunoglobulin A: Evidence for a stress-moderating effect of humor. *International Journal of Psychiatry in Medicine* 18:93–105.

Marvin, R. S., and R. C. Pianta. 1996. Mothers' reactions to their child's diagnosis: Relations with security of attachment. *Journal of Clinical Child Psychology* 25:436–445.

Melnyk, B. M. 1995. Coping with unplanned childhood hospitalization: The mediating functions of parental beliefs. *Journal of Pediatric Psychology* 20:299–312.

Murphy, R. F. 1990. *The body silent.* New York: W. W. Norton.

Myers, M. S. 1991. Extending the concept: Foster-family care applications with special applications. Unpublished paper. Royal Oak, Mich.: Judson Center.

Neef, N. A., S. Trachtenberg, J. Loeb, and K. Sterner. 1991. Video based training of respite care providers: An interactional analysis of presentation format. *Journal of Applied Behavior Analysis* 24:473–486.

Ostwald, S. K., B. Leonard, T. Choi, J. Keenan, K. Hepburn, and M. A. Aroskar. 1993. Caregivers of frail elderly and medically fragile children: Perceptions of ability to continue to provide home health care. *Home Health Care Services Quarterly* 14:55–80.

Patterson, K. L., and L. L. Ware. 1988. Coping skills for children undergoing painful medical procedures. *Issues in Comprehensive Pediatric Nursing* 11:113–143.

Pearlin, L. I., J. T. Mullan, S. J. Semple, and M. M. Skaff. 1990. Caregiving and the stress process: An overview of concepts and their measures. *Gerontologist* 30:583–594.

Perkins, M. T. 1993. Parent-nurse collaboration: Using the caregiver identity emergence phases to assist parents of hospitalized children with disabilities. *Journal of Pediatric Nursing* 8:2–9.

Peterson, K. E. 1992. The use of humor in AIDS prevention, in the treatment of HIV positive persons, and in the remediation of caregiver burnout. In *AIDS prevention and treatment: Hope, humor, and healing,* edited by M. R. Seligson and K. E. Peterson. New York: Hemisphere.

Pianta, R. C., R. S. Marvin, P. A. Britner, and K. C. Borowitz. 1996. Mothers' resolution of their children's diagnosis: Organized patterns of caregiving representation. *Infant Mental Health Journal* 17:239–256.

Price, R. H., M. V. Ryn, and A. D. Vinokur. 1992. Impact of a preventive job search intervention on the likelihood of depression among the unemployed. *Journal of Health and Social Behavior* 33:158–176.

Pringle, T. 1992. *This is the child.* Dallas: Southern Methodist University Press.

Reich, J. W., and A. J. Zautra. 1990. Dispositional control beliefs and the consequences of a control-enhancing intervention. *Journal of Gerontology* 45:46–51.

Sanders, M. R., R. W. Shepherd, G. Cleghorn, and H. Woolford. 1994. The treatment of recurrent abdominal pain in children: A controlled comparison of cognitive-behavioral family intervention and standard pediatric care. *Journal of Consulting and Clinical Psychology* 62:306–314.

Schulz, R., C. A. Tompkins, and M. T. Rau. 1988. A longitudinal study of the psychosocial impact of stroke on primary support persons. *Psychology and Aging* 3: 131–141.

Schulz, R., and G. M. Williamson. 1991. A two-year longitudinal study of depression among Alzheimer's caregivers. *Psychology and Aging* 6:569–578.

Shields, C. G. 1992. Family interaction and caregivers of Alzheimer's disease patients: Correlates of depression. *Family Process* 31:19–33.

Steinglass, P. 1987. Psychoeducational family therapy for schizophrenia: A review essay. *Psychiatry* 50:14–23.

Stewart, M. J. 1990. Expanding theoretical conceptualizations of self-help groups. *Social Science and Medicine* 31:1057–1066.

Stone, J. 1990. *In the country of hearts: Journeys in the art of medicine.* New York: Delta.

Stone, R. I., and P. Kemper. 1989. Spouses and children of disabled elders: How large a constituency for long-term care reform? *Milbank Quarterly* 67:485–506.

Tavris, C. 1992. *The mismeasure of woman.* New York: Simon and Schuster.

Thompson, S. C., N. I. Bundek, and A. Sobolew-Shubin. 1990. The caregivers of stroke patients: An investigation of factors associated with depression. *Journal of Applied Social Psychology* 20:115–129.

Thompson, S. C., and A. Sobolew-Shubin. 1993. Overprotective relationships: A nonsupportive side of social networks. *Basic and Applied Social Psychology* 14:363–383.

Townsend, A., L. Noelker, G. Deimling, and D. Bass. 1989. Longitudinal impact of interhousehold caregiving on adult children's mental health. *Psychology and Aging* 4:393–401.

Vaillant, G. E. 1977. *Adaptation to life.* Boston: Little Brown.

Vinokur, A. D., R. H. Price, and R. D. Caplan. 1991. From field experiments to program implementation: Assessing the potential outcomes of an experimental intervention program for unemployed persons. *American Journal of Community Psychology* 19:543–562.

Vitaliano, P. P., J. Russo, H. M. Young, L. Teri, and R. D. Maiuro. 1991. Predictors of burden in spouse caregivers of individuals with Alzheimer's disease. *Psychology and Aging* 6:392–402.

Wegner, D. M., D. J. Schneider, B. Knutson, and S. R. McMahon. 1991. Polluting the stream of consciousness: The effect of thought suppression on the mind's environment. *Cognitive Therapy and Research* 15:141–152.

Weiss, S. J. 1991. Personality adjustment and social support of parents who care for children with pervasive developmental disorders. *Archives of Psychiatric Nursing* 5:25–30.

Wellisch, D., M. Mosher, and C. Van Scoy. 1978. Management of family emotional stress: Family group therapy in a private oncology practice. *International Journal of Group Psychotherapy* 28:225–231.

Whitlatch, C. J., S. H. Zarit, and A. Von Eye. 1991. Efficacy of interventions with caregivers: A reanalysis. *Gerontologist* 31:9–14.

Williams, P. D., F. D. Lorenzo, and M. Borja. 1993. Pediatric chronic illness: Effects on siblings and mothers. *Maternal-Child Nursing Journal* 21:111–121.

Wood, J. V., and S. E. Taylor. 1991. Serving self-relevant goals through social comparison. In *Social comparison: Contemporary theory and research,* edited by J. Suls and T. A. Wills. Hillsdale, N.J.: Lawrence Erlbaum.

Wynne, L. C., C. G. Shields, and M. I. Sirkin. 1992. Illness, family theory, and family therapy: I. Conceptual issues. *Family Process* 31:3–18.

Zarit, S. H., and L. Teri. 1991. Interventions and services for family caregivers. In *Annual review of gerontology and geriatrics,* edited by K. W. Schaie and M. P. Lawton. New York: Springer.

Zarit, S. H., P. A. Todd, and J. M. Zarit. 1986. Subjective burden of husbands and wives as caregivers: A longitudinal study. *Gerontologist* 26:260–266.

CHAPTER 5    *Protecting Your Choices in Critical Care*

Asch, D. A., J. Hansen-Flaschen, and P. N. Lauken. 1995. Decisions to limit or continue life-sustaining treatment by critical care physicians in the United States: Conflicts between physicians' practices and patients' wishes. *American Journal of Respiratory and Critical Care Medicine* 151:288–292.

Asch, D. A., and N. A. Christakis. 1996. Why do physicians prefer to withdraw some forms of life support over others? *Medical Care* 34:103–111.

Barkin, R. L., T. R. Lubenow, S. Bruehl, B. Husfeldt, O. Ivankovich, and S. J. Barkin. 1996. Management of chronic pain. Part II. *Disease-A-Month* 42:457–507.

Bedell, S. E., D. Pelle, P. L. Maher, and P. D. Cleary. 1986. Do-not-resuscitate orders for critically ill patients in the hospital: How are they used and what is their impact? *Journal of the American Medical Association* 256:233–237.

Brock, D. W. 1994. Advance directives: What is it reasonable to expect from them? *Journal of Clinical Ethics* 5:57–60.

Burge, F. I. 1996. Dehydration and provision of fluids in palliative care. What is the evidence? *Canadian Family Physician* 42:2383–2388.

Bush, J. W. 1983. *Quality of well-being scale: Function status profile and symptom/problem complex questionnaire.* San Diego: University of California, Health Policy Project.

Caralis, P. V., B. Davis, K. Wright, and E. Marcial. 1993. The influence of ethnicity and race on attitudes toward advance directives, life-prolonging treatments, and euthanasia. *Journal of Clinical Ethics* 4:155–165.

Chambers, C. V., J. J. Diamond, R. L. Perkel, and L. A. Lasch. 1994. Relationship of advance directives to hospital charges in a Medicare population. *Archives of Internal Medicine* 154:541–547.

Christakis, N. A., and D. A. Asch. 1993. Biases in how physicians choose to withdraw life support. *Lancet* 342:642–646.

———. 1995. Physician characteristics associated with decisions to withdraw life support. *American Journal of Public Health* 85:367–372.

Cohen-Mansfield, J., B. A. Rabinovich, S. Lipson, A. Fein, B. Gerber, S. Weisman, and G. Pawlson. 1991. The decision to execute a durable power of attorney for health care and preferences regarding the utilization of life-sustaining treatments in nursing home residents. *Archives of Internal Medicine* 151:289–294.

Danis, M., L. I. Southerland, J. Garrett, and J. L. Smith. 1991. A prospective study of advance directives for life-sustaining care. *New England Journal of Medicine* 324:882–888.

Danis, M., J. Garrett, R. Harris, and D. L. Patrick. 1994. Stability of choices about life-sustaining treatments. *Annals of Internal Medicine* 120:567–573.

Devor, M., A. Wang, M. Renvall, D. Feigal, and J. Ramsdell. 1994. Compliance with social and safety recommendations in an outpatient comprehensive geriatric assessment program. *Journal of Gerontology* 49:M168–M173.

Diamond, E. L., J. A. Jernigan, R. A. Moseley, V. Messina, and R. A. McKeown. 1989. Decision-making ability and advance directive preferences in nursing home patients and proxies. *Gerontologist* 29:622–626.

Doukas, D. J., S. Lipson, and L. McCullough. 1989. Value history. In *Clinical aspects of aging,* edited by W. Reichel. Baltimore: Williams and Wilkins.

Doukas, D. J., and L. McCullough. 1991. The values history: The evaluation of the patient's values and advance directives. *Journal of Family Practice* 32:145–153.

Doukas, D. J., and D. W. Gorenflo. 1993. Analyzing the values history: An evaluation of patient medical values and advance directives. *Journal of Clinical Ethics* 4:41–45.

Dresser, R. 1994. Advance directives: Implications for policy. *Hastings Center Report* 24:S2–S5.

Druley, J. A., P. H. Ditto, K. A. Moore, and J. H. Danks. 1993. Physicians' predictions of elderly outpatients' preferences for life-sustaining treatment. *Journal of Family Practice* 37:469–475.

Emanuel, L. L., M. J. Barry, J. D. Stoeckle, and L. M. Ettelson. 1991. Advance directives for medical care: A case for greater use. *New England Journal of Medicine* 324:889–895.

Emanuel, E. J., and L. L. Emanuel. 1992. Proxy decision making for incompetent patients: An ethical and empirical analysis. *Journal of the American Medical Association* 267:2067–2071.

Emanuel, E. J., and A. S. Brett. 1993. How well is the patient self-determination act working?: An early assessment. *American Journal of Medicine* 95:619–628.

Emanuel, E. J., and L. L. Emanuel. 1994. The economics of dying: The illusion of cost savings at the end of life. *New England Journal of Medicine* 330:540–544.

Emanuel, L. L., E. J. Emanuel, J. D. Stoeckle, L. R. Hummel, and M. J. Barry. 1994. Advance directives: Stability of patients' treatment choices. *Archives of Internal Medicine* 154:209–217.

Emanuel, L. L., M. Danis, R. A. Pearlman, and P. A. Singer. 1995. Advance care planning as a process: Structuring the discussions in practice. *Journal of the American Geriatrics Society* 43:440–446.

Evans, S. H., and P. Clarke. 1993. Rethinking how we communicate about advance directives: Hidden errors in our assumptions about planning for care. In *Communications and the patient self-determination act: Strategies for meeting the educational mandate,* edited by F. Cate and B. Gill. Washington, D.C.: Annenberg Washington Program.

Everhart, M. A., and R. A. Pearlman. 1990. Stability of patient preferences regarding life-sustaining treatments. *Chest* 97:159–164.

Fainsinger, R. L., and E. Bruera. 1997. When to treat dehydration in a terminally ill patient? *Supportive Care in Cancer* 5:205–211.

Ferrell, B. A., ed. 1996. Pain management. *Clinics in Geriatric Medicine* 12.

Finucane, T. E., J. M. Shumway, R. L. Powers, and R. M. Alessandri. 1988. Planning with elderly outpatients for contingencies of severe illness: A survey and clinical trial. *Journal of General Internal Medicine* 3:322–325.

Gamble, E. R., P. J. Donald, and P. R. Lichstein. 1991. Knowledge, attitudes and behavior of elderly persons regarding living wills. *Archives of Internal Medicine* 151:277–280.

Garrett, J. M., R. P. Harris, J. K. Norburn, D. L. Patrick, and M. Danis. 1993. Life-sustaining treatments during terminal illness: Who wants what? *Journal of General Internal Medicine* 8:361–368.

Gillick, M. R., K. Hesse, and N. Mazzapica. 1993. Medical technology at the end of life: What would physicians and nurses want for themselves? *Archives of Internal Medicine* 153:2542–2547.

Hanson, L. C., M. Danis, J. M. Garrett, and E. Mutran. 1996. Who decides?: Physicians' willingness to use life-sustaining treatment. *Archives of Internal Medicine* 156:785–789.

Hare, J., and C. Nelson. 1991. Will outpatients complete living wills? A comparison of two interventions. *Journal of General Internal Medicine* 6:41–46.

———. 1992. Agreement between patients and their self-selected surrogates on difficult medical decisions. *Archives of Internal Medicine* 152:1049–1054.

Hastings Center. 1987. *Guideline on the termination of life-sustaining treatment and the care of the dying.* Bloomington: Indiana University Press.

High, D. M. 1989. Standards for surrogate decision making: What the elderly want. *Journal of Long-Term Administration* 17:8–13.

———. 1993a. Advance directives and the elderly: A study of intervention strategies to increase use. *Gerontologist* 33:342–349.

———. 1993b. Why are elderly people not using advance directives? *Journal of Aging and Health* 5:497–515.

———. 1994a. Families' roles in advance directives. *Hastings Center Report* 24:S16–S18.

———. 1994b. Surrogate decision making: Who will make decisions for me when I can't? In *Clinics in geriatric medicine,* edited by G. A. Sachs and C. K. Cassel. Philadelphia: Saunders.

Jacobson, J. A., B. E. White, M. P. Battin, L. P. Francis, D. J. Green, and E. S. Kasworm. 1994. Patients' understanding and use of advance directives. *Western Journal of Medicine* 160:232–236.

Joint Commission on Accreditation of Healthcare Facilities. 1992. *Accreditation manual for healthcare facilities.* Oak Brook, Ill.: Joint Commission on Accreditation of Healthcare Facilities.

Kohn, M., and G. Menon. 1988. Life prolongation: Views of elderly outpatients and health care professionals. *Journal of the American Geriatrics Society* 36:840–844.

Lambert, P., J. M. Gibson, and P. Nathanson. 1990. The values history: An innovation in surrogate medical decision making. *Law, Medicine, and Health Care* 18:202–212.

Layson, R. T., H. M. Adelman, P. M. Wallach, M. P. Pfeifer, S. Johnston, and R. A. McNutt. 1994. Discussions about the use of life-sustaining treatments: A literature review of physicians' and patients' attitudes and practices. *Journal of Clinical Ethics* 5:195–203.

Lubitz, J. D., and G. F. Riley. 1993. Trends in Medicare payments in the last year of life. *New England Journal of Medicine* 328:1092–1096.

Lundberg, G. D. 1993. American health care system management objectives: The aura of inevitability becomes incarnate. *Journal of the American Medical Association* 269:2554–2555.

Luptak, M. K., and C. Boult. 1994. A method for increasing elders' use of advance directives. *Gerontologist* 34:409–412.

Lurie, N., A. M. Pheley, S. H. Miles, and S. Bannick-Mohrland. 1992. Attitudes toward discussing life-sustaining treatments in extended care facility patients. *Journal of the American Geriatrics Society* 40:1205–1208.

Markson, L., and K. Steel. 1990. Using advance directives in the home-care setting. *Generations* 14:25–29.

Mold, J. W., S. W. Looney, N. J. Viviani, and P. A. Quiggins. 1994. Predicting the health-related values and preferences of geriatric patients. *Journal of Family Practice* 39:461–467.

Molloy, D. W., and G. H. Guyatt. 1991. A comprehensive health care directive in a home for the aged. *Canadian Medical Association Journal* 145:307–311.

Nightingale, S. D., and M. Grant. 1988. Risk preference and decision making in critical care situations. *Chest* 93:684–687.

O'Neill, W. M., P. O'Connor, and E. J. Latimer. 1992. Hospital palliative care services: Three models in three countries. *Journal of Pain and Symptom Management* 7:406–413.

Ouslander, J. G., A. J. Tymchuk, and B. Rahbar. 1989. Health care decisions among elderly long term care residents and their proxies. *Archives of Internal Medicine* 149:1367–1372.

Patrick, D. L., H. E. Starks, K. C. Cain, R. F. Uhlmann, and R. A. Pearlman. 1994. Measuring preferences for health states worse than death. *Medical Decision Making* 14:9–18.

Patrick, D. L., R. A. Pearlman, H. E. Starks, K. C. Cain, W. G. Cole, and R. F. Uhlmann. 1997. Validation of preferences for life-sustaining treatment: Implications for advance care planning. *Annals of Internal Medicine* 127:509–517.

Pearlman, R. A. 1994. Are we asking the right questions? *Hastings Center Report* 24:S24–S27.

Pearlman, R. A., K. C. Cain, D. C. Patrick, M. Appelbaum, H. E. Stanks, H. S. Jecker, and R. F. Uhlmann. 1993. Insights pertaining to patient assessments of states worse than death. *Journal of Clinical Ethics* 4:33–41.

Rhymes, J. A. 1996. Barriers to effective palliative care of terminal patients: An international perspective. *Clinics in Geriatric Medicine* 12:407–416.

Ripamonti, C., E. Zecca, and E. Bruera. 1997. An update on the clinical use of methadone for cancer pain. *Pain* 70:109–115.

Roth, P. 1991. *Patrimony: A true story.* New York: Simon and Schuster.

Rubin, S. M., W. M. Strull, M. F. Fialkow, S. J. Weiss, and B. Lo. 1994. Increasing the completion of the durable power of attorney for health care. *Journal of the American Medical Association* 271:209–212.

Sachs, G. A. 1994. Increasing the prevalence of advance care planning. *Hastings Center Report* 24:S13–S16.

Sachs, G. A., C. B. Stocking, and S. H. Miles. 1992. Empowerment of the older patient? A randomized, controlled trial to increase discussion and use of advance directives. *Journal of the American Geriatrics Society* 40:269–273.

Sam, M., and P. A. Singer. 1993. Canadian outpatients and advance directives: Poor knowledge and little experience but positive attitudes. *Canadian Medical Association Journal* 148:1497–1502.

Schneiderman, L. J., R. Kronick, R. M. Kaplan, J. P. Anderson, and R. D. Langer. 1992. Effects of offering advance directives on medical treatments and costs. *Annals of Internal Medicine* 117:599–606.

Schneiderman, L. J., R. A. Pearlman, R. M. Kaplan, J. P. Anderson, and E. M. Rosenberg. 1992. Relationship of general advance directive instructions to specific life-sustaining treatment preferences in patients with serious illness. *Archives of Internal Medicine* 152:2114–2122.

Schneiderman, L. J., N. S. Jecker, and A. R. Jonsen. 1996. Medical futility: Response to critiques. *Annals of Internal Medicine* 125:669–674.

Schofferman, J. 1993. Long-term use of opioid analgesics for the treatment of chronic pain of nonmalignant origin. *Journal of Pain and Symptom Management* 8:279–288.

Seckler, A. B., D. E. Meier, M. Mulvihill, and B. E. Paris. 1991. Substituted judgment: How accurate are proxy decisions? *Annals of Internal Medicine* 115:92–98.

Sehgal, A., A. Galbraith, M. Chesney, P. Schoenfeld, G. Charles, and B. Lo. 1992. How strictly do dialysis patients want their advance directives followed? *Journal of the American Medical Association* 267:59–63.

Shmerling, R. H., S. E. Bedell, A. Lilienfeld, and T. L. Delbanco. 1988. Discussing cardiopulmonary resuscitation: A study of elderly outpatients. *Journal of General Internal Medicine* 3:317–321.

Singer, P. A., S. Choudhry, J. Armstrong, E. M. Meslin, and F. H. Lowy. 1995. Public opinion regarding end-of-life decisions: Influence of prognosis, practice, and process. *Social Science and Medicine* 41:1517–1521.

Society of Critical Care Medicine. 1997. Consensus statement of the Society of Critical Care Medicine's Ethics Committee regarding futile and other possibly inadvisable treatments. *Critical Care Medicine* 25:887–891.

Solomon, M. Z., L. O'Donnell, B. Jennings, V. Guilfoy, S. M. Wolf, K. Nolan, R. Jackson, D. Koch-Weser, and S. Donnelley. 1993. Decisions near the end of life: Professional views on life-sustaining treatments. *American Journal of Public Health* 83:14–23.

Sonnenblick, M., Y. Friedlander, and A. Steinberg. 1993. Dissociation between the wishes of terminally ill parents and decisions by their offspring. *Journal of the American Geriatrics Society* 41:599–604.

Sulmasy, D. P., K. Haller, and P. B. Terry. 1994. More talk, less paper: Predicting the accuracy of substituted judgments. *American Journal of Medicine* 96:432–438.

Teno, J. M., J. Lynn, R. S. Phillips, D. Murphy, S. J. Youngner, P. Bellamy, A. F. Conners, Jr., N. A. Desbiens, W. Fulkerson, and W. A. Knaus. 1994. Do formal advance directives affect resuscitation decisions and the use of resources for seriously ill patients? *Journal of Clinical Ethics* 5:23–30.

Teno, J. M., H. L. Nelson, and J. Lynn. 1994. Advance care planning: Priorities for ethical and empirical research. *Hastings Center Report* 24:S32–S36.

Tomlinson, T., K. Howe, M. Notman, and D. Rossmiller. 1990. An empirical study of proxy consent for elderly persons. *Gerontologist* 30:54–64.

Trzcieniecka-Green, A., and A. Steptoe. 1996. The effects of stress management on the quality of life of patients following acute myocardial infarction or coronary bypass surgery. *European Heart Journal* 17:1663–1670.

Urba, S. G. 1996. Nonpharmacologic pain management in terminal care. *Clinics in Geriatric Medicine* 12:301–311.

Virmani, J., L. J. Schneiderman, and R. M. Kaplan. 1994. Relationship of advance directives to physician-patient communication. *Archives of Internal Medicine* 154:909–913.

von Gunten, C. F., and M. L. Twaddle. 1996. Terminal care for noncancer patients. *Clinics in Geriatric Medicine* 12:349–358.

Ward, S. E., N. Goldberg, V. Miller-McCauley, C. Mueller, A. Nolan, D. Pawlik-Plank, A. Robbins, D. Stormoen, and D. E. Weissman. 1993. Patient-related barriers to management of cancer pain. *Pain* 52:319–324.

Ward, S. E., P. E. Berry, and H. Misiewicz. 1996. Concerns about analgesics among patients and family caregivers in a hospice setting. *Research in Nursing and Health* 19:205–211.

Weeks, W. B., L. L. Kofoed, A. E. Wallace, and H. G. Welch. 1994. Advance directives and the cost of terminal hospitalization. *Archives of Internal Medicine* 154:2077–2083.

Weinstein, N. D. 1987. Unrealistic optimism about illness susceptibility: Conclusions from a community-wide sample. *Journal of Behavioral Medicine* 10:481–500.

Wetle, T. 1994. Individual preferences and advance directives. *Hastings Center Report* 24:S5–S8.

World Health Organization. 1986. *Cancer pain relief.* Geneva: World Health Organization.

Zenz, M., T. Zenz, M. Tryba, and M. Strumpf. 1995. Severe undertreatment of cancer pain: A 3-year survey of the German situation. *Journal of Pain and Symptom Management* 10:187–191.

Zweibel, N. R., and C. K. Cassel. 1989. Treatment choices at the end of life: A comparison of decisions by older patients and their physician-selected proxies. *Gerontologist* 29:615–621.

### Epilogue

Bandura, A., ed. 1995. *Self-efficacy in changing societies.* Cambridge: Cambridge University Press.

Francis, M. E., and J. W. Pennebaker. 1992. Putting stress into words: The impact of writing on physiological, absentee, and self-reported emotional well-being measures. *American Journal of Health Promotion* 6:280–287.

Greenberg, M. A. 1995. Cognitive processing of traumas: The role of intrusive thoughts and reappraisals. *Journal of Applied Social Psychology* 25:1262–1296.

Gregory, W. L., R. B. Cialdini, and K. M. Carpenter. 1982. Self-relevant scenarios as mediators of likelihood estimates and compliance: Does imagining make it so? *Journal of Personality and Social Psychology* 43:89–99.

Hughes, C. F., C. Uhlmann, and J. W. Pennebaker. 1994. The body's response to processing emotional trauma: Linking verbal text with autonomic activity. *Journal of Personality* 62:565–585.

Kobasa, S. C., S. R. Maddi, M. C. Puccetti, and M. A. Zola. 1985. Effectiveness of hardiness, exercise and social support as resources against illness. *Journal of Psychosomatic Research* 29:525–533.

Maddi, S. R., and S. C. Kobasa. 1991. The development of hardiness. In *Stress and coping,* edited by A. Monat and R. S. Lazarus. New York: Columbia University Press.

Pennebaker, J. W. 1993a. Overcoming inhibition: Rethinking the roles of personality, cognition, and social behavior. In *Emotion, inhibition, and health,* edited by H. C. Traue and J. W. Pennebaker. Seattle: Hogrefe & Huber.

———. 1993b. Putting stress into words: Health, linguistic, and therapeutic implications. *Behavioral Research and Therapy* 31:539–548.

Sherman, S. J., R. B. Cialdini, D. F. Schwartzman, and K. D. Reynolds. 1985. Imagining can heighten or lower the perceived likelihood of contracting a disease: The mediating effect of ease of imagery. *Personality and Social Psychology Bulletin* 11:118–127.

# INDEX

aberrant behavior, 160, 190. *See also* dementia

abortion, 218, 256

acid indigestion and reflux, 98

acupuncture, 11, 95

addiction to pain medication, fears about, 206, 207

advance directives, 4, 194, 195, 246; easily executed, 201; ethical basis for, 195, 202–203; and family communication, 195, 198–199, 217–218, 220–223; legal basis for, 197, 202; need to distribute, 201, 230–231; problems of, 198–207; professional advice about, 223–228; reasons for, 213; types of, 208–212. *See also* Living Will; Medical Directive; Medical Power of Attorney

advertising, health-related, 6

aerochamber, 51

affection, physical displays of, 136. *See also* handholding

agencies, commercial health-care, 153

agencies, commercial home-care, 153

agent, medical, 210, 217, 251, 255–256,
258, 259. *See also* health-care partner

AIDS: controlling uncertainty about, 101–103; patients' need for long-term support, 133; and stigma, 129

alcoholism, 117

allegories, in meaning of illness, 42

allergies, 51, 88

alopecia, *see* hair loss

alternative treatments, 3, 11, 18, 52, 78, 95–96; reasons for choosing, 95

altruism, 134

Alzheimer's disease, 152, 153, 157, 159, 194, 210, 214–215, 245, 246; caregivers of patients with, 183–184. *See also* dementia

ambiguity, 80–81, 100, 104

American Association of Critical-Care Nurses, 198, 203

American Association of Retired Persons (AARP), 53

American Diabetes Association, 49

American Medical Association (AMA), 203

amputation, 49, 224

analogies, in meaning of illness, 42

## ABOUT THE AUTHORS

PETER CLARKE is a Professor of Preventive Medicine and of Communication at the University of Southern California (USC) School of Medicine and the Annenberg School for Communication. He served as Dean of the Annenberg School for eleven years and has been on the faculties of the University of Michigan, the University of Wisconsin, and the University of Washington. His research has focused on communication and people's health, including patient education in cancer. He directs USC's Center for Health and Medical Communication. He received his Ph.D. from the University of Minnesota.

SUSAN H. EVANS is a Research Scientist at the University of Southern California School of Medicine's Institute for Health Promotion and Disease Prevention. She has conducted extensive research on ways to improve people's understanding of their health and coping with illness. Evans has received numerous awards for her projects using multimedia and new communication technologies for patient education. She received her Ph.D. from the University of Michigan.